Study Guide and Laboratory Manual

Jarvis

Physical Examination & Health Assessment

Fourth Canadian Edition

US Authors

Carolyn Jarvis, PhD, APRN, CNP
Professor of Nursing Emerita
Illinois Wesleyan University
Bloomington, Illinois
and
Family Nurse Practitioner
Bloomington, Illinois

Ann Eckhardt, PhD, RN
Associate Chair of Clinical Education and Clinical Associate Professor
College of Nursing and Health Innovation
University of Texas at Arlington
Arlington, Texas

Canadian Editors

Linda Van Pelt, MScN, NP-F
Senior Instructor
School of Nursing
University of Northern British Columbia
Prince George, British Columbia
and
Family Nurse Practitioner
Northern Health Authority
Prince George, British Columbia
(Situated as an uninvited settler on the unceded territory of the Lheidli T'enneh Peoples)
and
Clinical Faculty
Department of Family Medicine
University of British Columbia
Vancouver, British Columbia

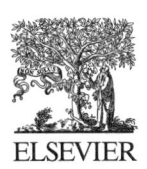

Lauren Irving, MN, NP(F)
Senior Lab Instructor
School of Nursing
University of Northern British Columbia
Prince George, British Columbia
and
Clinical Faculty
Department of Family Medicine
University of British Columbia
Vancouver, British Columbia

ELSEVIER

STUDY GUIDE AND LABORATORY MANUAL FOR JARVIS PHYSICAL
EXAMINATION & HEALTH ASSESSMENT, FOURTH CANADIAN EDITION   ISBN: 978-0-323-82742-3

Copyright © 2024 Elsevier, Inc. All Rights Reserved.
Previous edition copyrighted © 2019 Elsevier, Inc. and © 2014 by Elsevier Canada, a division of Reed Elsevier Canada, Ltd.

Adapted from *Study Guide & Laboratory Manual for Physical Examination & Health Assessment,* 9th edition, by Carolyn Jarvis and Ann Eckhardt. Copyright © 2024 by Elsevier, Inc. Copyright © 2020, 2016, 2012, 2008, 2004, 2000, 1996 by Saunders, an Imprint of Elsevier Inc. All rights reserved. ISBN: 9780323827805.

This adaptation of *Study Guide & Laboratory Manual for Physical Examination & Health Assessment,* 9th edition by Carolyn Jarvis and Ann Eckhardt is published by arrangement with Elsevier and has been undertaken by Elsevier Inc. at its sole responsibility.

No part of this publication may be reproduced or transmitted in any form or by any means, electronic or mechanical, including photocopy, recording, or any information storage and retrieval system, without permission in writing from the publisher. Reproducing passages from this book without such written permission is an infringement of copyright law.

Requests for permission to make copies of any part of the work should be mailed to: College Licensing Officer, access ©, 1 Yonge Street, Suite 1900, Toronto, ON M5E 1E5. Fax: (416) 868-1621. All other inquiries should be directed to the publisher, www.elsevier.com/permissions.

Every reasonable effort has been made to acquire permission for copyrighted material used in this text and to acknowledge all such indebtedness accurately. Any errors and omissions called to the publisher's attention will be corrected in future printings.

Notices

Practitioners and researchers must always rely on their own experience and knowledge in evaluating and using any information, methods, compounds or experiments described herein. Because of rapid advances in the medical sciences, in particular, independent verification of diagnoses and drug dosages should be made. To the fullest extent of the law, no responsibility is assumed by Elsevier, authors, editors or contributors for any injury and/or damage to persons or property as a matter of products liability, negligence or otherwise, or from any use or operation of any methods, products, instructions, or ideas contained in the material herein.

International Standard Book Number 978-0-323-82742-3

VP Education Content: Alyssa K. Fried
Senior Content Strategist, Canada Acquisitions: Roberta A. Spinosa-Millman
Content Development Specialist: Lenore Gray Spence
Publishing Services Manager: Deepthi Unni
Senior Project Manager: Manchu Mohan
Senior Designer: Brian Salisbury

Last digit is the print number: 9   8   7   6   5   4   3   2   1

Preface

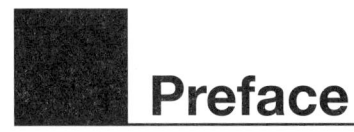

This *Study Guide and Laboratory Manual* is intended for you, the student, as a workbook to accompany the textbook *Physical Examination & Health Assessment*, 4th Canadian edition. You will use it in two places: in your own study area and in the skills laboratory.

As a study guide, this workbook highlights and reinforces the content from the text. Each chapter corresponds to a chapter in the textbook and contains activities and questions in varying formats to promote your mastery of content from the text. Fill out the lab manual chapter and answer the questions before coming to the skills laboratory. This will reinforce your lectures, expose any areas where you have questions for your clinical instructor, and prime you for the skills laboratory/clinical experience.

Once in the skills laboratory, use the *Study Guide and Laboratory Manual* as a direct clinical tool. A number of chapters contain assessment forms on perforated tear-out pages. Usually, you will work in pairs and perform the regional physical examinations on each other under the tutelage of your instructor. As you perform the examination on your peer, you can fill out the documentation sheet and assessment form to be handed in and checked by the instructor.

NEXT GENERATION NCLEX®

In the United States, the National Council for the State Boards of Nursing (NCSBN) is a not-for-profit organization whose members include nursing regulatory bodies. In empowering and supporting nursing regulators in their mandate to protect the public, the NCSBN is involved in the development of nursing licensure examinations, such as the NCLEX-RN®. The NCLEX-RN® was introduced in Canada in 2015 and is, as of the writing of this text, the recognized licensure exam required for practising RNs in Canada.

In 2023, the NCLEX-RN® is changing to ensure that its item types adequately and consistently measure clinical judgement, critical thinking, and problem-solving skills. The examination will incorporate the NCSBN Clinical Judgement Measurement Model (NCJMM), which the NCSBN created to measure a novice nurse's ability to apply clinical judgement in practice.

Clinical judgement has been a foundation underlying nursing education for decades, based on the work of a number of nursing theorists. The theory of clinical judgement that most closely aligns with that used in the NCJMM is Christine A. Tanner's model of clinical judgement in nursing.

The new version of the NCLEX-RN®, referred to as the "Next Generation NCLEX®" (or "NGN"), will feature the following:
- six key skills identified by the NCJMM—recognize cues, analyze cues, prioritize hypotheses, generate solutions, take action, and evaluate outcomes
- item types such as extended multiple response, drag and drop, highlight, matrix/grid, drop down, bowtie, and trend
- all new item types accompanied by mini-case studies with comprehensive patient information—some of it relevant to the question and some of it not
- case information for a single, unchanging moment in time (a "stand-alone" case study), accompanied by one to three questions
- case information for multiple moments in time as a patient's condition changes (an "unfolding" case study), accompanied by six questions

For further NCLEX-RN® examination preparation resources, see *Elsevier's Canadian Comprehensive Review for the NCLEX-RN® Examination*, 3rd edition, ISBN 978-0-323-81033-3.

Prior to preparing for any nursing licensure examination, refer to your provincial or territorial nursing regulatory body to determine which licensure examination is required in order for you to practise in your chosen jurisdiction.

STUDY GUIDE AND LABORATORY MANUAL FEATURES

Chapter 32, "Next Generation NCLEX® (NGN) Examination–Style Unfolding Case Studies," is a new chapter in this edition. It provides an opportunity to practice prioritizing, decision-making, and using clinical judgement skills.

Chapters 1 to 31 consist of two parts—cognitive and clinical—and contain:
- Purpose—a brief summary of the material you are learning in the chapter.
- Reading Assignment—the corresponding chapter from the *Physical Examination & Health Assessment*, 4th Canadian edition, and space for your instructor to assign journal articles, in addition to those in selected chapters.

- Glossary—important and specialized terms from the textbook chapter with accompanying definitions.
- Study Guide—specific short-answer and fill-in questions to help you highlight and learn content from the chapter. Important illustrations of human anatomy have been reproduced from the textbook with the labels deleted, so that you can identify and fill in the names of the structures yourself.
- Critical Thinking Exercises—exercises created to help you expand your thinking and apply your knowledge. These exercises will assist you to develop a variety of key nursing attributes, including diagnostic reasoning, professionalism, and a relational approach to practice.
- Review and Clinical Judgement Questions—multiple-choice questions, matching, and short-answer questions, with question items formatted similarly to those in the NCLEX-RN® examination. Questions requiring clinical judgement are interspersed among the review questions to help you monitor your own mastery of the material and begin preparing for your provincial or territorial licensing exam. Take the self-examination when you are ready, and then check your answers against the correct answers available on the Evolve site.
- Clinical Objectives—behavioural objectives that you should achieve during your peer practice in the regional examinations.
- Documentation Sheets—complete yet succinct physical examination forms that you can use in the skills laboratory or in the clinical setting. They serve as a memory prompt, listing key history questions and physical examination steps, and as a means of recording data during the patient encounter.
- Narrative Summary Forms—subjective, objective, assessment, plan (SOAP) format, so that you can learn to chart narrative accounts of the history and physical examination findings. These forms have accompanying sketches of regional anatomy and are an especially useful exercise for those studying for advanced-practice roles.

Learning the skills of history-taking and physical examination requires two kinds of practice: cognitive and clinical. It is our hope that this *Study Guide and Laboratory Manual* will help you achieve both of these learning and practice modalities.

Carolyn Jarvis
Ann Eckhardt
Linda Van Pelt
Lauren Irving

Acknowledgements

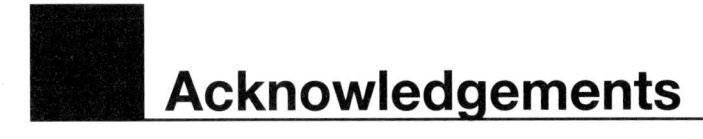

We are grateful to those on the team at Elsevier who worked on the US *Study Guide and Laboratory Manual*. Our thanks extend to Heather Bays-Petrovic, Content Strategist for organizing and reorganizing our new content; Danielle Frazier, Content Development Manager for hunting and acquiring material; Thoufiq Mohammed, Project Manager for patience and planning; Deepthi Unni, Publishing Services Manager; and Brian Salisbury, Book Designer. We are dependent on this wonderful team to bring our vision into print and to make it useful for our students.

Carolyn Jarvis
Ann Eckhardt

My deepest gratitude to those whose health care I am entrusted with, as well as to my colleagues, all of whom I am humbled by and learn from each and every day.

Linda Van Pelt

To all the nurses who work tirelessly every day making the world a better place, one patient at a time. To the trailblazers who pushed the limits of professional nursing practice and to those who continue to do so today. And to my nana, Isabel Carson, who graduated from St. Paul's Hospital School of Nursing in 1952 and who told me fantastic stories of her years in training and early career in Vanderhoof, BC.

Lauren Irving

Contents

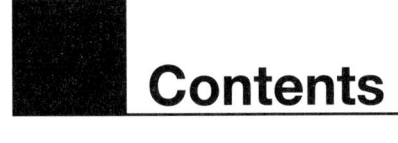

UNIT 1 ASSESSMENT OF THE WHOLE PERSON, 1
1. Critical Thinking and Evidence-Informed Assessment, **1**
2. Health Promotion in the Context of Health Assessment, **7**
3. A Relational Approach to Cultural and Social Considerations in Health Assessment, **11**
4. The Interview, **17**
5. The Complete Health History, **23**
6. Mental Health Assessment, **35**
7. Substance Use and Health Assessment, **45**
8. Interpersonal Violence and Health Assessment, **51**

UNIT 2 APPROACH TO THE CLINICAL SETTING, 57
9. Assessment Techniques and the Clinical Setting, **57**
10. General Survey, Measurement, and Vital Signs, **63**
11. Pain Assessment, **73**
12. Nutritional Assessment and Nursing Practice, **79**

UNIT 3 PHYSICAL EXAMINATION, 87
13. Skin, Hair, and Nails, **87**
14. Head, Face, and Neck, Including Regional Lymphatic System, **99**
15. Eyes, **107**
16. Ears, **119**
17. Nose, Mouth, and Throat, **129**
18. Breasts and Regional Lymphatic System, **137**
19. Thorax and Lungs, **149**
20. Heart and Neck Vessels, **159**
21. Peripheral Vascular System and Lymphatic System, **169**
22. The Abdomen, **181**
23. Anus, Rectum, and Prostate, **193**
24. Musculo-Skeletal System, **199**
25. Neurological System, **213**
26. Male Genitourinary System, **225**
27. Female Genitourinary System, **237**

UNIT 4 INTEGRATION OF THE HEALTH ASSESSMENT, 249
28. The Complete Health Assessment: Putting It All Together, **249**
29. Bedside Assessment and Reporting, **259**
30. Pregnancy, **265**
31. Assessment of the Older Adult, **281**
32. Next Generation NCLEX® (NGN) Examination–Style Unfolding Case Studies, **291**

Appendix, **299**
Answer Key—available on the text's Evolve site

UNIT 1 ASSESSMENT OF THE WHOLE PERSON

1 Critical Thinking and Evidence-Informed Assessment

PURPOSE

Learning to conduct systematic assessments and communicate assessment findings is foundational to nursing practice. This chapter discusses the key characteristics of systematic assessment: diagnostic reasoning, the nursing process, and critical thinking. Assessments are based in relational practice, to ensure respect is conveyed for the whole person and to avoid objectifying people. This chapter introduces the concept of evidenced-informed practice and highlights its significance in nursing practice. This chapter also introduces the concept of health, including the evolving definition of *health*; helps you understand that it is the definition of *health* that determines the kinds of factors that are assessed; and shows you how the data gathered during assessment will vary with the person's age, developmental state, physical condition, risk factors, and culture.

READING ASSIGNMENT

Jarvis: *Physical Examination and Health Assessment*, 4th Canadian ed., Chapter 1.

Suggested Reading

Registered Nurses' Association of Ontario. (2022). *Leading Change Toolkit*. https://rnao.ca/leading-change-toolkit
Woodbury, M. G., & Kuhnke, J. (2014). Evidence-based practice vs. evidence-informed practice: What's the difference? *Wound Care Canada, 12*(1), 18–21.

GLOSSARY

Study the following terms after reading the corresponding chapter in the text.

Assessment: the collection of data about an individual's health state for the purpose of making a judgement or diagnosis
Behavioural model: a model that moves health beyond treating disease to include secondary and primary preventions, with emphasis on changing behaviours and lifestyles
Biomedical model: the predominant model of the Canadian health care system, wherein health is the absence of disease; the focus is on diagnosis and treatment of disease
Complete (total health) database: a complete health history, full physical examination, laboratory studies, and other diagnostic tests
Critical thinking: a multidimensional thinking process by which nurses learn to assess and modify diagnoses and treatments, if indicated, before acting
Cue: an assessment finding: a piece of information, a sign or symptom, or a piece of laboratory data
Diagnostic hypothesis: a tentative explanation for a cue or a set of cues that can be used as a basis for further investigation
Diagnostic reasoning: a method of collecting and analyzing clinical information with the following components: (a) attending to initially available cues, (b) formulating diagnostic hypotheses, (c) gathering data relative to the tentative hypotheses, and (d) evaluating each hypothesis with the new data collected to arrive at a final diagnosis
Emergency database: it calls for a rapid collection of the data, often compiled while lifesaving measures are occurring
Episodic database: it is used for a limited or short-term problem; it concerns mainly one problem, one cue complex, or one body system
Evidence-informed practice (EIP): a systematic approach to making decisions about patient care and treatment that integrates the best available evidence with assessment data, the clinician's experience and expertise, and individual patient preferences and values, with the aim to improve outcomes
First-level priority problems: emergencies, life-threatening, and immediate, such as establishing an airway or supporting breathing.
Follow-up database: it is used in all settings to monitor short-term or chronic health problems

Health promotion: a comprehensive social and political process of enabling people to increase control over the determinants of health and thereby improve their health

Medical diagnosis: it is used to evaluate the cause and etiology of disease; focus is on the function or malfunction of a specific organ system

Nursing diagnosis: clinical judgement about the response of the whole person to actual or potential health problems, and identification of their health concerns, risks, and goals in response to the nurse's analysis of assessment data

Nursing process: a method of collecting and analyzing clinical information with the following components: (a) assessment, (b) nursing diagnosis, (c) planning, (d) implementation, and (e) evaluation

Objective data: what the health care provider observes by inspecting, percussing, palpating, and auscultating during the physical examination

Prevention: any action directed toward promoting health and preventing the occurrence of disease

Relational practice: it recognizes that health, illness, and the meanings they hold for a person are shaped by one's social, cultural, family, historical, and geographical contexts as well as one's age, sex, gender, ability, and other individual contexts

Second-level priority problems: those necessitating your prompt intervention to forestall further deterioration, such as mental status change, acute pain, acute urinary elimination problems, untreated medical problems, abnormal laboratory values, risks of infection, or risk to safety or security

Social determinants of health: the social, economic, and political conditions that shape the health of individuals, families, and communities

Socioenvironmental model: it incorporates sociological and environmental aspects of health as well as biomedical and behavioural aspects

Subjective data: what the person says about himself or herself during history-taking

Third-level priority problems: those that are important to the patient's health but can be addressed after more urgent health problems are addressed

STUDY GUIDE

After completing the reading assignment, you should be able to answer the following questions in the spaces provided.

1. The steps of the diagnostic reasoning process are listed below. Consider the clinical example given for "cue recognition," and fill in the remaining diagnostic reasoning steps.

Stage	Example
Cue recognition	A.J., a 62-year-old male, appears pale, diaphoretic, and anxious.
Hypothesis formulation	
Data gathering for hypothesis testing	
Hypothesis evaluation	

2. One of the critical thinking skills is identifying assumptions. Explain how the following statement contains an assumption. How would you get the facts in this situation?
   "Ellen, you have to break up with your boyfriend. He is too rough with you. He is no good for you."

3. Another critical thinking skill involves validation or checking the accuracy and reliability of data. Describe how you would validate the following data:
   Mr. Quinn tells you his weight this morning on the clinic scale was 75 kg.

The primary counsellor tells you Ellen is depressed and angry about being admitted to residential treatment in the clinic.

When auscultating the heart, you hear a blowing, swooshing sound between the first and second heart sounds.

4. Give one or two specific examples of data you might typically collect appropriate to each of the following health concepts:

   Biomedical model _____

   Behavioural model _____

   Socioenvironmental model _____

   Health promotion _____

5. Distinguish *subjective* data from *objective* data by placing an *S* or *O* after each of the following:

   complaint of sore shoulder _____; unconscious _____; blood in the urine _____; family has just moved to a new area _____; dizziness _____; sore throat _____; earache _____; weight gain _____.

6. How are medical diagnosis and nursing diagnosis similar?
   How are they different?

7. For the following situations, state the type of data collection you would perform (i.e., *complete* database, *episodic* or *problem-centred* database, *follow-up* database, *emergency* database).

   Barbiturate overdose _____; ambulatory, apparently well individual who presents at outpatient clinic with a rash _____; first visit to a health care provider for a "checkup" _____; recently placed on antihypertensive medication _____.

8. Discuss the effect that cultural and socioeconomic diversity of individuals has on the Canadian health care system.

9. Define each of the three levels of priority setting and give an example of each.

10. Give an example of a situation when you might question the consistency of data from the patient's history.

11. Evidence-informed practice depends on four factors. Name the factors and give an example of each.

REVIEW AND CLINICAL JUDGEMENT QUESTIONS

This test is for you to check your own mastery of the content. Answers are provided on the text's Evolve site.

1. The concept of health has expanded in the past 40 years. Select the phrase that reflects the narrowest description of health.
   a. the absence of disease
   b. incorporating sociological and environmental aspects of health
   c. changing behaviours and lifestyle
   d. prevention of disease

2. Select the best description of a complete database.
   a. subjective and objective data gathered by a health care provider from a patient
   b. objective data obtained from a patient through inspection, percussion, palpation, and auscultation
   c. a summary of a patient's record, including laboratory studies
   d. subjective and objective data gathered from a patient plus the results of any diagnostic studies completed

3. Nursing diagnoses, based on assessment of a number of factors, give nurses a common language with which to communicate nursing findings. The best description of a nursing diagnosis is
   a. an evaluation of the etiology of a disease.
   b. a pattern of coping.
   c. a concise description of actual or potential health problems or of wellness strengths.
   d. the patient's perception of and satisfaction with his or her own health status.

4. Depending on the clinical situation, the nurse may establish one of four kinds of database. An episodic database is described as
   a. including a complete health history and full physical examination.
   b. concerning mainly one problem.
   c. evaluation of a previously identified problem.
   d. rapid collection of data in conjunction with lifesaving measures.

5. Individuals should be seen at regular intervals for health care. The frequency of these visits
   a. is most efficient if performed on an annual basis.
   b. is not important. There is no recommendation for the frequency of health care.
   c. varies, depending on the age, gender, social context, and illness and wellness needs of the person.
   d. is based on the practitioner's clinical experience.

6. One of the central skills of relational practice is reflectivity, which is a process of
   a. enabling people to increase control over the determinants of health and therefore improve their health.
   b. developing a relationship between two people.
   c. repeating a patient's statement to clarify its meaning.
   d. continually examining how you view and respond to patients based on your own assumptions, sociohistorical background, past experiences, comfort or lack of comfort in particular situations, and so on.

7. Evidence-informed nursing practice can be described as
   a. combining clinical expertise with the use of nursing research to provide the best care for patients while considering the individual patient's values and circumstances.
   b. appraising and looking at the implications of one or two articles as they relate to the culture and ethnicity of the patient.
   c. completing a literature search to find relevant articles that utilize nursing research so as to encourage nurses to use good practices.
   d. finding value-based resources to justify nursing actions when working with patients of diverse cultural backgrounds.

8. What can be determined when the nurse clusters data as part of the critical thinking process?
   a. This identifies problems that may be urgent and require immediate action by the nurse.
   b. This step of the process involves recognizing inconsistencies in the data.
   c. The nurse recognizes patterns and relationships among the data.
   d. Risk factors can be determined so the nurse knows how to offer health teaching.

For questions 9 to 13, use the following information:

G.R. is a 75-year-old male who presents to the emergency department with chest pain and palpitations, and appears pale and diaphoretic. When the health history and physical examination are completed, the following problems emerge. Label them first (a), second (b), or third (c) level priority problems.

9. Blood pressure 74/50 mm Hg; heart rate: 148 bpm _____

10. Serum potassium 2.7 mmol/L (low); glucose 12.5 mmol/L (high) _____

11. Living alone, with no family in the area _____

12. Acute chest pain with radiation to jaw _____

13. Lack of familiarity with heart healthy dietary guidelines _____

14. Which of the following are objective data? (Select all that apply.)
    a. a 2-centimetre scar on the dorsal surface of the hand
    b. complaints of nausea
    c. clear breath sounds
    d. headache
    e. blood pressure 110/72 mm Hg

15. A.S. is a 35-year-old female who has come to your clinic today for a well visit. She recently moved to the area and is establishing a new primary care provider. What information would you include in the database for this new patient? (Select all that apply.)
    a. current health state
    b. lifestyle and risk factors
    c. subjective information only
    d. objective information only
    e. physical examination
    f. health maintenance behaviours
    g. your perception of the patient's health
    h. the patient's perception of current health

NOTES

NOTES

2 Health Promotion in the Context of Health Assessment

PURPOSE

This chapter introduces you to the role that Canada has played in health promotion; the foundational concepts of disease prevention and health promotion; and how nurses assess health-promoting behaviours in clinical settings.

READING ASSIGNMENT

Jarvis: *Physical Examination and Health Assessment*, 4th Canadian ed., Chapter 2.

Suggested Reading

Public Health Agency of Canada. (2020). *Social determinants and inequities in health for Black Canadians: A snapshot.* https://www.canada.ca/en/public-health/services/health-promotion/population-health/what-determines-health/social-determinants-inequities-black-canadians-snapshot.html#shr-pg0

Truth and Reconciliation Commission of Canada. (2015). *Honouring the truth, reconciling for the future: Summary of the final report of the Truth and Reconciliation Commission of Canada.* Montreal: McGill-Queen's University Press.

GLOSSARY

Study the following terms after reading the corresponding chapter in the text.

Health disparities: they occur when the combination and interaction of the social determinants of health result in differences in health status between segments of the population

Health inequities: they result when health disparities are avoidable, but outside the control of individuals

Health promotion: "... the process of enabling people to increase control over, and to improve their health. It moves beyond a focus on individual behaviour towards a wide range of social and environmental interventions." (World Health Organization, 2021)

"Moving upstream": a focus on the root causes of health conditions and taking action to avoid a problem before it occurs; it is the hallmark of primary prevention

Population Health Promotion Model: it provides a multifaceted approach to considering the social determinants of health in nursing health assessment

Primary prevention: the promotion of health and the prevention of illness by assisting individuals, families, and communities to prevent known health problems, protect existing states of health, and promote psychosocial wellness

Screening: early detection of a condition or disease; it is possible when a sensitive and effective tool for detection is available, when the natural history of the condition is adequately known and there is a detectable preclinical stage; and when a socially acceptable treatment method is available

Secondary prevention: early detection of disease, before symptoms emerge, often done through disease screening

Social determinants of health: they "refer to a specific group of social and economic factors within the broader determinants of health. These relate to an individual's place in society, such as income, education or employment. Experiences of discrimination, racism and historical trauma are important social determinants of health for certain groups such as Indigenous Peoples, LGBTQ and Black Canadians" (Public Health Agency of Canada, 2022, "Social determinants of health and health inequalities" web page)

Tertiary prevention: the prevention of complications when a condition or disease is present or has progressed

STUDY GUIDE

After completing the reading assignment, you should be able to answer the following questions in the spaces provided.

1. Define each of the three levels of disease prevention, and for each level give at least two examples of health-promoting strategies.

2. Describe at least one way in which each of the following social determinants might influence an individual's health:

   Education and literacy _____

   Access to health services _____

   Employment/working conditions _____

   Gender _____

   Income and social status _____

   Culture _____

3. Describe and compare *health disparities* and *health inequities* and give an example of each.

4. Describe screening and identify three conditions required for a screening measure to exist.

5. Describe the three major components of the Population Health Promotion Model, and at least one advantage of using this model.

6. Describe the three levels of disease prevention and give at least two examples of how health education and counselling might be used at each of the levels.

7. Describe the Looksee Checklist and identify when it should be used in the healthcare setting.

8. Identify at least four factors that will inform the health counselling that you offer a patient.

9. Briefly discuss what is meant by an "upstream approach" to health care.

REVIEW AND CLINICAL JUDGEMENT QUESTIONS

This test is for you to check your own mastery of the content. Answers are provided on the text's Evolve site.

1. Effective and concrete public participation and directing action on the social determinants of health are health promotion principles identified by the
   a. Looksee Checklist.
   b. the Population Health Promotion Model.
   c. "moving upstream" approach.
   d. World Health Organization.

2. You are teaching an adolescent girls' group about safer sexual practices. This is an example of which level of disease prevention?
    a. primary prevention
    b. secondary prevention
    c. tertiary prevention
    d. disease screening

3. The purpose of the Looksee Checklist screening instrument is to
    a. provide epidemiological data.
    b. form an intelligence test.
    c. detect developmental delays.
    d. reduce risk factors.

4. The *Lalonde Report* (1974) was important because it
    a. laid the foundation for developmental screening in infants.
    b. shifted traditional thinking about health from socioenvironmental influences to better understanding health as a biomedical response.
    c. shifted traditional thinking about health from biomedical responses to the influences of lifestyle, human biology, and the social environment.
    d. laid out clear disease-screening guidelines.

5. You are part of a group working to find housing for homeless people. This is an example of which health promotion principle?
    a. involving the population as a whole in the context of their everyday lives
    b. directing action toward the social determinants of health
    c. combining diverse but complementary methods
    d. aiming at effective and concrete public participation

6. An example of a "moving upstream" approach would be
    a. starting up an early childhood development program.
    b. ensuring that adolescents have access to sexually transmitted infection screening.
    c. initiating a school lunch program.
    d. providing foot care to diabetic older adults.

7. You are providing nutritional counselling to a woman living with diabetes who resides in a remote Indigenous community. You advise her to include more fresh vegetables in her diet, but she tells you that vegetables are very expensive in the community and that she can't afford to buy them. This is an example of
    a. secondary prevention.
    b. the *Ottawa Charter for Health Promotion*.
    c. tertiary prevention.
    d. a social determinant of health.

8. The Canadian Paediatric Society recommends the use of a universal, structured developmental assessment tool
    a. at the 18-month well-baby visit.
    b. at the 12-month well-baby visit.
    c. at each health visit under age 2 years.
    d. only when parents express a concern about their baby's development.

CLINICAL JUDGEMENT EXERCISE 1

Consider the following clinical situations. What is your reaction to each? How would you handle the situation if you were part of the conversation or overheard the conversation?

- **Situation 1:** You receive a report on a new admission who has pancreatitis. The report indicates that the woman has alcohol use disorder, and the emergency department has started the alcohol withdrawal protocol. After you share this information with the admitting physician, the physician states, "Oh, great! I hope this patient isn't drunk when she gets to the floor! Hopefully she has brought someone with her to help look after her. These people ALWAYS have large families. What do you think her blood alcohol level is? What's your best guess?"

- **Situation 2:** You are at the nurses' station and overhear the following conversation:
  Person 1: "I need to know which patient is going home so that I can write discharge orders."

  Person 2: "The Indian patient."

  Person 1 (laughing): "Indian how? Red dot or red feather?"

- **Situation 3:** A nurse is visibly upset and crying at the nurses' station. She tells you: "The patient in 3201 is going to die! She is experiencing postpartum hemorrhage, but she won't accept a blood transfusion because of her religion. I wish I could convince her to get the transfusion. I don't understand why she's worried about it."

- **Situation 4:** The emergency department nurse calls to give report on a new admission. This is the information you receive: John, or wait he goes by something else now—I mean she (snickering). He . . . she . . . I don't know . . . I'll just say they have a penis, but also breasts. You cannot put this patient in with a male or female patient!

CLINICAL JUDGEMENT EXERCISE 2

With a partner or in a small group, discuss common stereotypes you have heard, seen, or believed. Be open and honest in your discussion. Where do the stereotypes come from? How might a negative stereotype impact the care you provide to a patient? How can being aware of stereotypes potentially enhance patient care?

NOTES

3 A Relational Approach to Cultural and Social Considerations in Health Assessment

PURPOSE

This chapter reviews concepts that are central to understanding cultural and social considerations in health assessment. It also reviews cultural sensitivity, cultural competence, and cultural safety, and their implications for nursing practice; examples of ethnocultural diversity; and trends in health, social, and gender inequities in Canada. As well, it provides guidelines for assessing culturally based understandings and the social and economic contexts of people's lives.

READING ASSIGNMENT

Jarvis: *Physical Examination and Health Assessment*, 4th Canadian ed., Chapter 3.

Suggested Reading
Cottrell, D. B. (2019). Fostering sexual and gender minority status disclosure in patients. *The Nurse Practitioner, 44*(7), 43–48.

GLOSSARY

Study the following terms after reading the corresponding chapter in the text.

Complementary and alternative health care (CAHC): an umbrella term that describes numerous therapies including acupuncture, chiropractic, naturopathy, massage, herbal medicine, yoga, and healing touch

Critical cultural perspective: understanding culture as a relational aspect of individuals that shifts and changes over time depending on an individual's history, social context, gender identity, past experiences, professional identity, and so on

Cultural competence: the knowledge, skills, attitudes, or personal attributes health care workers utilize to develop and maintain respectful relationships with patients and co-workers of diverse cultures

Cultural safety: both a process and an outcome whose goal is to promote greater equity by focusing on the root causes of power imbalances and inequitable social relationships in health care, including racism and other forms of discrimination. Cultural safety is increasingly being incorporated into nursing, medicine, and other health care professions

Cultural sensitivity: the idea that people have culturally based understandings, practices, and customs, and that health care providers should be aware of and accommodate those understandings in a way that does not stereotype people for the ways in which they may be different from the dominant cultural norm

Culturalism: the process of conceptualizing culture in narrow terms, or assuming that people act in particular ways because of their culture

Culture: more than shared beliefs, knowledge, and customs; a dynamic, relational process that is lived and created between people within particular historical, social, political, economic, physical, and linguistic contexts

Discrimination: the systemic inequitable treatment of individuals or groups based on stratified classifications, the process by which individuals or members of a group are denied equitable treatment and opportunities with respect to education, housing, health care, employment, and so on

Ethnicity: a social construct used to categorize people based on multiple different aspects such as country of origin or ancestry, family history, languages spoken, and in some cases religious identity, or certain physical characteristics

Health inequality: a generic term used to designate differences, variations, and disparities in the health status of individuals, groups, and populations

Health inequities: those inequalities in health that are unnecessary and avoidable, and differences that are considered unfair and unjust

Immigrant: a term that applies to all people who are, or have ever been, a landed immigrant, and have been granted the right to permanently reside in Canada by Immigration, Refugees and Citizenship Canada

***Indian Act*:** legislation that contains all the federal policies and regulations pertaining to "registered status Indians"; it classifies First Nations people into registered status Indians or nonstatus Indians, to distinguish people who receive legal recognition as First Nations citizens in Canada from those who do not

Indigenous peoples: In Canada, Indigenous peoples include First Nations, Métis, and Inuit. Although the term *Aboriginal* is commonly used (e.g., by Statistics Canada), and the colonial term *Indian* is still used in federal policy documents (e.g., the *Indian Act*), in many parts of Canada, the term *First Nations* is viewed as more respectful.

Race: a socially constructed category used to classify humankind according to common ancestry and reliant on differentiation by physical characteristics such as colour of skin, hair texture, stature, and facial characteristics. Science has long established that the concept of "race" has no biological basis; therefore, it has no meaning independent of its social definitions

Racialization: the social process by which people are labelled according to particular physical characteristics or presumed ethnocultural or "racial" categories and then treated in accordance with misinformed beliefs related to those labels

Relative poverty: a situation in which individuals lack the necessary resources (i.e., income) to carry out or participate in the activities associated with the average standard of living in a country

Visible minority: defined in Canada by Statistics Canada as "persons, other than Aboriginal peoples, who are non-Caucasian in race or non-white in colour." This definition is revealing of the conflation of "race" and ethnicity in Canada.

STUDY GUIDE

After completing the reading assignment, you should be able to answer the following questions in the spaces provided.

1. Describe the main principles of cultural safety.

2. Describe four current trends in the demographic profile of Canada.

3. Describe the key areas to pay attention to during health assessments.

4. Describe the inequities in health status experienced by many Indigenous peoples in Canada.

5. Describe Canada's demography and shifting demographic trends.

6. Describe three factors that contribute to the pattern of declining health status that is prevalent in nonEuropean immigrants to Canada.

7. Identify at least four determinants of health associated with poverty and describe their relative impact on health status.

8. Differentiate among the terms *sex*, *gender*, and *gender identity*, and describe the potential effects of stigma attached to gender diversity.

9. Describe the seven Truth and Reconciliation Commission "calls to action" that relate specifically to health.

REVIEW AND CLINICAL JUDGEMENT QUESTIONS

This test is for you to check your own mastery of the content. Answers are provided on the text's Evolve site.

1. Cultural competence involves developing knowledge in all of the following areas, *except*
    a. your own personal ethnocultural and social background.
    b. the significance of social, economic, and cultural contexts.
    c. the construction of racial categories.
    d. the culture of the health care system.

2. Federal legislation containing the policies and regulations pertaining to First Nations people is
    a. the *Indian Act*, originally developed in 1976.
    b. the *Indian Act*, originally developed in 1876.
    c. the *Multiculturalism Act*, originally developed in 1985.
    d. the *Aboriginal Act*, originally developed in 1907.

3. The majority of the population of Canada live in the following major cities:
    a. Toronto, Montreal, and Calgary.
    b. Toronto, Montreal, and Ottawa.
    c. Toronto, Montreal, and Vancouver.
    d. Toronto, Vancouver, and Ottawa.

4. All of the following statements are true, *except*
    a. Poverty is a primary cause of poor health among Canadians.
    b. People who come from the same country will have the same cultural, social, and linguistic backgrounds.
    c. People who immigrate to Canada often experience difficulties getting the help they need from health care providers, hospitals, and other health care agencies.
    d. The concept of race has no basis in biological reality.

5. Which of the following groups are more likely to become ill and less likely to receive appropriate health care services?
    a. lone mothers in low-income brackets
    b. older women
    c. people with severe or persistent mental illnesses or addictions
    d. refugees and some immigrant groups
    e. all of the above

6. All of the following questions convey respect while exploring people's varying health practices, *except*
   a. "Which church do you attend?"
   b. "Have you found any treatments, supplements, practices, or medications that have worked for you in the past?"
   c. "Did you use any treatments, supplements, practices, or medications in your home country that seemed to work for you?"
   d. "Do you have any religious beliefs or practices that you would like me to know about in relation to your health?"

7. Which factors are important during an interview? (Select all that apply.)
   a. equal status seating
   b. leading questions
   c. active listening
   d. distancing
   e. social responses
   f. avoidance language
   g. providing privacy
   h. professional jargon

8. Which of the following statements/questions need to be rewritten to avoid heterosexist language?
   a. What type of birth control do you use?
   b. Are you in a relationship?
   c. What is your marital status?
   d. What is your pronoun?
   e. Please circle your gender: Male   Female

9. You work in the emergency department, and an 88-year-old Punjabi-speaking patient was just brought by ambulance with chest pain. You do not speak Punjabi, and there is no in-person interpreter available. Your best option to ensure communication is to
   a. identify a friend or family member who can provide interpreter services. It's better to have someone in person.
   b. leverage technology to ensure communication. Your hospital recently invested in video interpreter services.
   c. use gestures, simple words, and a loud voice to work through the history and physical examination.
   d. call another floor and see if they have anyone who knows Punjabi. The patient can probably wait for a while.

10. Nonverbal behaviours are just as important as verbal behaviours. Please mark the following behaviours as positive or negative.

Behaviour	Positive	Negative
Tapping a pen rhythmically on the table		
A warm smile while leaning slightly forward		
A moderate tone of voice and rate of speech		
Frequently crossing and uncrossing legs		
Arms crossed over chest		
Standing by the patient's bed		

CRITICAL THINKING EXERCISE

Techniques for appropriate communication are important, but knowing yourself is equally important—your beliefs, your culture, your biases. You must quickly establish rapport with patients, and you need to make sure that you can adequately meet their needs in a safe, nonjudgemental way. Negative facial expression or other negative nonverbal messages can break communication and shatter the rapport you have established. By knowing yourself and your personal biases, you may be able to control your nonverbal expressions. Most people have beliefs about subjects like teen pregnancy and alcohol or other substance use. Awareness of personal prejudices can help you maintain neutrality when faced with difficult patient situations.

Answer the following questions or complete the following statements openly and honestly without editing your thoughts in an effort to get to know yourself better.

1. What do I believe about gender roles?

2. What is my definition of health?

3. When I take care of a person from a different religion, I feel . . .

4. When I meet someone new, I make the following assumptions . . .

5. I am most fearful of working with . . .

6. When I see a same-sex couple, I feel . . .

7. I have the following assumptions/stereotypes about people who are
    a. homeless.
    b. unemployed.
    c. teen mothers.
    d. drug addicts.
    e. Catholic.
    f. Muslim.
    g. Christian.
    h. Jewish.
    i. sexual and gender minorities.

NOTES

4 The Interview

PURPOSE

This chapter reviews the process of communication: techniques of interviewing, including open-ended versus closed questions; the eight types of examiner responses; the 10 "traps" of interviewing; and nonverbal communication skills. It also considers variations in technique that are necessary for interviewing individuals of different ages, for those with special needs, and across differing ethnocultural and sociohistorical backgrounds.

READING ASSIGNMENT

Jarvis: *Physical Examination and Health Assessment*, 4th Canadian ed., Chapter 4.

GLOSSARY

Study the following terms after reading the corresponding chapter in the text.

Active listening: the skill of listening with your complete attention and engagement, both to what the patient tells you and to the way the patient tells his or her story
Avoidance language: the use of euphemisms to avoid reality or to hide feelings
Clarification: an examiner's response when the patient's word choice is ambiguous or confusing, or a discrepancy is noted
Closed question: it asks for specific information that elicits a short, one- or two-word answer, a "yes" or "no," or a forced choice
Distancing: the use of impersonal speech to put space between a threat and the self
Empathy: it means viewing the world from the other person's inner frame of reference while remaining yourself; recognizing and accepting the other person's feelings, without criticism
Explanation: an examiner's statements that inform the patient; the examiner shares factual and objective data
Facilitation: an examiner's response that encourages the patient to say more, to continue with the story
Geographical privacy: a private room or space with only examiner and patient present
Interpretation: an examiner's statement that is not based on direct observation but is based on the examiner's inference or conclusion that links events, makes associations, or implies cause
Interview: a meeting between examiner and patient with the goal of gathering a complete health history
Jargon: using medical vocabulary with a patient in an exclusionary and paternalistic way
Leading question: a question that implies that one answer is "better" than another
Nonverbal communication: a message conveyed through body language—posture, gestures, facial expression, eye contact, foot tapping, touch, hand movements, and even where a person places their chair
Open-ended question: it asks for narrative information; it is unbiased and leaves patients free to answer in any way, and to express themselves fully
Reflection: an examiner's response that echoes the patient's words; it involves repeating part of what the patient has just said to encourage the patient to elaborate
Summary: a final review of what the examiner understands the patient has said; it condenses facts and presents a survey of the examiner's perception of the patient's health problem or need
Verbal communication: messages sent through spoken words, vocalizations, and tone of voice

STUDY GUIDE

After completing the reading assignment, you should be able to answer the following questions in the spaces provided.

1. Describe the points to consider when preparing the physical setting for the interview.

2. List the pros and cons of note-taking during the interview.

3. Contrast open-ended with closed questions, and explain the purpose of each during the interview.

4. List the eight types of examiner responses that could be used during the interview, and give a short example of each.

5. List the 10 "traps" of interviewing, and give a short example of each.

6. State at least seven types of nonverbal behaviours that an interviewer could use.

7. State a useful phrase to use as a closing when ending the interview.

8. Discuss special considerations when interviewing the older adult.

9. Formulate a response to a patient who has spoken to you in ways you interpret as sexually aggressive.

10. Discuss how relational practice enhances communication across cultures.

11. List at least five points to consider when using an interpreter during an interview.

REVIEW AND CLINICAL JUDGEMENT QUESTIONS

This test is for you to check your own mastery of the content. Answers are provided on the text's Evolve site.

1. The practitioner, entering the examining room to meet a patient for the first time, states: "Hello, I'm M.M., and I'm here to gather some information from you and to perform your examination. This will take about 30 minutes. D.D. is a student working with me. If it's all right with you, D.D. will remain during the examination." Which of the following must be added to cover all aspects of the interview?
   a. a statement regarding confidentiality, patient costs, and the expectation of each person
   b. the purpose of the interview and the role of the examiner
   c. the time and place of the interview and a confidentiality statement
   d. the explicit purpose of the interview and a description of the physical examination, including diagnostic studies

2. An accurate understanding of the other person's feelings within a communication context is an example of
   a. empathy.
   b. liking others.
   c. facilitation.
   d. a nonverbal listening technique.

3. You have come into a patient's room to conduct an admission interview. Because you are expecting a phone call, you stand near the door during the interview. A more appropriate approach would be to
   a. arrange to have someone page you so you can sit on the side of the bed.
   b. have someone else answer the phone so you can sit facing the patient.
   c. use this approach given the circumstances; it is correct.
   d. arrange for a time free of interruptions until the initial physical examination is complete.

4. Students frequently ask teachers, "May I ask you a question?" This is an example of
   a. an open-ended question.
   b. a reflective question.
   c. a closed question.
   d. a double-barrelled question.

5. During a patient interview, you recognize the need to use interpretation. This verbal response
   a. is the same as clarification.
   b. is a summary of a statement made by a patient.
   c. is used to focus on a particular aspect of what the patient has just said.
   d. is based on the interviewer's inference from the data that have been presented.

6. A good rule for an interviewer is to
   a. stop the patient each time something is said that is not understood.
   b. spend more time listening to the patient than talking.
   c. consistently think of your next response so the patient will know you have understood what has been said.
   d. use "why" questions to seek clarification of unusual symptoms or behaviour.

7. During an interview, a patient denies having any anxiety. The patient frequently changes position in the chair, holds their arms folded tightly against their chest, and has little eye contact with the interviewer. The interviewer should
   a. use clarification to bring the discrepancy between verbal and nonverbal behaviour to the patient's attention.
   b. proceed with the interview. Usually patients are truthful with a health care provider.
   c. make a mental note to discuss the behaviour after the physical examination is completed.
   d. proceed with the interview and examination as outlined on the agency assessment form. The patient's behaviour is appropriate for the circumstances.

8. Touch should be used during the interview
   a. only with individuals who speak English.
   b. as a way of establishing contact with the person and communicating empathy.
   c. only with patients of the same sex.
   d. only if the interviewer knows the person well.

9. Children are usually brought for health care by a parent or caregiver. At about what age should the interviewer begin to question the child instead of the parent or caregiver regarding presenting symptoms?
   a. age 5
   b. age 7
   c. age 9
   d. age 11

10. Because of adolescents' developmental level, not all interviewing techniques can be used with them. The two to be avoided are
    a. facilitation and clarification.
    b. clarification and explanation.
    c. empathy and interpretations.
    d. silence and pause after question.

11. Mr. B. tells you, "Everyone here ignores me." You respond, "Ignores you?" This technique is best described as
    a. clarification.
    b. selective listening.
    c. reflecting.
    d. validation.

12. Active listening skills include all of the following, *except*
    a. taking detailed notes during the interview.
    b. watching for clues in body language.
    c. repeating the person's statements to make sure you have understood what has been said.
    d. asking open-ended questions to explore the person's perspective.

13. When interviewing patients who do not speak English or have limited English proficiency, the examiner should
    a. take advantage of family members who are readily available and willing to assist.
    b. use a qualified medical interpreter who is culturally literate.
    c. seek as much information as possible, and then continue with the physical examination.
    d. ask the patient in the next bed and who speaks the same language as the patient, if he or she would mind interpreting.

14. The mother of a 2-year-old toddler tells the nurse that her son has an ear infection. What would be the most appropriate response?
    a. "Maybe he is just teething, but we will look in his ears later."
    b. "Does he have a history of frequent ear infections? It could just be teething."
    c. "Are you sure he is really having ear pain and not something else?"
    d. "Describe what he is doing that makes you think he has an ear infection."

15. You are preparing for an initial interview with a 15-year-old patient. To establish rapport, you
    a. begin the interview by immediately discussing the health concern. Adolescents do not want to make small talk and want to finish as quickly as possible.
    b. begin the interview by completing the full health history and discussing drug/alcohol use. Adolescents want to finish as quickly as possible.
    c. begin the interview by asking open, friendly questions about school and hobbies. Adolescents appreciate the opportunity to discuss themselves.
    d. begin the interview by asking open-ended questions that explore the health history. Adolescents are knowledgeable, and you can speak to them like adults.

16. Which of the following factors are important during an interview? (Select all that apply.)
    a. equal status seating
    b. leading questions
    c. active listening
    d. distancing
    e. social responses
    f. avoidance language
    g. providing privacy
    h. professional jargon

CRITICAL THINKING EXERCISE

Practice is an important part of developing communication skills. With a partner, record a patient and nurse interaction. Have your partner pretend to be a patient seeking health care at a local clinic. The partner should create a character, such as a single mother who describes vague symptoms in an attempt to get a prescription for her children; an older woman who focuses the interview on the student nurse's personal life instead of answering questions; a patient who is angry about having to wait 30 minutes to be seen; an Indigenous woman with systems trauma due to repeated experiences of racism, discrimination, and colonization in health care settings; or a gender-diverse youth that is worried about sharing their gender identity with a health care provider.

You can create your own character, but that character should be someone who poses a communication challenge. You may want to ask your instructor for other potential vignettes. Entering the interview, you will not know the reason for the visit and must rely on therapeutic communication skills to figure out how to effectively communicate with the patient. The interviews should last no more than 10 minutes and will likely be much shorter. Once you have been the nurse, pick a new scenario and switch roles. After completing the interactions, analyze the recording with special attention to

- therapeutic communication techniques, verbal and nonverbal
- nontherapeutic communication techniques, verbal and nonverbal
- areas for improvement
- skills at which you excelled

A video recording of this exercise is ideal so you can analyze the interaction. Pay special attention to your nonverbal behaviour, including a tendency to fidget. Although you may be nervous to record yourself, a recording provides the best opportunity to analyze your skills and will help you in your future interactions with patients. What you said during the interaction is not as important as your analysis of the interaction.

SKILLS LABORATORY/CLINICAL SETTING

Note that the clinical component of this chapter is the gathering of the complete health history. The history forms are included in Chapter 5.

NOTES

NOTES

5 The Complete Health History

PURPOSE

This chapter reviews the elements of a complete health history; how to interview a patient to gather the data for a complete health history; how to analyze patient data; and how to record the history accurately.

READING ASSIGNMENT

Jarvis: *Physical Examination and Health Assessment*, 4th Canadian ed., Chapter 5.

Suggested Readings

Dewell, S., Benzies, K., & Ginn, C. (2020). Precision health and nursing: Seeing the familiar in the foreign. *Canadian Journal of Nursing Research*, *52*(3), 199–208. https://doi.org/10.1177/0844562120945159

Provincial Health Services Authority. (n.d.) *Gender inclusive language—Clinical settings with new clients.* http://www.phsa.ca/transcarebc/Documents/HealthProf/Gender_Inclusive_Language_Clinical.pdf

Sexual Orientation and Gender Identity Nursing. (2021). https://soginursing.ca

STUDY GUIDE

After completing the reading assignment, you should be able to answer the following questions in the spaces provided.

1. State the purpose of the complete health history.

2. List and define the critical characteristics used to explore each symptom the patient identifies.

3. Define the elements of the health history: biographical data; reason for seeking care; current health or history of current illness; past health history; family health history; review of systems; functional assessment.

4. Discuss the rationale for obtaining a family history.

5. Discuss the rationale for obtaining a review of systems.

6. Describe the items included in a functional assessment.

7. Describe the additional questions you would ask of people who are newcomers.

REVIEW AND CLINICAL JUDGEMENT QUESTIONS

This test is for you to check your own mastery of the content. Answers are provided on the text's Evolve site.

1. When reading a medical record, you see the following notation: "Patient states, 'I've had a cold for about a week, and now I'm having difficulty breathing.'" This is an example of
   a. past history.
   b. a review of systems.
   c. a functional assessment.
   d. a reason for seeking care.

2. You are working in a primary care clinic. As you conduct a history for a 68-year-old patient you are seeing for a diabetes chronic disease visit, you have reason to question the reliability of the information being provided by the patient. One way to verify the reliability within the context of the interview is to
   a. rephrase the same questions later in the interview.
   b. review the patient's previous medical records.
   c. call the person identified as an emergency contact to verify the data provided.
   d. provide the patient with a printed history to complete and then compare the data provided.

3. The statement "reason for seeking care" has replaced the "chief complaint." This change is significant because
   a. "chief complaint" is really a diagnostic statement.
   b. the newer term allows another individual to supply the necessary information.
   c. the newer term incorporates wellness needs.
   d. "reason for seeking care" can incorporate the history of present illness.

4. During an initial interview, the examiner says, "Mrs. J., tell me what you do when your headaches occur." With this question, the examiner is seeking information about
   a. the patient's perception of the problem.
   b. aggravating or relieving factors.
   c. the frequency of the problem.
   d. the severity of the problem.

5. You are working in the emergency department and are taking a history for a 77-year-old female patient presenting with chest pain. Which of the following is an appropriate recording of the patient's reason for seeking health care?
   a. angina pectoris, duration 2 hours
   b. substernal pain radiating to left axilla, 1-hour duration
   c. "grabbing" chest pain for 2 hours
   d. pleurisy, 2 days' duration

6. You are preceptoring a nursing student and ask them to go ahead and begin taking a history for your patient. Given the patient's diagnosis of a hereditary genetic condition, you ask the student to create a genogram. The genogram is used specifically for the
   a. past health history
   b. past health history, specifically hospitalizations
   c. family history
   d. social history

7. Select the best description of "review of systems" as part of the health history.
   a. the evaluation of the past and current health state of each body system
   b. a documentation of the problem as described by the patient
   c. the recording of the objective findings of the practitioner
   d. a statement that describes the overall health state of the patient

8. A 26-year-old patient on the surgical ward rings their call ball. Upon arrival to the room, the patient tells you they have a new onset of abdominal pain that started 2 hours ago. You conduct an assessment and note a temperature of 38.5°C (101°F), a heart rate of 96 bpm, and blood pressure of 137/91 mm Hg. Which of the following is subjective?
   a. temperature of 38.5°C (101°F)
   b. heart rate of 96 bpm
   c. blood pressure of 137/91 mm Hg
   d. pain lasting 2 hours

9. The nurse asks a patient about his reason for seeking care and the signs and symptoms he is experiencing. Which of the following is an example of a symptom? (Select all that apply.)
   a. chest pain
   b. clammy skin
   c. fatigue
   d. serum potassium level 4.2 mmol/L
   e. cyanosis around lips
   f. a temperature of 37.8°C (100°F)
   g. numbness in fingers

10. Functional assessment measures how a person manages day-to-day activities. The impact of a disease on the daily activities of older adults is referred to as
    a. interpersonal relationship assessment.
    b. instrumental activities of daily living.
    c. reason for seeking care.
    d. disease burden.

11. When completing the health history on a young child, additional information is collected. Identify whether the following information is collected regardless of age or only collected on children.

Information	Always Collected	Children Only
Perinatal history		
Reason for seeking care		
Immunization status		
Medications		
Developmental milestones		
Family history		

12. As you complete the health history, the patient appears nervous and avoids eye contact. It is unclear whether he is a reliable source of information, and you begin to question whether he is being truthful during the interview. Your best option is
    a. continue with the interview, but note the nervous appearance and avoidance of eye contact.
    b. confront the patient. Let him know that you are concerned he is not a reliable source of his health information.
    c. continue with the interview, but ask the same question in a different way to determine reliability.
    d. ask the person if there is someone else who can serve as a secondary contact to ensure information is correct.

CRITICAL THINKING EXERCISE

Visit https://cbiit.github.io/FHH/html/index.html and complete the "My Family Health Portrait." After completion, consider the following questions:

1. How difficult was it for you to obtain the information necessary to complete the health portrait?

2. Were there questions that you could not answer even after consulting with other family members? How did that make you feel?

3. Did you identify unknown health risks through completion of your personal genogram?

4. How will completing your genogram impact the way in which you describe the importance of family history when interacting with patients?

SKILLS LABORATORY/CLINICAL SETTING

You are now ready for the clinical component of the interview and health history chapters. The purpose of the clinical component is to practise conducting a complete health history on a peer in the skills laboratory and to achieve the following.

Clinical Objectives

1. Demonstrate knowledge of interviewing skills by arranging a private, quiet, comfortable setting; introduce yourself and state your goals for the interview; pose open-ended and direct questions appropriately; listen to the patient in an attentive, nonjudgemental manner; choose appropriate vocabulary that the patient understands.

2. Demonstrate knowledge of the components of a health history by recording the reason for seeking care in the person's own words; elicit all the critical characteristics to describe the patient's symptom(s); gather pertinent data for the past history, family history, and systems review; identify self-care behaviours and risk factors from the functional assessment.

3. Record the history data accurately and as a reflection of what the patient believes the true health state to be.

Instructions

Work in pairs, and obtain a complete health history from a peer. Although you already know each other as student colleagues, play your role straight as "examiner" or "patient" for the best learning experience. Be aware that some of the history questions cover personal content. When you are acting as the patient, you have the right to withhold an answer if you do not feel comfortable with the amount of material you will be asked to divulge. Your own rights to privacy must coexist with the goals of the learning experience.

Familiarize yourself with the following history form, and practise phrasing your questions ahead of time. Note that the language on this form is intended as a prompt for the examiner and must be translated into clear and appropriate phrases for the patient. As a beginning examiner, you will need to use one copy of the form as a worksheet during the actual interview and use a fresh copy of the form for your rewritten formal record.

DOCUMENTATION—HEALTH HISTORY

Date _____

Examiner _____

I. **Biographical Data**

Name _____ Phone _____

Address _____ Preferred pronouns _____

Birthdate _____ Birthplace _____

Other recent countries of residence _____

Age _____ Sex _____ Gender _____ Relationship status _____

Current occupation _____ Usual occupation _____

Employer _____

Primary language _____ Preferred language _____

Authorized representative, if any _____

II. **Source and Reliability**

III. **Reason for Seeking Care**

IV. **Current Health or History of Current Illness**

V. **Past Health History**

General health _____
_____

Childhood illnesses _____
_____

Accidents or injuries _____
_____

Serious or chronic illnesses _____

_____

Hospitalizations _____

_____

Operations _____

_____

Obstetrical history _____

_____

Gravida _____ Term _____ Preterm _____
(# Pregnancies)   (# Term pregnancies)   (# Preterm pregnancies)

Ab/incomplete _____ Children living _____
(# Abortions/Miscarriages)

Course of pregnancy _____

(Date of delivery; length of pregnancy; length of labour; baby's weight and sex; vaginal delivery or Caesarean section; complications; baby's condition; postpartum course)

Immunizations _____

Most recent examination date _____

Allergies _____ Reaction _____

Current medications _____

_____

VI. **Family Health History**
Ages and health or cause of death for blood relatives
Ask specifically:

Heart disease _____

High blood pressure _____

Stroke _____

Diabetes _____

Blood disorders _____

Breast cancer _____

Cancer (other) _____

Sickle cell _____

Arthritis _____

Allergies _____

Asthma _____

Obesity _____

Alcoholism _____

Mental health concerns or illness _____

Seizure disorder _____

Kidney disease _____

Tuberculosis _____

Construct genogram below.

VII. **Review of Systems**
Include both past health problems that have been resolved and current problems, including date of onset. (Circle if present.) (Comment, if needed.)

General overall health state: Current weight gain or loss, how much, period of time, by diet or other factors; fatigue, weakness or malaise, fever, chills, sweats, or night sweats

Skin: History of skin disease (eczema, psoriasis, hives), pigment or colour change, change in mole, excessive dryness or moisture, pruritus, excessive bruising, rash, or lesion

Hair: Recent loss, change in texture

Nails: Change in shape, colour, or brittleness
   Health promotion: Amount of sun exposure, method of self-care for skin and hair

Head: Any unusually frequent or severe headache, any head injury, dizziness (syncope), or vertigo

Eyes: Changes to or difficulty with vision (decreased acuity, blurring, blind spots), eye pain, diplopia (double vision), redness or swelling, watering or discharge, glaucoma, or cataracts
   Health promotion: Wears glasses or contacts; most recent vision check or glaucoma test; how coping with loss of vision, if any

Ears: Earaches, infections, discharge and its characteristics, tinnitus, or vertigo
   Health promotion: Hearing loss, hearing aid use, how loss affects daily life, any exposure to environmental noise, use of earplugs or other noise reducing devices, method of cleaning ears

Nose and sinuses: Discharge and its characteristics, any unusually frequent or severe colds, sinus pain, nasal obstruction, nosebleeds, allergies or hay fever, or change in sense of smell

Mouth and throat: Mouth pain, frequent sore throat, bleeding gums, toothache, lesion in mouth or tongue, dysphagia, hoarseness or voice change, tonsillectomy, altered taste
  Health promotion: Pattern of daily dental care, use of prostheses (dentures, bridge), most recent dental checkup, smoking, use of chewing tobacco

Neck: Pain, limitation of motion, lumps or swelling, enlarged or tender nodes, goitre

Axilla: Pain, lump or swelling, rash

Upper Body: Pain, lump, nipple discharge, rash, history of breast disease, any surgery on breasts
  Health promotion: Knowledge of personal risk factors for breast cancer, most recent mammogram and results, recommendations for doing routine self-examination, clinical examination

Respiratory system: History of lung disease (asthma, emphysema, bronchitis, pneumonia, tuberculosis), sleep apnea, chest pain with breathing, wheezing or noisy breathing, shortness of breath, how much activity produces shortness of breath, cough, sputum (colour, amount), hemoptysis, toxin or pollution exposure
  Health promotion: Most recent chest X-ray, tuberculin skin test; use of CPAP machine

Cardiovascular system: Precordial or retrosternal pain, palpitation, cyanosis, dyspnea on exertion (specify amount of exertion that triggers dyspnea), orthopnea, paroxysmal nocturnal dyspnea, nocturia, edema, history of heart murmur, hypertension, coronary artery disease, anemia
  Health promotion: Date of last electrocardiogram or other heart tests, and results; usual physical activity and exercise, "heart-healthy diet awareness"

Peripheral vascular system: Coldness, numbness, tingling, swelling of legs (time of day, activity), discoloration in hands or feet (bluish-red, pallor, mottling, associated with position, especially around feet and ankles), varicose veins or complications, intermittent claudication, thrombophlebitis, ulcers
  Health promotion: If work involves long-term sitting or standing, avoid crossing legs at the knees, wear support hose, get up and move around every 20 minutes

Gastro-intestinal system: Appetite, food intolerance, dysphagia, heartburn, indigestion, pain (associated with eating), other abdominal pain, pyrosis (esophageal and stomach burning sensation with sour eructation), nausea and vomiting (character), vomiting blood, history of abdominal disease (ulcer, liver or gallbladder, jaundice, appendicitis, colitis), flatulence, frequency of bowel movement, any recent change, stool characteristics, constipation or diarrhea, black stools, rectal bleeding, rectal conditions (hemorrhoids, fistula)
  Health promotion: Use of antacids, laxatives; dietary history; maintaining adequate hydration and nutrition

Urinary system: Frequency, urgency, nocturia (the number of times the person awakens at night to urinate, recent change), dysuria, polyuria or oliguria, hesitancy or straining, narrowed stream, urine colour (cloudy or presence of hematuria), incontinence, history of urinary disease (kidney disease, kidney stones, urinary tract infections, prostate), pain in flank, groin, suprapubic region, or low back
  Health promotion: Measures to avoid or treat urinary tract infections; use of Kegel exercises after childbirth

External genitals: Penis or testicular pain, sores or lesions, penile discharge, lumps, hernia. Vulvar sores or lesions, vulvar or vaginal itching, discharge and its characteristics
  Health promotion: Perform testicular self-examination? how frequently?

Internal genitals: Menstrual history (age at menarche, most recent menstrual cycle and duration, any amenorrhea or menorrhagia, premenstrual pain or dysmenorrhea, intermenstrual spotting), vaginal itching, discharge and its characteristics, age at menopause, menopausal signs or symptoms, postmenopausal bleeding
  Health promotion: Last gynecological checkup; most recent Pap test and results; changes associated with perimenopause (as appropriate to age and life stage)

Sexual health: Currently in a relationship involving intercourse? Are aspects of sexual intimacy satisfactory to patient and partner, any dyspareunia (for a patient with a vagina), any changes in erection or ejaculation (for a patient with a penis), use of contraceptive, is contraceptive method satisfactory? Use of condoms, how consistently? Aware of any contact with partner who has a sexually transmitted infection (STI; e.g., gonorrhea, herpes, chlamydia, venereal warts, human immunodeficiency virus/acquired immunodeficiency syndrome [HIV/AIDS], syphilis)?
  Health promotion: Knowledge of safer sexual practices; signs and symptoms of STIs

Musculo-skeletal system: History of arthritis or gout. In the joints: any pain, stiffness, swelling (location, migratory nature), deformity, limitation of motion, and noise with joint motion. In the muscles: any pain, cramps, weakness, gait problems, or problems with coordinated activities. In the back: any pain (location and radiation to extremities), stiffness, limitation of motion, or history of back pain or disc disease
  Health promotion: How much walking per day? What is the effect of limited range of motion on daily activities, such as on grooming, feeding, toileting, and dressing? Any mobility aids used? For patients with mobility concerns or older adults, ask about fall-prevention strategies

Neurological system: History of seizure disorder, stroke, fainting, blackouts. In motor function: weakness, tic or tremor, paralysis, or coordination problems. In sensory function: numbness and tingling (paresthesia). In cognitive function: memory disorder (recent or distant, disorientation). In mental status: any nervousness, mood change, depression, or any history of mental health dysfunction or hallucinations
  Health promotion: Data about interpersonal relationships and coping patterns can be placed in this section

Hematological system: Bleeding tendency of skin or mucous membranes, excessive bruising, lymph node swelling, exposure to toxic agents or radiation, blood transfusion and reactions

Endocrine system: History of diabetes or symptoms of diabetes (polyuria, polydipsia, polyphagia), history of thyroid disease, intolerance to heat or cold, change in skin pigmentation or texture, excessive sweating, relationship between appetite and weight, abnormal hair distribution, nervousness, tremors, and need for hormone therapy
  Health promotion: Depending on the diabetic patient's health history, ask about use of appropriate footwear to prevent foot sores or ulcers

FUNCTIONAL ASSESSMENT (INCLUDING ACTIVITIES OF DAILY LIVING)

Remember to ask about and document self-care behaviours as you work through each section of the Functional Assessment.

Self-concept, self-esteem: Education (last grade completed, other significant training) _____

Financial status (income adequate for lifestyle and/or health and social concerns) _____

Value or belief system (religious or spiritual practices and perception of personal strengths) _____

Activity and mobility: Daily profile, usual pattern of a typical day _____

Independent or needs assistance with activities of daily living (ADLs): feeding, bathing, hygiene, dressing, toileting, bed-to-chair transfer, walking, standing, climbing stairs _____
Use of wheelchair, prostheses, or mobility aids _____
Leisure activities _____

Exercise pattern (type, amount per day or week, method of warm-up session, method of monitoring body's response to exercise) _____

Sleep and rest: Sleep patterns, insomnia, night awakenings, snoring, daytime naps, any sleep aids used, CPAP machine
_____
_____

Nutrition and elimination: Record 24-hour diet recall; note meal pattern _____
_____
_____

Is this diet and meal pattern typical of most days? _____

Who buys food? _____ Who prepares food? _____

Does the patient have difficulty preparing food? Why? _____

Difficulties chewing or swallowing? _____

Finances adequate for food? _____

Home environment adequate for meal preparation? (e.g., water, appliances, utilities) _____

Who is present at mealtimes? _____

Interpersonal relationships and resources: Who does the patient live with? Family, pet, roommate? _____
_____

Is living arrangement satisfactory? _____

If the patient lives alone, what social contacts are there? How often? Satisfactory? _____

Describe patient's role in family (e.g., caregiver, meal preparation, housework) _____
_____

Tensions or conflicts with family, friends, co-workers, classmates? _____

Financial, physical, or social strains? _____

Seeks support for a problem from _____

How much daily time spent alone? Is this pleasurable or isolating? _____
_____

Spiritual resources: Does religious faith or spirituality play an important part in the patient's and family's life? Does it influence their health or health care decisions? If yes, is there a preference for how religious and spiritual matters are addressed within the context of their health care? _____
_____

Coping and stress management: Describe current stresses in life _____
_____

Significant life changes or losses in past year _____

Methods used to relieve stress _____

Are these methods helpful? _____

Tobacco use history:

Tobacco use (cigarettes, pipe, vaporizer, e-cigarettes, chewing tobacco, snuff)? _____

Frequency of use (number of packs, pipes, cartridges, or chews) per day _____

Daily use? _____ For how many years _____ Age started _____

Ever tried to cut down? _____ How did it go? _____

Alcohol: Refer to Chapter 7 in the Jarvis 4th Canadian ed. textbook for guidelines on how to inquire about alcohol and substance use in effective, respectful ways.

Drink alcohol? _____ Frequency of alcohol use _____

Date of last alcohol use _____

Amount of alcohol that episode _____

Out of the last 30 days, on how many days was alcohol consumed? _____

Ever felt drinking was a problem? Ever been in treatment for alcohol use? _____
_____

Substance use: Depending on the patient's personal context, and the extent to which you have established rapport with the patient, you may ask about specific substance use: that is, marihuana, cocaine, crack cocaine, fentanyl, amphetamines, barbiturates, benzodiazepines, crystal methamphetamine, LSD, heroin, methadone, methylenedioxymethamphetamine (Ecstasy), phencyclidine hydrochloride (PCP), other.

Frequency of use _____ Duration of use _____

Has usage ever affected the patient's work, relationships, family, or economic circumstances? _____
_____

Ever been in treatment for drug use? _____

Environmental hazards: Housing and neighbourhood (type of structure, live alone, know neighbours) ____
_____

Safety of area _____

Adequate heat and utilities _____

Access to transportation _____

Involvement in community services _____

Hazards at workplace or home _____

Use of seatbelts and helmets _____

Geographical or occupational exposures _____

Travel to, or residence in other countries (including military service) _____

Intimate partner violence (IPV):*

How are things at home? School? Work? _____

How are things at home, school, and work affecting your health? _____

Is your home, school, or work environment safe? _____

Occupational health: Please describe your job. _____

Work with any health hazards (e.g., asbestos, inhalants, chemicals, repetitive motion)? _____
_____

Any protective equipment used at work to reduce your exposure? _____

Any work programs designed to monitor your exposure? _____

Any health problems that you think are related to your job? _____

What do you like or dislike about your job? _____

Perception of health: What does it mean to you to be healthy? _____

View of own health now _____

What are your concerns? _____

What do you expect will happen to your health in the future? _____
_____

Your health goals _____

What are your expectations of your health care providers? _____
_____

*If you sense that violence is an issue, use the strategies discussed in the 4th Canadian ed. of the Jarvis textbook, Chapter 8, for guidelines on how to inquire about IPV in effective, respectful ways.

6 Mental Health Assessment

PURPOSE

This chapter helps you to learn the components of a mental health assessment. You will learn how to interview a patient to gather data for a mental health history; assess the person's appearance, behaviour, cognitive functions, thought processes, and perceptions; analyze patient data; and document the mental health assessment accurately.

READING ASSIGNMENT

Jarvis: *Physical Examination and Health Assessment*, 4th Canadian ed., Chapter 6.

Suggested Reading

Fazel, S., & Runeson, B. (2020). Suicide. *New England Journal of Medicine, 382,* 266–274.

GLOSSARY

Study the following terms after reading the corresponding chapter in the text.

Abstract reasoning: the ability to think conceptually; to comprehend meaning beyond the concrete, factual, and literal; and to analyze information and problem-solve complex information
Affect: a display of feelings or state of mind
Appearance: general presentation to others
Attention: concentration, ability to focus on one specific thing
Consciousness: being aware of one's feelings, thoughts, and environment
Delirium: an acute confusional change or loss of consciousness and perceptual disturbance; it may accompany acute illness and usually resolves when the underlying cause is treated
Delusion: a false belief that occurs when abnormal significance is attached to a genuine perception without rational or emotional justification
Dementia: newly named *mild or major neurocognitive disorder* by the DSM-5; a progressive degenerative disease caused by damage to the brain cells, symptoms include memory loss and a deterioration of cognitive performance and function, physical capacity, and personality features
Dysarthria: distorted speech, including misuse of words; omitting letters, syllables, or words; and transposing words
Dysphonia: abnormal volume and pitch when speaking
Hallucination: a perception occurring while awake and conscious that has no source in the external world
Illusion: misinterpretation of a true optical, auditory, tactile, or olfactory sensation
Insight: awareness of the reality of the situation
Judgement: the ability to choose a logical course of action
Memory: the ability to lay down and store experiences and perceptions for later recall
Mental disorder: constellations of co-occurring symptoms that may involve alterations in thought, experience, and emotion serious enough to cause distress and impair functioning, cause difficulties in sustaining interpersonal relationships and performing jobs, and sometimes lead to self-destructive behaviour and suicide; it is defined and diagnosed in Canada via criteria specified in the American Psychiatric Association's *Diagnostic and Statistical Manual of Mental Disorders*, 5th ed., (2013)
Mental health: the capacity to feel, think, express emotions, and behave in ways that enhance personal capacity to manage challenges, adapt successfully to a range of demands, and enjoy life
Mental illness: a biological condition of the brain that causes alterations in thinking, mood, or behaviour (or any combination thereof); it is associated with significant distress and impaired daily functioning
Mental status: an aspect of mental health that involves emotional and cognitive functioning
Mental status examination: a structured way of observing and describing a person's current state of mind, under the domains of appearance, behaviour, cognition, and thought processes
Mood: a sustained emotion the patient is experiencing
Orientation: awareness of the objective world in relation to the self

Perception: awareness of objects through any of the five senses
Speech: using language and the voice to communicate one's thoughts and feelings
Thought content: *what* the person thinks—specific ideas, beliefs, use of words
Thought process: the *way* a person thinks—the logical train of thought

STUDY GUIDE

After completing the reading assignment, you should be able to answer the following questions in the spaces provided.

1. Define the term *mental health*.

2. List four situations in which it would be necessary to perform a full mental health assessment.

3. Explain four factors that could affect a patient's response to the mental status examination but have nothing to do with mental disorders.

4. Distinguish *dysphonia* from *dysarthria*.

5. Describe the Global Assessment of Functioning test.

6. Identify convenient ways to assess a person's recent memory within the context of the initial health history, and list two possible causes of recent memory deficits.

7. Which mental function is the Four Unrelated Words Test intended to test?

8. List at least three questions you could ask a patient that would screen for suicidal ideation.

9. Describe the patient response level of consciousness that would be graded as follows:

Lethargic or somnolent _____

Obtunded _____

Stupor or semicoma _____

Coma _____

Acute confusional state (delirium) _____

REVIEW AND CLINICAL JUDGEMENT QUESTIONS

This test is for you to check your own mastery of the content. Answers are provided on the text's Evolve site.

1. Although a full mental status examination may not be required, the examiner must be aware of the four main headings of the assessment while performing the interview and physical examination. These headings are
    a. mood, affect, consciousness, and orientation.
    b. memory, attention, thought content, and perceptions.
    c. language, orientation, attention, and abstract reasoning.
    d. appearance, behaviour, cognition, and thought processes.

2. Select the finding that most accurately describes the appearance of a patient.
    a. tense posture and restless activity; clothing clean but not appropriate for the season (patient wearing T-shirt and shorts in cold weather)
    b. oriented ×3; affect is appropriate for circumstances
    c. alert and responds to verbal stimuli; tearful when diagnosis discussed
    d. laughing inappropriately; oriented ×3

3. The ability to lay down new memories is part of the assessment of cognitive functions. One way to accomplish this is by
    a. noting whether the patient completes a thought without wandering.
    b. a test of general knowledge.
    c. a description of past medical history.
    d. use of the Four Unrelated Words Test.

4. To accurately plan for discharge teaching, additional assessments may be required for the patient with aphasia. This may be accomplished by asking the patient to
    a. calculate serial sevens.
    b. name his or her grandchildren and their birthdays.
    c. demonstrate word comprehension by naming articles in the room or on the body as you point to them.
    d. interpret a proverb.

5. During an interview with a patient newly diagnosed with a seizure disorder, the patient states, "I plan to be an airline pilot." If the patient continues to have this career goal after teaching regarding seizure disorders has been provided, the practitioner might question the patient's
    a. thought processes.
    b. judgement.
    c. attention span.
    d. recent memory.

6. On a patient's second day in an acute care hospital, the patient complains about the "bugs" on the bed. The bed is clean. This would be an example of altered
    a. thought process.
    b. orientation.
    c. perception.
    d. higher intellectual function.

7. One way to detect dementia and delirium and to differentiate these from psychiatric mental illness is
   a. the Proverb Interpretation Test.
   b. the Montreal Cognitive Assessment (MoCA).
   c. the Four Unrelated Words Test.
   d. the Older Adult Behavioural Checklist.

8. The Pediatric Symptom Checklist, completed by a parent, is used to assess the emotional and behavioural wellness of
   a. infants.
   b. children ages 1 to 5 years.
   c. children ages 4 to 18 years.
   d. adolescents.

9. A major characteristic of dementia is
   a. impairment of short- and long-term memory.
   b. hallucinations.
   c. the sudden onset of symptoms.
   d. substance induced.

10. A patient with a MoCA score of 21 may be expected to have
    a. no cognitive impairment.
    b. mild cognitive impairment.
    c. moderate cognitive impairment.
    d. severe cognitive impairment.

11. You are asked to complete a full mental status examination of a patient who is being seen for increasing "forgetfulness." Put the steps below in the correct order by numbering them 1 to 5.

    _____ Check hearing and vision.

    _____ Ask orientation questions.

    _____ Conduct a supplemental mental status examination (e.g., Mini-Cog, MMSE, MoCA).

    _____ Note general appearance.

    _____ Give patient four words to remember for the Four Unrelated Words Test.

12. Consider each item below and specify whether it is an indicator of dementia, delirium, or depression. Some characteristics may be associated with more than one disease process.

	Delirium	Dementia	Depression
Sudden onset			
Impaired memory			
Level of consciousness not altered			
Characterized by rapid emotional swings			
Reversible with proper treatment			

Match column A to column B.

Column A—Definition

13. Lack of emotional response
14. Loss of identity
15. Excessive well-being
16. Apprehension from the anticipation of a danger whose source is unknown
17. Annoyed, easily provoked
18. Loss of control
19. Sad, gloomy, dejected
20. Rapid shift of emotions
21. Worried about known external danger

Column B—Type of Mood and Affect

a. Depression
b. Anxiety
c. Flat affect
d. Euphoria
e. Lability
f. Rage
g. Irritability
h. Fear
i. Depersonalization

22. Write a narrative account of a mental status assessment with normal findings.

CRITICAL THINKING EXERCISE

Use the Montreal Cognitive Assessment (MoCA) on the next page to complete a cognitive screen on a partner. Switch partners and complete the Mini-Cog (https://mini-cog.com) on a different partner. Compare and contrast the differences between the screening tools. Which seemed more appropriate for use in an outpatient clinic? The hospital? Were you comfortable providing instructions and scoring each instrument? What questions do you have about scoring?

Next, use the MoCA and Mini-Cog in a clinical setting. Complete the MoCA and Mini-Cog on different older adults (>65 years). Did you have to change your delivery with an older adult? Discuss the experience with classmates to identify differences found with different patients and in different settings.

NOTES

MONTREAL COGNITIVE ASSESSMENT (MoCA)
Version 7.1 Original Version

NAME:
Education: Date of birth:
Sex: DATE:

VISUOSPATIAL / EXECUTIVE

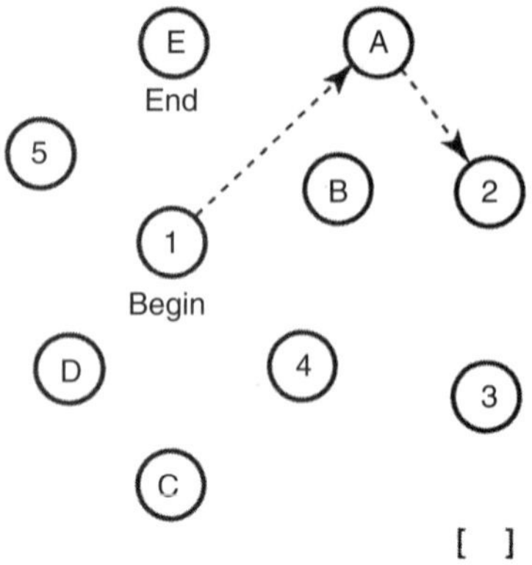

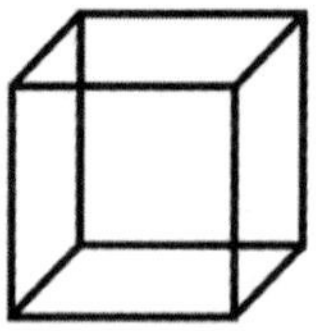

Trail-making task: points labeled 1, 2, 3, 4, 5 and A, B, C, D, E with "Begin" at 1 and "End" at E. Dashed arrows show path 1 → A → 2.

Copy cube [ ]

Draw CLOCK (Ten past eleven) (3 points) [ ] Contour   [ ] Numbers   [ ] Hands

___/5

NAMING

[ ] lion   [ ] rhinoceros   [ ] camel

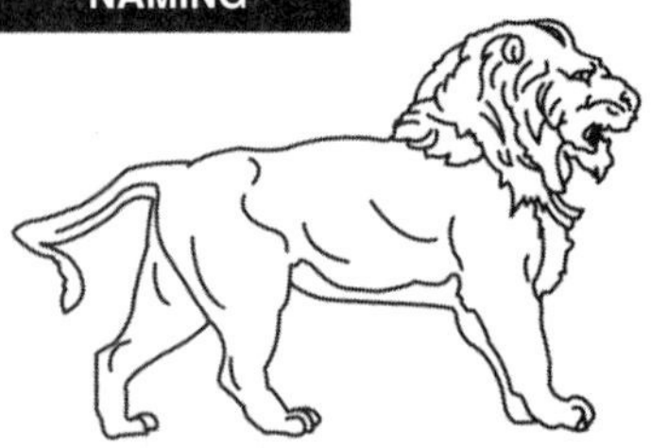

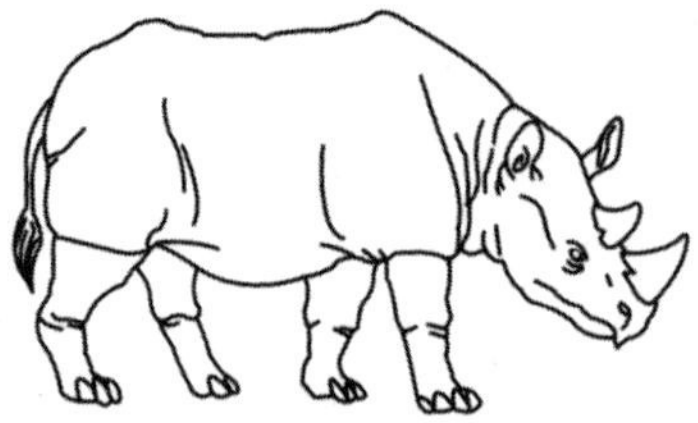

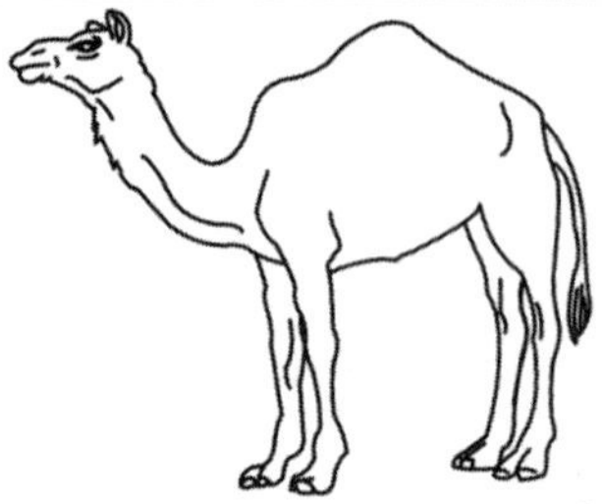

___/3

MEMORY

Read list of words, subject must repeat them. Do 2 trials, even if 1st trial is successful. Do a recall after 5 minutes.

	FACE	VELVET	CHURCH	DAISY	RED
1st trial					
2nd trial					

No points

ATTENTION

Read list of digits (1 digit/sec.).
Subject has to repeat them in the forward order   [ ] 2 1 8 5 4
Subject has to repeat them in the backward order   [ ] 7 4 2

___/2

Read list of letters. The subject must tap with his hand at each letter A. No points if ≥2 errors
[ ] F B A C M N A A J K L B A F A K D E A A A J A M O F A A B

___/1

Serial 7 subtraction starting at 100   [ ] 93   [ ] 86   [ ] 79   [ ] 72   [ ] 65
4 or 5 correct subtractions: **3 pts**, 2 or 3 correct: **2 pts**, 1 correct: **1 pt**, 0 correct: **0 pt**

___/3

LANGUAGE

Repeat: I only know that John is the one to help today. [ ]
The cat always hid under the couch when dogs were in the room. [ ]

___/2

Fluency/Name maximum number of words in one minute that begin with the letter F   [ ] _____ (N ≥ 11 words)

___/1

ABSTRACTION

Similarity between e.g. banana - orange = fruit   [ ] train – bicycle   [ ] watch – ruler

___/2

DELAYED RECALL

Has to recall words WITH NO CUE	FACE [ ]	VELVET [ ]	CHURCH [ ]	DAISY [ ]	RED [ ]	Points for UNCUED recall only
Optional Category cue						
Multiple choice cue						

___/5

ORIENTATION

[ ] Date   [ ] Month   [ ] Year   [ ] Day   [ ] Place   [ ] City

___/6

© Z.Nasreddine MD   www.mocatest.org   Normal ≥ 26/30   TOTAL ___/30
Administered by: _____   Add 1 point if ≤12 yr edu

Copyright © Z. Nasreddine, MD. Reproduced with permission. Copies are available at http://www.mocatest.org

SKILLS LABORATORY/CLINICAL SETTING

You are now ready for the clinical component of the mental status examination. The purpose of the clinical component is to achieve beginning competency with the administration of the mental status examination and with the supplemental MoCA.

Practise the steps of the full mental status examination on a peer or a patient in the clinical setting, giving appropriate instructions as you proceed. Formulate ahead of time your questions to pose to the patient. Record your findings using the documentation sheet that follows.

Next, practise the steps of the MoCA. It is used frequently in clinical and research settings.

NOTES

NOTES

DOCUMENTATION—MENTAL STATUS EXAMINATION

Date _____

Examiner _____

Patient _____ Age _____ Gender _____

Occupation _____

Mental Status
Before testing, tell the person the four words you want them to remember and to recall in a few minutes for the Four Unrelated Words Test.

1. **Appearance** _____

    Body movements _____

    Dress _____

    Grooming and hygiene _____

2. **Behaviour** _____

    Level of consciousness _____

    Facial expression _____

    Speech:

        Quality _____

        Pace _____

        Word choice _____

    Mood and affect _____

3. **Cognitive Functions**

    Orientation:

        Time _____

        Place _____

        Person _____

    Attention span _____

    Recent memory _____

    Remote memory _____

    New learning—Four Unrelated Words Test _____

    Additional testing for aphasia:

    Word comprehension

        Reading _____

        Writing _____

        Judgement _____

4. Thought Processes and Perceptions _____

    Thought processes _____

    Thought content _____

    Perceptions _____

    Suicidal thoughts _____

7 Substance Use and Health Assessment

PURPOSE

The purpose of this chapter is to provide nurse–clinicians with knowledge of substance use to integrate into health assessments across a range of practice contexts with patients across the life span.

READING ASSIGNMENT

Jarvis: *Physical Examination and Health Assessment*, 4th Canadian ed., Chapter 7.

SUGGESTED READINGS

Danda, M. (2021, November 22). We've lost sight of the ongoing substance use crisis; Here's what nurses should do about it. *Canadian Nurse*. https://www.canadian-nurse.com/blogs/cn-content/2021/11/22/weve-lost-sight-of-the-ongoing-substance-use-crisi

Government of Canada. (2022, June 24). *Data, surveillance and research on opioids and other substances.* https://www.canada.ca/en/health-canada/services/opioids/data-surveillance-research.html

Mackavey, C., & Kearney, K. (2020). Substance use disorder: Screening adolescents in primary care. *The Nurse Practitioner, 45*(5), 25–33.

GLOSSARY

Study the following terms after reading the corresponding chapter in the text.

Dependence: a label for compulsive, out-of-control substance use; it has been problematic and confusing to clinicians and has resulted in patients with normal tolerance and withdrawal being labelled as addicts. Accordingly, the term *dependence* is limited to physiological dependence, which is an expected, anticipated, and normal response to repeated doses of many medications

Harm reduction: policies, programs, and practices that aim primarily to reduce the adverse health, social, and economic consequences of the use of legal and illegal psychoactive substances, without necessarily reducing drug consumption. Harm reduction benefits people who use substances as well as their families and the community

Interpersonal violence: includes physical, psychological, sexual, and other forms of violence, including child maltreatment, sexual assault and intimate partner violence

Intoxication: a condition that follows the administration of a psychoactive substance and results in disturbances in the level of consciousness, cognition, perception, judgement, affect, or behaviour, or other psychophysiological functions and responses

Physiological dependence: a normal physiological response to repeated doses of many medications, including beta-blockers, antidepressants, opioids, antianxiety agents, and other drugs and substances, which produce symptoms upon discontinuation of use

Substance use: use of certain substances, such as tobacco, alcohol, opiates, benzodiazepines, amphetamines, nonprescribed prescription drugs, and marijuana, that may cause family, personal, work, or legal problems

Tolerance: defined by a need for markedly increased amounts of the substance to achieve intoxication or the desired effect

Withdrawal: physiological symptoms that occur when the medication or drug is withdrawn, requiring care to manage and mitigate withdrawal symptoms

STUDY GUIDE

After completing the reading assignment, you should be able to answer the following questions in the spaces provided.

1. Describe how the use of the terms *addiction* and *dependence* has been problematic for health care providers and patients.

2. Outline the social contexts and factors that influence the public perception of specific drugs or substances.

3. Describe Canada's current policy with respect to drugs and other substances.

4. Provide a summary of the findings of the 2017 Canadian Tobacco, Alcohol and Drugs Survey.

5. List three of the factors that contribute to and influence substance use.

6. List the five *A*s for integrating knowledge of substance use in a health assessment.

7. Outline ways in which health care providers can examine their own attitudes toward substance use.

8. Describe the method of asking progressively more detailed questions related to substance use during the health assessment process.

9. Describe the CAGE and TWEAK screening tools.

10. Identify the key considerations for providers when assessing for substance use in a pregnant person.

REVIEW AND CLINICAL JUDGEMENT QUESTIONS

This test is for you to check your own mastery of the content. Answers are provided on the text's Evolve site.

1. You are working in primary care and are scheduled to see a 29-year-old female for a wound assessment. When you greet your patient, you notice that she appears dishevelled and fatigued. She has a wound on her right antecubital fossa that you suspect may be from IV drug use. What is an appropriate response? (Select all that apply.)
   a. "It's important to use clean needles when injecting drugs."
   b. "Do you use substances? If so, what substances are you using? How do you use them? How often and how much do you use?"
   c. "You need help. I think you should check yourself into detox ASAP."
   d. "Are you interested in discussing treatment options for substance use disorders today?"
   e. "Have you ever had an overdose? Would you like a Narcan kit today?"

2. Muscle pain is a symptom of opiate withdrawal.
   a. true
   b. false

3. The TWEAK tool assesses which of the following?
   a. tolerance, worry, eye-opener, amnesia, k(c)ut down
   b. tolerance, worry, eye-opener, aggression, k(c)ut down
   c. tremors, worry, eye-opener, aggression, k(c)ut down
   d. tolerance, withdrawal, eye-opener, amnesia, k(c)ut down

4. When health care providers reflect on their own values related to substance use, they should consider all of the following *except*
   a. their own family values and attitudes.
   b. if judgements arise when they care for people who use substances.
   c. what social issues they see as influencing people's substance use patterns.
   d. if they themselves have used substances.

5. *Canada's Guidance on Alcohol and Health: Final Report* (https://ccsa.ca/sites/default/files/2023-01/Canada%27s%20 Guidance%20on%20Alcohol%20and%20Health%20Final%20Report_l.pdf) states that people should drink no more than 1-2 standard drinks per week to maintain a low risk drinking profile and thus likely avoid alcohol-related consequences for themselves and others.
   a. true
   b. false

6. Health care providers can assess for substance use in a more respectful way by
   a. being clear about why they are gathering information and conveying the reasons for the assessment.
   b. learning about the context and population being served.
   c. not gathering information that is not needed or not going to be used.
   d. starting history-taking with the least intrusive questions.
   e. all of the above.

7. You are screening your patient for alcohol and substance use. The patient reports drinking alcohol, but he reports abstaining from illicit substance use. When you complete the CAGE questionnaire, the patient reports that he sometimes thinks he should cut down on his drinking and that he finds himself occasionally needing to have a drink in the morning to get going. Based on this assessment, you tell the patient:
   a. "While I don't think you should drink in the morning, your drinking doesn't seem to be impacting your work or home life. You might consider cutting down, though."
   b. "I would recommend keeping a journal of how much you drink. That way, when you come back, we can have a discussion on drinking patterns."
   c. "I believe you may have an alcohol use disorder. I'm here to help. Would you like to discuss some treatment options?"
   d. "I believe you have an alcohol use disorder. You must stop drinking now or you will likely die early."

8. The relationship between all forms of interpersonal violence, including child maltreatment, sexual assault and intimate partner violence, and increased and/or harmful substance use has been shown consistently across age groups.
   a. true
   b. false

9. You are screening for alcohol use in a 45-year-old female who reports an increase in drinking after being laid off. Which of the following statements would be indicative of exceeding the moderate risk limit? Check all that apply?
   a. "I used to go out after work on Fridays with my friends. Now I drink one beer on two nights a week."
   b. "I used to go out after work on Fridays with my friends. Now I have three or four beers most nights."
   c. "I used to go out after work on Fridays with my friends. Now I don't drink at all since I don't go out after work."
   d. "I used to go out after work on Fridays with my friends. Now I have two beers most nights."

10. As per *Canada's Guidance on Alcohol and Health: Final Report* (https://ccsa.ca/sites/default/files/2023-01/Canada%27s%20Guidance%20on%20Alcohol%20and%20Health%20Final%20Report_1.pdf), which of the following is a standard drink? (Select all that apply)
    a. 142 mL (5 oz) glass of wine
    b. 43 mL (1.5 oz) shot glass of spirits (e.g., gin, vodka, whiskey)
    c. 473 mL (16 oz) can of malt liquor
    d. One martini
    e. 341 mL (12 oz) of beer
    f. Pint of beer
    g. 1/2 bottle of a standard table wine (750 mL bottle)
    h. 341 mL (12 oz) of cooler, cider, or ready-to-drink beverage

11. For each substance below, specify the associated characteristic(s) of intoxication. Some characteristics may apply to more than one substance.

Characteristic	Alcohol	Marijuana	Opiates	Cocaine
Pinpoint pupils				
Reddened eyes				
Pupillary dilation				
Loss of balance				
Slurred speech				
Talkativeness				

12. For each substance below, specify the associated characteristic(s) of withdrawal. Some characteristics may apply to more than one substance.

Characteristic	Alcohol	Marijuana	Opiates	Cocaine
Irritability				
Dilated pupils				
Hallucinations				
Fatigue				
Hand tremors				

CRITICAL THINKING EXERCISES

Over recent years, opioid and other substance-related deaths and harms have continued to rise significantly across Canada. In response, the Government of Canada created a website with links to evidence guiding the government's response to the overdose crisis. Take a moment to visit https://www.canada.ca/en/health-canada/services/opioids/data-surveillance-research.html. Reflecting on where you reside in Canada, review the provincial and territorial information on the website. How does your province or territory compare to others? What differences do you notice among the provinces and territories? What might explain these differences?

SKILLS LABORATORY/CLINICAL SETTING

Pair up with a classmate and interview each other using the TWEAK questionnaire. Keep your answers confidential—the interviews are not to be turned in to the instructor. Record the score at the end of each line and then total; the maximum total is 7. A score of 2 or more indicates a risk for a drinking problem. Once you have completed this interview, switch to the CAGE questionnaire and repeat the process. Record the score at the end of each line and then total; the maximum total is 4. An answer of "yes," "sometimes," or "often" to 2 or more questions indicates a risk for a drinking problem. How does it feel asking these questions to another person? Which questionnaire did you prefer?

NOTES

NOTES

8 Interpersonal Violence and Health Assessment

PURPOSE

This chapter reviews intimate partner violence (IPV), elder abuse, child abuse, and other forms of interpersonal violence. It also reviews how to assess the extent of abuse, physical and psychological harm (including injury), and how to document IPV appropriately.

READING ASSIGNMENT

Jarvis: *Physical Examination and Health Assessment*, 4th Canadian ed., Chapter 8.

Suggested Readings

Jack, S. M., Munro-Kramer, M. L., Williams, J. R., et al. (2021). Recognising and responding to intimate partner violence using telehealth: Practical guidance for nurses and midwives. *Journal of Clinical Nursing, 30*(3–4), 588–602. https://doi.org/10.1111/jocn.15554

Roney, L. N., & Villano, C. E. (2020). Recognizing victims of a hidden crime: Human trafficking victims in your pediatric trauma bay. *Journal of Trauma Nursing, 27*(1), 37–41.

GLOSSARY

Study the following terms after reading the corresponding chapter in the text.

Child emotional abuse: any pattern of behaviour that harms a child's emotional development or sense of self-worth; it includes frequent belittling, rejection, threats, and withholding of love and support

Child maltreatment: "the abuse and neglect that occurs to children under 18 years of age. It includes all types of physical and/or emotional ill-treatment, sexual abuse, neglect, negligence and commercial or other exploitation, which results in actual or potential harm to the child's health, survival, development or dignity in the context of a relationship of responsibility, trust or power. Child maltreatment includes neglect, physical, sexual and emotional abuse, and fabricated or induced illness" (WHO, 2019)

Child neglect: failure to provide for a child's basic needs (physical, educational, medical, and emotional)

Child physical abuse: physical injury due to punching, beating, kicking, biting, burning, shaking, or otherwise harming a child. Even if the parent or caretaker did not intend to harm the child, such acts are considered abuse when done purposefully.

Child sexual abuse: it includes fondling a child's genitals, incest, penetration, rape, sodomy, indecent exposure, and commercial exploitation through prostitution or the production of pornographic materials

Elder abuse: violence, mistreatment, or neglect that older adults living in either private residences or institutions experience at the hands of their spouses, children, other family members, caregivers, service providers, or other individuals in positions of power

Human trafficking: "compelling or coercing a person to provide labour or services, or to engage in commercial sex acts" (US Department of Justice, 2020). If the victim is a minor, commercial sex acts are considered trafficking whether coercion is present. Human trafficking does not require movement of the person from one place to another

Intimate partner violence (IPV): physical or sexual violence (use of physical force) or both, or threat of such violence; also psychological or emotional abuse or coercive tactics when there has been prior physical or sexual violence between spouses or nonmarital partners current or former ("partners" includes dates or boyfriend and girlfriend)

Mandatory reporting of abuse: a situation in which a specified group of people (e.g., health care providers, social workers) is required by law to report abuse (of a specified nature against specified people) to a governmental agency (e.g., protective services, the police)

Psychological abuse: the infliction of emotional or mental anguish by humiliation, coercion, and threats or lack of social stimulation. Examples include yelling, threats of harm, threats of withholding basic medical or personal care, and leaving the person alone for long periods

Sexual assault: forced sexual activity with or without physical injury; it is considered a crime under the Canadian *Criminal Code*

Spousal abuse: physical or sexual violence, psychological violence, or financial abuse within current or former marital or common-law relationships, including same-sex spousal relationships

STUDY GUIDE

After completing the reading assignment, you should be able to answer the following questions in the spaces provided.

1. Identify the most common chronic physical health problems that result from intimate partner violence (IPV).

2. Identify the most common mental health problems that result from IPV.

3. Distinguish between abuse and neglect.

4. Identify three principles to follow when assessing for IPV.

5. Identify important elements of assessment for an abused person.

6. List five risk factors associated with homicides in IPV situations.

7. Discuss bruising in children and how it relates to their developmental level.

8. Identify some of the important elements of the child's medical history when assessing for suspected child maltreatment.

9. Discuss some of the long-term consequences of child maltreatment.

10. Identify risk factors that may contribute to child maltreatment.

REVIEW AND CLNICAL JUDGEMENT QUESTIONS

This test is for you to check your own mastery of the content. Answers are provided on the text's Evolve site.

1. Which of the following are examples of IPV?
   a. an ex-boyfriend stalking his ex-girlfriend
   b. marital rape
   c. hitting a date
   d. all of the above

2. Which one of the following is *not* accurate concerning the challenges associated with routine screening for violence when women come for health care?
   a. There may be potential harm to women from routine screening programs.
   b. Routine screening results in decreased exposure to violence.
   c. Detecting abuse through routine screening does not necessarily result in meaningful responses.
   d. Women may fear that responses from health care providers will increase their risks.

3. Mental health problems associated with IPV include
   a. hallucinations.
   b. suicidality.
   c. schizophrenia.
   d. attention-deficit/hyperactivity disorder (ADHD).

4. Gynecological problems *not* associated with IPV include
   a. pelvic pain.
   b. ovarian cysts.
   c. sexually transmitted infections (STIs).
   d. vaginal tearing.

5. Risk factors for intimate partner homicide include
   a. abuse during pregnancy.
   b. victim substance abuse.
   c. victim unemployment.
   d. history of victim childhood sexual assault.

6. Elder abuse includes
   a. willful infliction of force.
   b. withholding prescription medications without medical orders.
   c. threatening to place someone in a long-term care facility.
   d. all of the above.

7. When assessing an injury on a child, which of the following should be considered?
   a. the child's developmental level
   b. the child's medical and medication history
   c. the history of how the injury occurred
   d. all of the above

8. Known risk factors for child maltreatment include which of the following?
   a. substance abuse
   b. IPV
   c. physical disability or intellectual disability in the child
   d. all of the above

9. Bruising in a child who is not yet cruising
   a. is a common finding from normal infant activity.
   b. must be further evaluated for either an abusive or a medical explanation.
   c. is commonly seen on the buttocks.
   d. cannot be reported until a full medical evaluation is completed.

10. Which of the following should be routinely included when evaluating a possible case of elder abuse?
    a. corroborative interview from a caregiver
    b. baseline laboratory tests
    c. testing for STIs
    d. tuberculosis skin test

11. During an examination, you notice a patterned injury on a 10-year-old patient's back. There are linear ecchymoses on the back, but no other signs of bruising and no history of blood dyscrasia. The parents tell you that their child has a bad cold with a high fever and that they have been working to release the negative energies associated with the illness using coining. Given your knowledge of cultural practices, you recognize that
    a. coining is practised in Chinese and Southeast Asian cultures and is not considered effective unless it leaves bruises.
    b. coining is a form of child abuse because it has no medical benefit, so the parents should be reported immediately for abuse.
    c. coining is a cultural practice, but it should not leave bruises on the skin. The child needs to be evaluated for abuse.

12. You are caring for an adolescent female in an urgent care clinic. Her boyfriend checked her in and filled out paperwork. You note that she is listed as 18 years old, but appears younger. She is at the clinic due to pelvic pain, and her boyfriend has requested a pregnancy test. You notice that the boyfriend appears be in his late 20s or early 30s. She is withdrawn, does not answer questions, and seems unable to answer basic demographic information including her address and phone number. To complete a full assessment, you do the following. Select only the steps that are appropriate.
    a. Defer to the boyfriend to answer questions, since he seems to know what is happening.
    b. Complete a physical assessment noting any bruising or other signs of trauma.
    c. Provide a pregnancy test.
    d. Screen for STIs.
    e. Separate the patient and her boyfriend to get a more thorough history from the patient.
    f. Allow the boyfriend to stay in the room to avoid making the patient uncomfortable.

13. Documentation of suspected abuse should include which of the following? (Select all that apply.)
    a. photographic evidence
    b. subjective descriptions of injuries
    c. objective descriptions of injuries
    d. appropriate forensic terminology
    e. a paraphrased account of the victim statement without direct quotes
    f. appropriate direct quotes with some paraphrasing
    g. direct quotes that remove expletives or potentially offensive language

CRITICAL THINKING EXERCISES

1. Reflect on media stories that are related to intimate partner (domestic) violence and elder abuse, including stories about intimate partner or elder homicide, or child maltreatment that you may have seen recently. Notice the details of the story, including if there is subtle "victim blaming," various myths about abuse that are apparent, or precipitating factors that are identified.

2. Recall whether you were asked about IPV at your last encounter as a patient in the health care system. Check to see if your health care provider has any posters about domestic violence or brochures in the washrooms or other accessible areas.

3. Research a local intimate partner (domestic) violence shelter in your area. Take note of what health care services are offered to women and children who are staying there.

4. Research adult protective services or child protective services in your area. As a nurse, how would you file a report if this is every required of you? Research what happens when a nurse makes a report about elder abuse or child abuse.

NOTES

NOTES

UNIT 2   APPROACH TO THE CLINICAL SETTING

9 Assessment Techniques and the Clinical Setting

PURPOSE

This chapter helps you learn the physical assessment techniques of inspection, palpation, percussion, and auscultation. It also covers the equipment needed for a complete physical examination and age-specific modifications you would make for the examination of individuals throughout the life cycle.

READING ASSIGNMENT

Jarvis: *Physical Examination and Health Assessment*, 4th Canadian ed., Chapter 9.

Suggested Reading

Perkins, R., Ingebretson, E., Holifield, L., & Bergeron, A. (2021). A nurse's guide to COVID-19: An evidence-based review of the care of hospitalized adults with this disease. *American Journal of Nursing, 121*(3), 28–38.

GLOSSARY

Study the following terms after reading the corresponding chapter in the text.

Amplitude: (or intensity) indicates degree of loudness or softness of a sound
Auscultation: listening to sounds produced by parts of the body, usually using a stethoscope
Bimanual palpation: using both hands during palpation to envelop or capture certain body parts or organs—such as the kidneys, uterus, or adnexa—for more precise delimitation
Direct percussion: tapping in which the striking hand directly contacts the body wall, yielding a sound
Duration: the length of time a percussion sound lingers
Health care–associated infection: an infection acquired during hospitalization
Indirect percussion: tapping that involves both hands, where the striking hand contacts the stationary hand fixed on the person's skin, yielding a sound and a subtle vibration
Inspection: close, careful scrutiny, first of the individual as a whole and then of each body system
Ophthalmoscope: an instrument that illuminates the internal eye structures, enabling the examiner to look through the pupil at the fundus (background) of the eye
Otoscope: an instrument that illuminates the ear canal, enabling the examiner to look at the ear canal and tympanic membrane
Palpation: using touch to assess texture, temperature, moisture, and organ location and size, as well as any swelling, vibration or pulsation, rigidity or spasticity, crepitation, presence of lumps or masses, and presence of tenderness or pain
Percussion: tapping the person's skin with short, sharp strokes to yield a palpable vibration and a characteristic sound that depicts the location, size, and density of the underlying structures
Pitch: (or frequency) the number of vibrations (or cycles) per second of a percussion sound
Quality: (or timbre) a subjective difference in a percussion sound due to the sound's distinctive overtones

STUDY GUIDE

After completing the reading assignment, you should be able to answer the following questions in the spaces provided.

1. Define and describe the technique of the four physical examination skills:

    Inspection _____
    _____

    Palpation _____
    _____

    Percussion _____
    _____

    Auscultation _____
    _____

2. Define the characteristics of the following percussion notes:

Characteristic	Pitch	Amplitude	Quality	Duration
Resonant				
Hyperresonance				
Tympany				
Dull				
Flat				

3. Distinguish between direct percussion and indirect percussion.

4. Relate the parts of the hands to palpation techniques used in assessment.

5. Distinguish among light, deep, and bimanual palpation.

6. Name the two endpieces of the stethoscope and the conditions for which each is best suited.

7. Describe the environmental conditions to consider in preparing the examination setting.

8. List 21 basic items of equipment necessary to conduct a complete screening physical examination on an adult.

9. Describe your own preparation as you encounter the patient for examination: your own dress, your demeanour, safety and universal precautions, sequence of examination steps, and instructions to patient.

10. Differentiate standard and transmission-based precautions. Provide examples of when to use each.

11. What age-specific considerations would you make for the examination of each of the following age groups:

   Infants _____

   Toddlers _____

   Preschool-age children _____

   School-age children _____

   Adolescents _____

   Older adults _____

   Acutely ill people _____

Note that tables summarizing growth and development milestones for infancy through adolescence can be found in Appendices A through E of this study guide and laboratory manual, for your reference.

REVIEW AND CLINICAL JUDGEMENT QUESTIONS

This test is for you to check your own mastery of the content. Answers are provided on the text's Evolve site.

1. Various parts of the hands are used during palpation. The part of the hand used for the assessment of vibration is (are) the
   a. fingertips.
   b. index finger and thumb in opposition.
   c. dorsum of the hand.
   d. ulnar surface of the hand.

2. When performing indirect percussion, the stationary finger is struck
   a. at the ulnar surface.
   b. at the middle joint.
   c. at the distal interphalangeal joint.
   d. wherever it is in contact with the skin.

3. The best description of the pitch of a sound wave obtained by percussion is
   a. the intensity of the sound.
   b. the number of vibrations per second.
   c. the length of time the note lingers.
   d. the overtones of the note.

4. The bell of the stethoscope
   a. is used for soft, low-pitched sounds.
   b. is used for high-pitched sounds.
   c. is held firmly against the skin.
   d. magnifies sound.

5. The ophthalmoscope has five apertures. Which aperture would be used to assess the eyes of a patient with undilated pupils?
   a. grid
   b. slit
   c. small
   d. large

6. At the conclusion of the examination, the examiner should
   a. document findings before leaving the examining room.
   b. have findings confirmed by another practitioner.
   c. relate objective findings to the subjective findings for accuracy.
   d. summarize findings to the patient.

7. When the practitioner enters the examining room, the infant patient is asleep. The practitioner would best start the examination with
   a. height and weight.
   b. blood pressure.
   c. heart, lung, and abdomen.
   d. temperature.

8. The sequence of an examination changes from beginning with the thorax to that of head to toe with what age child?
   a. the infant
   b. the preschool-age child
   c. the school-age child
   d. the adolescent

9. When inspecting the ear canal, the examiner chooses which speculum for the otoscope?
   a. a short, broad one
   b. the narrowest for a child
   c. the longest for an adult
   d. the largest that will comfortably fit

10. A health care–associated infection is one that is acquired
    a. in a hospital setting.
    b. in a public facility.
    c. by the fecal–oral route.
    d. through airborne contaminants.

11. Palpation can be used for which of the following? (Select all that apply.)
    a. position of an organ
    b. size of a mass
    c. density of an organ
    d. deep tendon reflex
    e. pulsation
    f. vibration

12. When percussing over the lungs of a patient, the nurse notices a dull sound. The nurse should
    a. consider this a normal finding and continue the assessment.
    b. palpate this area for an underlying mass.
    c. reposition the hands and attempt to percuss in this area again to confirm the finding.
    d. move on with the assessment so as not to alarm the patient.

13. An examiner is preparing to assess a patient who reports changes in skin pigmentation. The best option for lighting is
    a. natural daylight.
    b. overhead lighting.
    c. tangential lighting.
    d. a sun lamp.

14. Extra heart sounds and murmurs are described as low-pitched sounds. Given your knowledge of the stethoscope, you know that low-pitched sounds are best heard with
    a. the bell endpiece held firmly to the skin.
    b. the bell endpiece held lightly against the skin.
    c. the diaphragm endpiece held firmly to the skin.
    d. the diaphragm endpiece held lightly to the skin.

15. To assess a patient's abdomen by palpation, how should the nurse proceed?
    a. Avoid palpation of reported "tender" areas because this may cause the patient pain.
    b. Quickly palpate a tender area to avoid any discomfort that the patient may experience.
    c. Begin the assessment with deep palpation, encouraging the patient to relax and take deep breaths.
    d. Start with light palpation to detect surface characteristics and to accustom the patient to being touched.

16. You are preparing to assess a 99-year-old gentleman who is in the emergency department due to shortness of breath. His respirations appear rapid and laboured. Complete the following sentences by selecting the correct phrases/words for blanks 1, 2, and 3.

    The best position for this patient is _____1_____. To complete the assessment, you should _____2_____ and _____3_____.
    a. supine
    b. a high Fowler's position
    c. dorsal recumbent
    d. proceed in head-to-toe format
    e. complete a focused assessment
    f. pause as necessary and provide breaks
    g. complete the assessment as quickly as possible
    h. complete a full head-to-toe assessment
    i. avoid taking breaks to complete the examination quickly

17. You are preparing to enter the room of a patient with suspected pertussis. To protect yourself and others, what should you do? (Select all that apply.)
    a. Use standard precautions.
    b. Use contact precautions.
    c. Use droplet precautions.
    d. Use airborne precautions.
    e. Use hand sanitizer.
    f. Wash your hands with soap and water if visibly soiled.
    g. Always wash your hands instead of using hand sanitizer.

SKILLS LABORATORY/CLINICAL SETTING

Note that the clinical component of this chapter is combined with Chapter 10. Instructions and documentation forms are listed at the end of Chapter 10.

NOTES

10 General Survey, Measurement, and Vital Signs

PURPOSE

This chapter helps you learn the method of gathering data for a general survey on a patient and the techniques for measuring height, weight, and vital signs.

READING ASSIGNMENT

Jarvis: *Physical Examination and Health Assessment*, 4th Canadian ed., Chapter 10.

Suggested Readings

Canadian Society for Exercise Physiology. (2021). *Canadian 24-hour movement guidelines; an integration of physical activity, sedentary behaviour, and sleep.* https://csepguidelines.ca

Elias, M. F., & Goodless, A. L. (2021). Human errors in automated office blood pressure measurement: Still room for improvement. *Hypertension, 77,* 6–15.

Hypertension Canada. (2021). *A practical guide informed by the Hypertension Canada guidelines for the prevention, diagnosis, risk assessment, and treatment of hypertension.* https://guidelines.hypertension.ca

GLOSSARY

Study the following terms after reading the corresponding chapter in the text.

Auscultatory gap: a brief time period when Korotkoff's sounds disappear during auscultation of blood pressure (BP); it is common with hypertension
Bradycardia: a heart rate less than 50 beats/min in the adult
Bradypnea: a decreased respiratory rate; typically, fewer than 8–12 breaths/min in the adult
Diastolic pressure: the elastic recoil, or resting, pressure that the blood exerts constantly between each contraction
Korotkoff's sounds: the components of a blood pressure reading consisting of phases I, IV, and V.
Mean arterial pressure (MAP): the pressure forcing blood into the tissues, averaged over the cardiac cycle.
Pulse pressure: the difference between the systolic and diastolic pressures; it reflects the stroke volume
Sinus arrhythmia: a common normal arrhythmia in children and young adults where the heart rate varies with the respiratory cycle, speeding up at the peak of inspiration and slowing to normal with expiration.
Sphygmomanometer: an instrument for measuring arterial blood pressure
Stroke volume: an amount of blood pumped out of the heart and into the aorta with each heartbeat
Symmetry: equal bilateral appearance of body parts
Systolic pressure: the maximum pressure felt on the artery during left ventricular contraction, or systole
Tachycardia: a heart rate of over 95 beats/min to 100 beats/min in the adult
Tachypnea: rapid respiratory rate; a respiratory rate above 25 breaths/min in the adult

STUDY GUIDE

After completing the reading assignment, you should be able to answer the following questions in the spaces provided.

1. List the significant information considered in each of the four areas of a general survey: physical appearance, body structure, mobility, and behaviour.

2. Describe the normal posture and body build.

3. Note aspects of normal gait.

4. Describe the clinical appearance of the following variations in stature:

   Hypopituitary dwarfism _____

   Gigantism _____

   Acromegaly _____

   Achondroplastic dwarfism _____

   Marfan syndrome _____

   Endogenous obesity (Cushing's syndrome) _____

   Anorexia nervosa _____

   Bulimia nervosa _____

5. State the normal weight range for an adult who is 175 cm tall.

6. Define *serial weight measurements* and describe when patients should be instructed to conduct them.

7. Describe the technique for measuring head circumference and chest circumference on an infant.

8. Describe normal changes in height and in weight distribution for an adult in their 80s and 90s.

9. Describe the tympanic membrane thermometer, and compare its use to other forms of temperature measurement.

10. Describe four qualities to consider when assessing the pulse.

11. Relate the qualities of normal respirations to the appropriate approach to counting them.

12. Define and describe the relationships among the terms *blood pressure, systolic pressure, diastolic pressure, pulse pressure*, and *mean arterial pressure*.

13. List factors that affect blood pressure.

14. Relate the use of an improperly sized blood pressure cuff to the possible findings that may be obtained.

15. Explain the significance of phase I, phase IV, and phase V Korotkoff's sounds during blood pressure measurement.

16. State the expected range for oral temperature, pulse, respiratory rate, and blood pressure for an apparently healthy 20-year-old adult.

17. List the diagnostic criteria for hypertension.

18. List the health-promoting behaviours recommended by Hypertension Canada for hypertension control.

REVIEW AND CLINICAL JUDGEMENT QUESTIONS

This test is for you to check your own mastery of the content. Answers are provided on the text's Evolve site.

1. The four areas to consider during the general survey are
   a. ethnicity, sex, age, and socioeconomic status.
   b. physical appearance, sex, ethnicity, and affect.
   c. dress, affect, nonverbal behaviour, and mobility.
   d. physical appearance, body structure, mobility, and behaviour.

2. During the general survey part of the examination, gait is assessed. When walking, the base is usually
   a. varied, depending upon the height of the person.
   b. equal to the length of the arm.
   c. as wide as the shoulder width.
   d. half of the height of the person.

3. An 18-month-old pediatric patient is brought in for a routine health screening visit. To assess the height of the child,
   a. use a tape measure.
   b. use a horizontal measuring board.
   c. have the child stand on the upright scale.
   d. measure arm span to estimate height.

4. You are working on the labour and delivery unit as a student nurse. A newborn you are assigned to care for was delivered by Caesarean section at 38 weeks of gestation because of fetal distress. She weighed 2.8 kg. This weight
   a. is appropriate for gestational age.
   b. is small for gestational age.
   c. is large for gestational age.
   d. cannot be determined from available data.

5. During the eighth and ninth decades of life, what changes occur in height and weight?
   a. both increase
   b. weight increases, height decreases
   c. both decrease
   d. both remain the same as during the 70s

6. During an initial home visit, the patient's temperature is noted to be 36.3°C (97.3°F). This temperature
   a. cannot be evaluated without knowledge of the person's age.
   b. is below normal. The person should be assessed for possible hypothermia.
   c. should be retaken by the rectal route because this best reflects core body temperature.
   d. should be reevaluated at the next visit before a decision is made.

7. Select the best description of an accurate assessment of a patient's pulse.
   a. Count for 15 seconds if pulse is regular
   b. Begin counting with 0; count for 30 seconds
   c. Count for 30 seconds, and multiply by 2 for all cases
   d. Count for 1 full minute; begin counting with 0

8. After assessing the patient's pulse, the practitioner determines the pulse force to be "normal." This would be recorded as follows:
   a. 3+
   b. 2+
   c. 1+
   d. 0

9. Select the best description of an accurate assessment of a patient's respirations.
   a. Count for a full minute before taking the pulse.
   b. Count for 15 seconds and multiply by 4.
   c. Count after informing the patient where you are in the assessment process.
   d. Count for 30 seconds following pulse assessment.

10. Pulse pressure is
    a. the difference between the systolic and diastolic pressure.
    b. a reflection of the viscosity of the blood.
    c. another way to express the systolic pressure.
    d. a measure of vasoconstriction.

11. The examiner is going to assess for coarctation of the aorta. In an individual with coarctation, the thigh pressure would
    a. be higher than in the arm.
    b. be equal to that in the arm.
    c. show no constant relationship; findings are highly individual.
    d. be lower than in the arm.

12. Mean arterial pressure is
    a. the arithmetic average of systolic and diastolic pressures.
    b. the driving force of blood during systole.
    c. diastolic pressure plus one-third pulse pressure.
    d. corresponding to phase III Korotkoff.

13. You are assessing a 5-month-old with known increased intracranial pressure and cranial enlargement. Which finding would you expect?
    a. The infant's head circumference would be 2 cm larger than the chest circumference.
    b. The infant's head circumference and chest circumference would measure equally.
    c. The infant's head circumference would be 5 cm larger than the chest circumference.
    d. The infant's head circumference would be 2 cm smaller than the chest circumference.

14. M.L. is a 16-year-old male who is 205.7 cm tall with an arm span that is greater than his height and a long pubis-to-sole measurement. He is thin with a narrow face and hyperextensible joints. Based on the general survey, M.L. may have
    a. Marfan syndrome
    b. gigantism
    c. acromegaly
    d. hyperpituitarism

15. A patient is being seen in the clinic after experiencing "fainting episodes that started last week." How should you proceed with the examination?
    a. Take the blood pressure in both arms and thighs to determine whether coarctation of the aorta is present.
    b. Ask the person to walk a few paces and then take the blood pressure. Compare the reading to the resting blood pressure.
    c. Record the blood pressure in the lying, sitting, and standing positions to determine whether orthostatic hypotension is the cause.
    d. Record the blood pressure in the lying and sitting positions and average these numbers to obtain a mean blood pressure.

16. Indicate whether each finding is normal or abnormal.

Finding	Normal	Abnormal
Rectal temperature: 37.7°C (99.86°F)		
Respiratory rate: 20/min, even		
Respiratory rate: 9/min		
Pulse: 80 bpm, 2+, irregular		
Temperature: 35°C (95°F)		

17. You are assessing the vital signs of a 22-year-old male athlete who reports playing soccer since he was 3 years old. You record the following vital signs: T 36.5°C (97.7°F), pulse 50 bpm, RR 16/min, BP 100/64 mm Hg. Which statement is true about these results?
    a. The patient is experiencing tachycardia and tachypnea.
    b. These are normal vital signs for a healthy, athletic adult.
    c. The patient's pulse rate is bradycardic. His physician should be notified.
    d. On the basis of today's readings, the patient should return for follow-up.
    e. Follow-up is needed due to low BP and pulse in this patient.

18. Highlight or circle the correct answer for each bolded pair of words.

    The nurse should recognize that temperature regulation **improves/declines** with normal aging. Older adult patients often have **lower/higher** normal temperatures than their younger counterparts and are **more/less** likely to have a fever with an infection.

19. E.W. is a 2-month-old at your clinic for a routine checkup. Given your knowledge of developmental needs, what is the best way to proceed with vitals signs?
    a. Proceed in the same order for all patients: temperature, pulse, respiratory rate, and blood pressure. Make sure to count the pulse for a full minute.
    b. Consider the infant's age and begin with the respiratory rate and pulse, counting each for a minute. Then take the blood pressure and temperature.
    c. Consider the infant's age and begin with the respiratory rate and pulse, counting each for a minute. Then take the temperature. Blood pressure is not routinely assessed in infants.
    d. Disrobe the infant and lay him on the table to make counting respirations easier. Count the respiratory rate and pulse, and then take the temperature.

20. A 4-year-old female presents at the clinic for a checkup. Her parents recently moved to the area and reports she has not visited a primary care provider in a few years. Her mother reports an uneventful prenatal course. She was born at term and does not have any pre-existing conditions. You obtain the following vital signs: T 37°C (98.6°F); pulse 90 bpm; RR 26/min; BP 158/78 mm Hg, right arm, sitting. Given these vital signs, the best next steps would be as follows:
    a. Notify a pediatrician immediately. Consider possible essential hypertension.
    b. Obtain blood pressure in the left arm and thigh pressure before notifying the provider.
    c. Obtain blood pressure in the left arm, and repeat the right arm pressure. Then notify the provider.
    d. Check instrument calibration and get a different blood pressure cuff. She should not have high blood pressure.
    e. The most likely explanation is user error. Have another nurse obtain bilateral blood pressure readings.

CRITICAL THINKING EXERCISE

Analyze the following vital sign values. Are they normal or abnormal? If they are abnormal, try to determine why this may be the case. Make sure to note any additional information you need to fully analyze the values.
- 55-year-old woman: T 37°C (98.6°F), RR 18/min, pulse 160 bpm, BP 90/60 mm Hg
- 2-year-old boy: T 37°C (98.6°F), RR 18/min, pulse 130 bpm
- 89-year-old woman: T 36°C (96.8°F), RR 12/min, pulse 55 bpm, BP 140/98 mm Hg
- 25-year-old man: T 39°C (102.2°F), RR 26/min, pulse 113 bpm, BP 100/60 mm Hg

SKILLS LABORATORY/CLINICAL SETTING

You are now ready for the clinical component of Chapter 10. The purpose of the clinical component is to practise the general survey and vital signs portion of the examination on a peer in the skills laboratory and to achieve the following.

Clinical Objectives

1. Using the general survey, observe and describe the significant characteristics of a peer.

2. Measure height and weight, and determine whether findings are within normal range.

3. Gather vital signs data.

4. Record the physical examination findings accurately.

Instructions

Practise the steps of gathering data for a general survey, for height and weight, and vital signs on a peer. Make sure you are familiar with the equipment you will be using. If available, practise with both a balance scale and digital scale. Record your findings using the documentation sheet that follows. The first section of the sheet—the general survey—is intended as a worksheet. The second section of the sheet provides instructions on writing the general survey summary; this statement will serve as an introduction for the complete physical examination documentation.

NOTES

NOTES

DOCUMENTATION—GENERAL SURVEY, MEASUREMENT, AND VITAL SIGNS

Date _____

Examiner _____

Patient _____ **Age** _____ **Gender** _____

Occupation _____

I. Physical Examination
   A. General survey
   1. Physical appearance

   Age _____

   Gender _____

   Level of consciousness _____

   Skin colour _____

   Facial features _____

   2. Body structure

   Stature _____

   Nutrition _____

   Symmetry _____

   Posture _____

   Position _____

   Body build, contour _____

   Any physical deformity _____

   3. Mobility

   Gait _____

   Range of motion _____

   4. Behaviour

   Facial expression _____

   Mood and affect _____

   Speech _____

   Dress _____

   Personal hygiene _____

   B. Measurement

   1. Height cm _____   4. Waist circumference (cm) _____

   2. Weight (kg) _____   5. Waist ratio _____

   3. Body mass index _____

C. Vital signs

1. Temperature_____

2. Pulse _____

   Rate _____

   Rhythm _____

3. Respirations_____

4. Blood pressure: R arm _____ L arm _____

II. Summary

Write a summary of the general survey, including height, weight, and vital signs. This statement will serve as an introduction for the complete physical examination documentation.

_____ **NOTES** _____

11 Pain Assessment

PURPOSE

This chapter reviews the structure and function of pain pathways; the process of nociception; the rationale for and methods of pain assessment; and the accurate recording of the findings.

READING ASSIGNMENT

Jarvis: *Physical Examination and Health Assessment*, 4th Canadian ed., Chapter 11.

Suggested Readings

Canada's Drug and Health Technology Agency. (2021). Models of care for chronic pain: An environmental scan. *CADTH Health Technology Review*. https://www.cadth.ca/models-care-chronic-pain-environmental-scan

Delgado, S.A. (2020). Managing pain in critically ill adults: A holistic approach. *American Journal of Nursing, 120*(5), 34–43.

GLOSSARY

Study the following terms after reading the corresponding chapter in the text.

Acute pain: pain that is short term and self-limiting; it follows a predictable trajectory and dissipates after an injury heals
Cutaneous pain: pain originating from skin surface or subcutaneous structures
Modulation: the last phase of nociception, when the pain message is inhibited
Neuropathic pain: the abnormal processing of the pain message; often described as burning or shooting pain
Nociception: the process whereby noxious stimuli are perceived as pain
Nociceptive pain: pain caused by tissue injury that is well-localized and often described as aching or throbbing
Nociceptors: specialized nerve endings that detect painful sensations
Pain: "An unpleasant sensory and emotional experience associated with, or resembling that associated with, actual or potential tissue damage." (International Association for the Study of Pain)
Perception: conscious awareness of a painful sensation
Persistent (chronic) pain: persistent or recurring pain lasting longer than 3 months
Referred pain: pain felt at a particular site but one that originates from another location
Somatic pain: pain derived from muscle, bone, joints, tendons, or blood vessels
Transduction: the first phase of nociception, whereby the painful stimulus is changed into a pain message (or action potential)
Transmission: the second phase of nociception, whereby the pain impulse moves from the spinal cord to the brain
Visceral pain: pain originating from the larger internal organs, such as the gallbladder or stomach

STUDY GUIDE

After completing the reading assignment, you should be able to answer the following questions in the spaces provided.

1. Describe the process of nociception using the four phases:

   Transduction _____

   Transmission _____

   Perception _____

   Modulation _____

2. Identify the differences between nociceptive and neuropathic pain.

3. List various sources of pain.

4. Explain how acute and chronic pain differs in terms of nonverbal behaviours.

5. Identify the most reliable indicator of a person's pain.

6. Recall the OPQRSTUV questions for an initial pain assessment.

7. Name the pain assessment tools that are appropriate for adults, children, infants, and premature infants.

8. Describe physical examination findings that may indicate pain.

9. Explain how poorly controlled acute and persistent (chronic) pain adversely affects physiological, social, and cognitive functioning.

10. What would you say to a colleague who remarks that the individual with Alzheimer's disease does not feel pain and therefore does not require an analgesic?

11. Fill in the labels indicated on the following illustration.

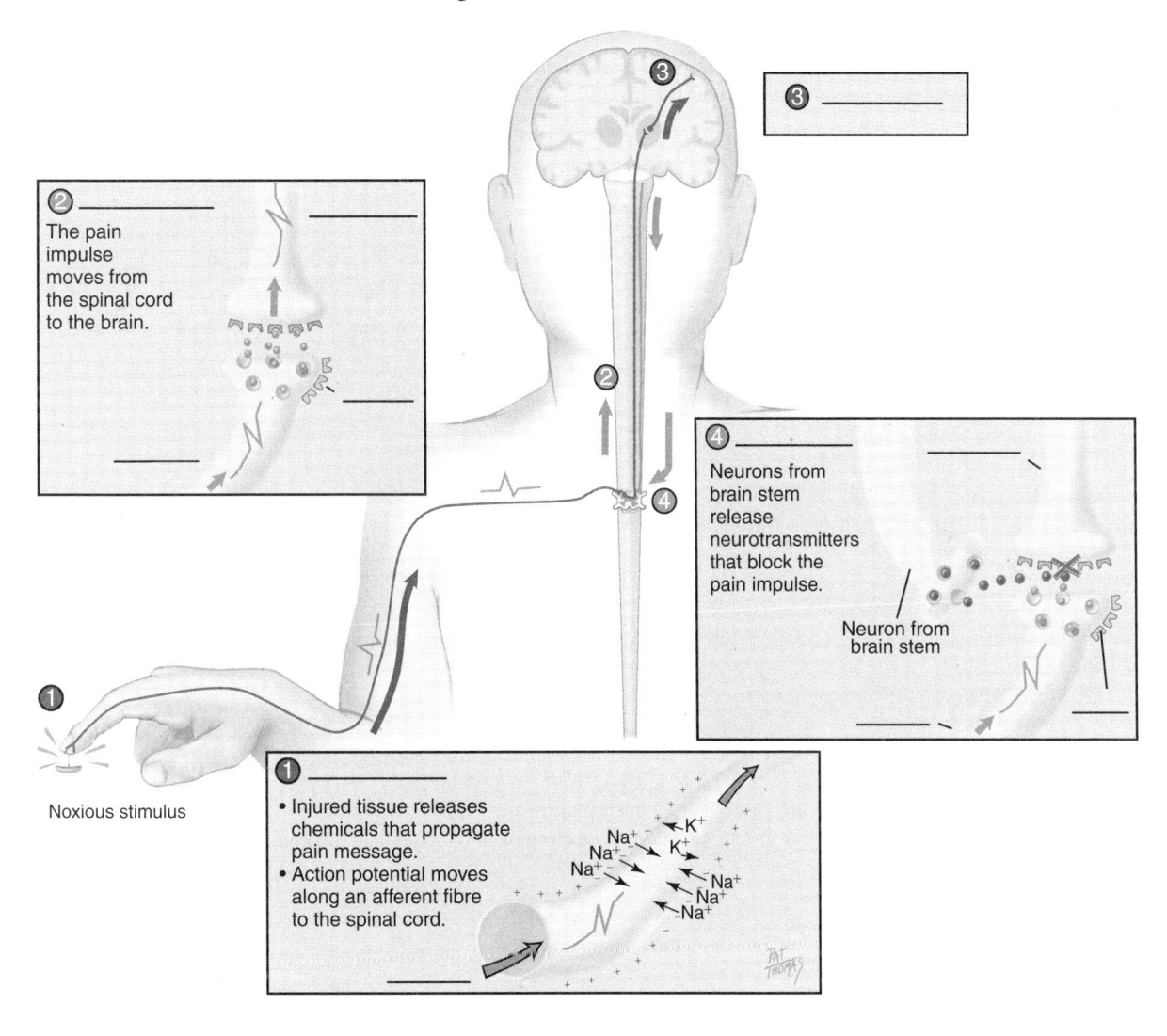

② _____
The pain impulse moves from the spinal cord to the brain.

③ _____

④ _____
Neurons from brain stem release neurotransmitters that block the pain impulse.

Neuron from brain stem

① _____
- Injured tissue releases chemicals that propagate pain message.
- Action potential moves along an afferent fibre to the spinal cord.

Noxious stimulus

REVIEW AND CLINICAL JUDGEMENT QUESTIONS

This test is for you to check your own mastery of the content. Answers are provided on the text's Evolve site.

1. At what phase during nociception does the individual become aware of a painful sensation?
   a. modulation
   b. transduction
   c. perception
   d. transmission

2. While you are taking a history, the patient describes a burning, painful sensation that moves around his toes and bottoms of his feet. These symptoms are suggestive of
   a. nociceptive pain.
   b. neuropathic pain.

3. During the physical examination, your patient is diaphoretic and pale, and complains of pain directly over the left upper quadrant (LUQ) of the abdomen. This would be categorized as
   a. cutaneous pain.
   b. somatic pain.
   c. visceral pain.
   d. psychogenic pain.

4. While caring for a preterm infant, you are aware that
   a. inhibitory neurotransmitters are in sufficient supply by 15 weeks' gestation.
   b. the fetus has less capacity to feel pain.
   c. repetitive blood draws have minimal long-term consequences.
   d. the preterm infant is more sensitive to painful stimuli.

5. The most reliable indicator of pain in the adult is
   a. degree of physical functioning.
   b. nonverbal behaviours.
   c. magnetic resonance imaging findings.
   d. the patient's self-report.

6. For examining a broken arm of a 4-year-old boy, select the appropriate assessment tool to evaluate his pain status.
   a. 0–10 Numeric Rating Scale
   b. Faces Pain Scale
   c. simple Descriptor Scale
   d. 0–5 Numeric Rating Scale

7. When a person presents with acute pain of the abdomen, following the initial examination, it is best to withhold analgesia until diagnostic testing is completed and a diagnosis is made.
   a. true
   b. false

8. For older adult postoperative patients, poorly controlled acute pain places them at higher risk for
   a. atelectasis.
   b. increased myocardial oxygen demand.
   c. impaired wound healing.
   d. all of the above.

9. A 30-year-old female reports having persistent intense pain in her right arm related to trauma sustained from a car accident 5 months ago. She states that the slightest touch or clothing can exacerbate the pain. This report is suggestive of
   a. referred pain.
   b. psychogenic pain.
   c. complex regional pain syndrome.
   d. cutaneous pain.

10. The PACSLAC-II is an appropriate pain assessment tool for
    a. seniors with limited ability to communicate.
    b. children ages 2 to 8 years.
    c. infants.
    d. premature infants.

11. A pain problem should be anticipated in a cognitively impaired older adult with a history of
    a. diabetes.
    b. peripheral vascular disease.
    c. chronic obstructive pulmonary disease (COPD).
    d. Parkinson's disease.

12. You are caring for a 36-year-old male who presents to the emergency department with acute right lower quadrant (RLQ) pain rated at 10 out of 10 on the Numeric Rating Scale. The patient is tachycardic, tachypneic, grimacing, and curled in the fetal position. During the workup, the provider refuses to order any pain medication. You should do the following:
    a. Advocate for the patient to receive pain medication. It will be easier to complete the workup if the patient is comfortable.
    b. Let the patient know that no pain medication can be given until the workup is complete, as the medication may mask symptoms.
    c. Recognize that the provider understands the need for the patient to feel the pain so he can adequately describe it.
    d. Call your supervisor to intervene. The patient should have pain medication ordered immediately.

13. A patient has osteoarthritis in her hips and knees. She can move around in her room this morning and has offered no complaints. When asked, she states that her pain is "bad this morning" and rates the pain at an 8 on a 10-point scale. The nurse suspects that the patient
    a. is addicted to her pain medication and cannot obtain relief from small doses.
    b. does not want to trouble anyone with her complaints.
    c. is not in severe pain but would like pain medication.
    d. has experienced pain for years and adapted to the chronic pain.

14. Acute and chronic pain result in a variety of physiological changes. Mark the changes that may result from acute pain and chronic pain.

	Acute Pain	Chronic Pain
Depression		
Nausea		
Fear		
Isolation		
Limited functioning		
Tachycardia		

15. When caring for a patient with advanced dementia, which of the following categories are included in the PAINAD scale? (Select all that apply.)
    a. breathing independent of vocalization
    b. yelling
    c. body language
    d. consolability
    e. activity
    f. negative vocalization
    g. positive vocalization
    h. facial expression
    i. face
    j. vital signs

CRITICAL THINKING EXERCISES

1. What conditions are more likely to produce pain in the older adult?

2. How would you modify your examination when the patient reports having abdominal pain?

3. How would you assess for pain in an individual with dementia?

4. What would you say to someone who tells you that infants do not remember pain and that they are too little for the pain to have any damaging effect?

SKILLS LABORATORY/CLINICAL SETTING

You are now ready for the clinical component of the pain assessment. The purpose of the clinical component is to practise the examination on a peer in the skills laboratory or on a patient in the clinical setting and to achieve the following.

Clinical Objectives

1. Perform an initial pain assessment on a classmate or patient.

2. Demonstrate a physical examination on a painful area and identify abnormal findings.

3. Select appropriate pain assessment tools for further follow-up and monitoring.

4. Document the history and physical examination findings accurately, assess the nature of the pain, and develop an appropriate plan of care.

NOTES

12 Nutritional Assessment and Nursing Practice

PURPOSE

This chapter reviews the components of the nutritional assessment, including how to assess dietary intake and nutritional status of individuals; how to identify the possible occurrence, nature, and extent of impaired nutritional status (ranging from undernutrition to overnutrition); and how to accurately record the assessment.

READING ASSIGNMENT

Jarvis: *Physical Examination and Health Assessment*, 4th Canadian ed., Chapter 12.

Suggested Readings

Graf, M.D., Karp, S.M., Lutenbacher, M., et al. (2021). Clinical strategies for addressing obesity in infants and toddler. *The Nurse Practitioner, 46*(2), 28–34.
Obesity Canada. (2022). *Bariatric friendly healthcare.* https://obesitycanada.ca/resources/bariatric-friendly/#

GLOSSARY

Study the following terms after reading the corresponding chapter in the text.

24-hour recall: an individual is asked to recall everything eaten within the past 24 hours
Android obesity: excess body fat that is localized predominantly within the abdomen and upper body, as opposed to the hips and thighs
Anthropometry: the measurement of and evaluation of growth, development, and body composition; for example, height, weight, circumferences, skinfold thickness
Body mass index (BMI): weight in kilograms divided by height in metres squared (W/H^2); a value of 30 or more indicates obesity; a value of less than 18.5 indicates undernutrition
Central obesity: body fat that collects deep within the central abdominal area of the body, called *visceral fat*
Diet history: a detailed record of dietary intake obtainable from 24-hour recalls, food frequency questionnaires, food diaries, and similar methods
Dietary Reference Intakes (DRIs): recommended amounts of nutrients to prevent deficiencies, reduce the risk of chronic disease, and avoid toxicity
Food diaries: individual records of everything consumed for a certain period of time (usually for three days—two working days and one nonworking day)
Food frequency questionnaire: information collected related to how many times per day, week, or month an individual eats particular foods; it does not quantify the amount of food eaten
Gynoid obesity: excess body fat that is placed predominantly within the hips and thighs
Malnutrition: it may mean any nutrition disorder but usually refers to long-term nutritional inadequacies or excesses
Nitrogen balance: a condition in which nitrogen losses from the body are equal to nitrogen intake; the expected state of the healthy adult
Nutrition screening: a process used to identify individuals at nutritional risk or with nutritional problems
Obesity: excessive accumulation of body fat with body mass index (BMI: weight/height^2) exceeding 30 kg/m^2 and is subclassified into class 1 (BMI 30 to 34.9), class 2 (BMI 35 to 39.9), and class 3 (BMI >40)
Protein-calorie malnutrition (PCM): inadequate consumption of protein and energy, resulting in a gradual body wasting and increased susceptibility to infection
Serum proteins: proteins present in serum that are indicators of the body's visceral protein status (e.g., albumin, prealbumin, transferrin)
Waist–hip ratio (WHR): the waist or abdominal circumference divided by the hip or gluteal circumference; a method for assessing fat distribution

STUDY GUIDE

After completing the reading assignment, you should be able to answer the following questions in the spaces provided.

1. Define nutritional status.

2. Describe the unique nutritional needs for various developmental periods throughout the life cycle.

3. Describe the role cultural heritage and values may play in an individual's nutritional intake.

4. State three purposes of a nutritional assessment.

5. State the purpose of nutrition labelling of food products, and define the term *percent daily value*.

6. Describe four sources of error that may occur when using the 24-hour diet recall.

7. Explain the clinical concerns associated with the following terms:
   Obesity _____
   Central obesity _____
   Diabetes _____
   Metabolic syndrome _____
   Celiac disease _____

REVIEW AND CLINICAL JUDGEMENT QUESTIONS

This test is for you to check your own mastery of the content. Answers are provided on the text's Evolve site.

1. The balance between nutrient intake and nutrient requirements is described as
   a. undernutrition.
   b. malnutrition.
   c. nutritional status.
   d. overnutrition.

2. To support the synthesis of maternal and fetal tissue during pregnancy, a weight gain of how many kilograms is recommended?
   a. 11.5 to 16 kg
   b. 12.5 to 18 kg
   c. 7 to 11 kg
   d. Recommendation depends on BMI of mother at the start of the pregnancy.

3. All of the following are normal physiological changes in older adults that directly affect nutritional status, *except*
   a. poor dentition.
   b. decreased visual acuity.
   c. increased gastro-intestinal absorption.
   d. diminished olfactory and taste sensitivity.

4. Which of the following data would be obtained as part of a nutritional screening?
   a. temperature, pulse, and respiration
   b. blood pressure and genogram
   c. weight and nutrition intake history
   d. serum creatinine levels

5. The 24-hour recall of dietary intake is
   a. an anthropometric measure of calories consumed.
   b. a questionnaire or interview of everything eaten within the last 24 hours.
   c. the same as a food frequency questionnaire.
   d. a form of food diary.

6. The nutritional needs of a patient with trauma or major surgery
   a. are met by fat reserves in obese individuals.
   b. may be two to three times greater than normal.
   c. can be met with intravenous fluids, supplemented with vitamins and electrolytes.
   d. are met by glycogen reserves.

7. M.J. is a 15-year-old female who has come in for an assessment. During the health history, she tells you that menarche has not occurred. An explanation to be explored is
   a. nutritional deficiency.
   b. alcohol intake.
   c. smoking history.
   d. possible elevated blood sugar.

8. Older adults are at risk for alteration in nutritional status. From the individuals described below, select the individual(s) who appear(s) least at risk.
   a. an 80-year-old widow who lives alone
   b. a 65 year old widower who visits a long-term care facility with a meal program 5 days a week
   c. a 70-year-old with poor dentition who lives with a son
   d. a 73-year-old couple with low income and no transportation

9. Body weight as a percentage of ideal body weight is calculated to assess for malnutrition. Severe malnutrition is diagnosed when current body weight is
   a. 80% to 90% of ideal weight.
   b. 70% to 80% of ideal weight.
   c. less than 75% of ideal body weight.
   d. 120% of ideal body weight.

10. You are completing an initial assessment for a patient being admitted to a long-term care facility. The patient is unable to stand for a measurement of height. To obtain this important anthropometric information, the examiner may
    a. measure the waist-to-hip circumference.
    b. estimate the BMI.
    c. measure arm span.
    d. obtain a mid-upper arm muscle circumference to estimate skeletal muscle reserve.

11. Which assessment finding indicates nutrition risk?
    a. BMI = 24
    b. serum albumin = 30 g/L
    c. current weight = 90 kg
    d. BMI = 19

12. Which BMI category in adults is indicative of obesity?
    a. 18.5 to 24.9
    b. 25.0 to 29.9
    c. 30.0 to 39.9
    d. <18.5

13. H.S. is a 5-month-old infant living in Saskatchewan. She is exclusively breastfed. How much vitamin D should she be taking daily?
    a. 600 IU
    b. none, breast milk provides all the nutrients that a healthy infant needs
    c. 400 IU
    d. 100 mcg

14. In the following patient scenario, underline the findings that are concerning for the patient.

    A.L., a 9-year-old female, is being seen in the clinic today for a well-child visit. A.L. reports that she has a good appetite and enjoys a variety of foods. Her parents confirm access to fresh fruits and vegetables. They also confirm adequate resources to provide nutritious meals. A.L. is 137 cm tall and weighs 42 kg. Vital signs: HR 85 bpm, resp 20/min, BP 110/80 mm Hg. Her BMI is 22.4, which puts her in the 96th percentile.

15. Based on the information in question 14:
    a. A.L. has pediatric metabolic syndrome. This puts her at a higher risk for cardiovascular disease and early mortality. She should be treated immediately for hypertension, high cholesterol, and obesity.
    b. A.L. has concerning assessment findings. Counselling to promote lifestyle modifications and close monitoring are necessary.
    c. A.L. is undernourished. She should be started on a multivitamin and return for assessment in 1 year.
    d. A.L. is a growing child. While her findings are not within normal limits, they are not concerning until she is at least 16 years old. The health care team will continue to monitor for any changes.

16. In the following patient scenario, underline the assessment findings that place the person at risk for metabolic syndrome.

    K.L. is a 52-year-old female who comes to the clinic today for her annual checkup. During the history, she reports no recent changes to diet and has no acute concerns. Her current medications include simvastatin (Zocor) for high cholesterol, metformin (Glucophage) to lower blood glucose levels, a calcium supplement, a fish oil supplement, and a multivitamin. Weight is 93 kg, height is 165 cm, BMI is 35.2, and waist circumference is 104 cm. Vital signs: HR 89 bpm, resp 20/min, BP 138/90 mm Hg. Lungs are clear to auscultation. Mild edema is present in bilateral lower extremities. All lab values are within normal limits.

17. Based on the information in question 16, K.L. should
    a. be diagnosed with metabolic syndrome (MetS). She is on medication for cholesterol and glucose. Her blood pressure is high and her waist circumference is ≥88 cm.
    b. be diagnosed with MetS. Her blood pressure, BMI, and waist circumference are all indicative of MetS in an adult.
    c. be counselled on lifestyle modification. Her BP and BMI are high, but her lab values are all within normal limits, so she is low risk.
    d. be counselled on lifestyle modification. By reducing her weight and waist circumference, she can avoid the diagnosis of MetS.

18. J.H. is in the clinic for a checkup. He is an 89-year-old widower who lost his wife 8 months ago. He has two children who live approximately 8 hours away. He lives alone and no longer drives. He has lost 4 kg in the previous 6 months but denies trying to lose weight. Select all appropriate questions related to J.H.'s nutritional status.
    a. Do you currently wear dentures? If yes, do they fit appropriately?
    b. Who do you eat with for meals?
    c. What did you eat for dinner last night?
    d. Can you tell me everything you ate in the last 24 hours, including drinks?
    e. Do you go grocery shopping yourself? If not, who buys your groceries?
    f. Is your income adequate to purchase food?
    g. What medications do you take? I only need to know about prescription medications.

CRITICAL THINKING EXERCISE

Weight bias refers to negative attitudes and views about obesity and about people with obesity. Unfortunately, our current health care system has room for improvement in providing bariatric friendly health care. People-first language is an example of how we can improve respectful interactions with our patients. Instead of stating "obese patient," use "patient with obesity." This small change reinforces that obesity is a chronic disease and not a characteristic. Visit the Obesity Canada website listed at the beginning of this chapter. Reflect on your student clinical experiences. Have you witnessed weight bias in health care? What steps can you take to help decrease weight bias in health care?

SKILLS LABORATORY/CLINICAL SETTING

You are now ready for the clinical component of the nutritional assessment. The purpose of the clinical component is to practise the steps of the assessment on a peer in the skills laboratory and to achieve the following.

Clinical Objectives

1. Identify people at risk for developing malnutrition.

2. Develop an appreciation for cultural influences on nutritional status.

3. Use anthropometric measures and laboratory data to assess the nutritional status of an individual.

4. Use nutritional assessment in the provision of health care.

5. Record the assessment findings accurately.

Instructions

Practice the steps of the *Admission Nutrition Screening Tool* on a peer in the skills laboratory. This will familiarize you with the appropriate nutrition history. Following your history, being mindful of people's sensitivities around their body image and weight, with consent, practice measuring the height, weight, waist–hip ratio, and waist circumference of your peer and then calculate their BMI. Record your findings using the assessment form that follows. In addition to the *Admission Nutrition Screening Tool*, review the Canadian Nutrition Screening Tool and complete the malnutrition screening tool below.

See also the following learning resource: Health Canada. (2019). *Food guide snapshot— other languages.* https://www.canada.ca/en/health-canada/services/canada-food-guide/resources/snapshot/languages.html

ADMISSION NUTRITION SCREENING TOOL

A. Diagnosis

If the patient has at least ONE of the following diagnoses, circle and proceed to section E to consider the patient AT NUTRITIONAL RISK, and stop here:
- Anorexia nervosa/bulimia nervosa
- Malabsorption (celiac sprue, ulcerative colitis, Crohn's disease, short bowel syndrome)
- Multiple trauma (closed-head injury, penetrating trauma, multiple fractures)
- Decubitus ulcers
- Major gastro-intestinal surgery within the past year
- Cachexia (temporal wasting, muscle wasting, cancer, cardiac)
- Coma
- Diabetes

- End-stage liver disease
- End-stage renal disease
- Nonhealing wounds

B. Nutrition Intake History

If the patient has at least ONE of the following symptoms, circle and proceed to section E to consider the patient AT NUTRITIONAL RISK, and stop here:
- Diarrhea (>500 mL × 2 days)
- Vomiting (more than 5 days)
- Reduced intake (less than half normal intake for more than 5 days)

C. Average Body Weight Standards (BMI)

Determine the patient's current BMI by measuring his or her height and weight, and compare it to the World Health Organization (WHO) standards for average weight. (Refer to Fig. 10.1 of the text for a body mass index chart, and Chapter 12 for BMI calculation instructions.)

If the patient's BMI is <18.5, proceed to section E to consider the patient AT NUTRITIONAL RISK, and stop here.

D. Weight History

Any recent unplanned weight loss? No _____ Yes _____ Amount (lb or kg) _____
If yes, within the past _____ weeks or _____ months
Current weight (lb or kg) _____
Usual weight (lb or kg) _____
Height (ft, in., or cm) _____
Find percentage of weight lost:

$$\frac{\text{Usual wt} - \text{Current wt}}{\text{Usual wt}} \times 100 = \% \text{ wt loss}$$

Compare the % wt loss with the chart values, and circle the appropriate value:

Length of Time	Significant (%)	Severe (%)
One week	1–2	>2
Two to three weeks	2–3	>3
One month	4–5	>5
Three months	7–8	>8
Five months or longer	10	>10

If the patient has experienced a significant or severe weight loss, proceed to section E and consider the patient AT NUTRITIONAL RISK.

E. **Nurse Assessment**
   Using the above criteria, what is this patient's nutritional risk? (Circle one.)
   LOW NUTRITIONAL RISK
   AT NUTRITIONAL RISK

CANADIAN NUTRITION SCREENING TOOL (CNST)
Identify patients who are at risk for malnutrition

Ask the patient the following questions*	Date: Admission		Date: Rescreening	
	Yes	No	Yes	No
Have you lost weight in the past 6 months WITHOUT TRYING to lose this weight? If the patient reports a weight loss but gained it back, consider it as NO weight loss.				
Have you been eating less than usual FOR MORE THAN A WEEK?				
Two "YES" answers indicate nutrition risk†				

* If the patient is unable to answer the questions, a knowledgeable informant can be used to obtain the information. If the patient is uncertain regarding weight loss, ask if clothing is now fitting more loosely.

† If a patient is not at risk, rescreen within a week. Only consider weight change in the past week.

From Canadian Malnutrition Task Force. (2022). *Canadian Nutrition Screening Tool (CNST)*. http://nutritioncareincanada.ca/sites/default/uploads/files/CNST.pdf

NOTES

NOTES

UNIT 3 PHYSICAL EXAMINATION

13 Skin, Hair, and Nails

PURPOSE

This chapter reviews the structure and function of the skin and its appendages; the rationale for and methods of inspection and palpation of the skin; and the accurate recording of the assessment.

READING ASSIGNMENT

Jarvis: *Physical Examination and Health Assessment*, 4th Canadian ed., Chapter 13.

Suggested Readings

Oozageer Gunowa, N., Brooke, J., Hutchinson, M., et al. (2020). Embedding skin tone diversity into undergraduate nurse education: Through the lens of pressure injury. *Journal of clinical nursing, 29*(21–22), 4358–4367. https://doi.org/10.1111/jocn.15474

O'Sullivan, D. E., Brenner, D. R., Demers, P. A., et al. (2019). Indoor tanning and skin cancer in Canada: A meta-analysis and attributable burden estimation. *Cancer epidemiology, 59*, 1–7. https://doi.org/10.1016/j.canep.2019.01.004

GLOSSARY

Study the following terms after reading the corresponding chapter in the text.

Alopecia: (baldness) hair loss
Annular: a circular shape to skin lesion
Apocrine glands: are located mainly in the axillae, anogenital area, nipples, and navel and are vestigial in humans and produce a thick, milky secretion and open into the hair follicles
Basal cell layer: a cell layer within the epidermis that form new skin cells
Bulla: an elevated cavity containing free fluid in epidermis, >1 cm diameter
Confluent: skin lesions that merge together
Crust: thick, dried-out exudate left on skin when vesicles or pustules burst or dry up
Cyanosis: a dusky or bluish mottled discoloration of skin or mucous membranes due to increased amount of unoxygenated hemoglobin
Eccrine glands: a type of sweat gland that is coiled tubules that open directly onto the skin surface and produces a dilute saline solution called *sweat*
Erosion: a scooped-out, shallow depression in skin
Erythema: an intense redness of the skin due to excess blood in dilated superficial capillaries, as in fever, local inflammation, or emotional reactions
Excoriation: a self-inflicted abrasion on skin due to scratching
Fissure: a linear crack in skin extending into dermis
Furuncle: a boil; a suppurative inflammatory skin lesion due to infected hair follicle
Hemangioma: a skin lesion due to benign proliferation of blood vessels in the dermis
Iris: target shape of skin lesion
Jaundice: yellow colour to skin, palate, and sclera due to excess bilirubin in the blood
Keloid: a hypertrophic scar, elevated beyond site of original injury
Lichenification: tightly packed set of papules that thickens skin; caused by prolonged intense scratching
Lipoma: benign fatty tumour, composed of mature fat cells
Macule: a flat skin lesion with only a colour change
Nevus: a mole; a circumscribed skin lesion due to excess melanocytes
Nodule: an elevated skin lesion, >1 cm diameter
Pallor: excessively pale, whitish pink colour to lightly pigmented skin

Papule: a palpable skin lesion of <1 cm diameter
Plaque: a skin lesion in which papules coalesce or come together
Pruritus: itching
Purpura: a red to purple skin lesion due to blood in tissues from breaks in blood vessels
Pustule: an elevated cavity containing thick, turbid fluid
Scale: compact desiccated flakes of skin from shedding of dead skin cells
Telangiectasia: a skin lesion due to permanently enlarged and dilated blood vessels that are visible
Ulcer: sloughing of necrotic inflammatory tissue that causes a deep depression in skin, extending into dermis
Vesicle: an elevated cavity containing free fluid up to 1 cm diameter
Wheal: a raised red skin lesion due to interstitial fluid
Zosteriform: a linear shape of skin lesion along a nerve route

STUDY GUIDE

After completing the reading assignment, you should be able to answer the following questions in the spaces provided.

1. List the three layers associated with the skin, and describe the contents of each layer.

2. Define two types of human hair.

3. Differentiate between sebaceous, eccrine, and apocrine glands.

4. List at least five functions of the skin.

5. Describe the appearance of pallor, erythema, cyanosis, and jaundice, both in light-skinned and in dark-skinned people. State common causes of each.

6. List causes of changes in skin temperature, texture, moisture, mobility, and turgor.

7. Describe each grade on the four-point grading scale for pitting edema.

8. Distinguish the terms *primary* versus *secondary* in reference to skin lesions.

9. The white linear markings that normally are visible through the nail and on the pink nail bed are termed _____.

10. Describe the following findings, which are common variations on the infant's skin:

    Congenital dermal melanocytosis _____

    Café au lait spot _____

    Erythema toxicum _____

    Cutis marmorata _____

    Physiological jaundice _____

    Milia _____

11. Describe the following findings, which are common variations on the older adult's skin:

    Lentigines _____

    Seborrheic keratosis _____

    Actinic keratosis _____

    Acrochordons (skin tags) _____

    Sebaceous hyperplasia _____

12. Differentiate between these purpuric lesions: petechiae, ecchymosis, and hematoma.

13. Differentiate between the appearance of the skin rash of these childhood illnesses: measles (rubeola); German measles (rubella); chicken pox (varicella).

14. Contrast a furuncle with an abscess.

15. Describe the appearance of these conditions of the nails: paronychia, Beau's lines, splinter hemorrhages, onychomycosis, and clubbing.

16. a. Define and give an example of the following primary skin lesions: macule; papule; plaque; nodule; tumour; wheal; vesicle; pustule.

   b. Define and give an example of the following secondary lesions: crust; scale; fissure; erosion; ulcer; excoriation; scar; atrophic scar; lichenification; keloid.

17. Fill in the labels indicated on the following illustrations.

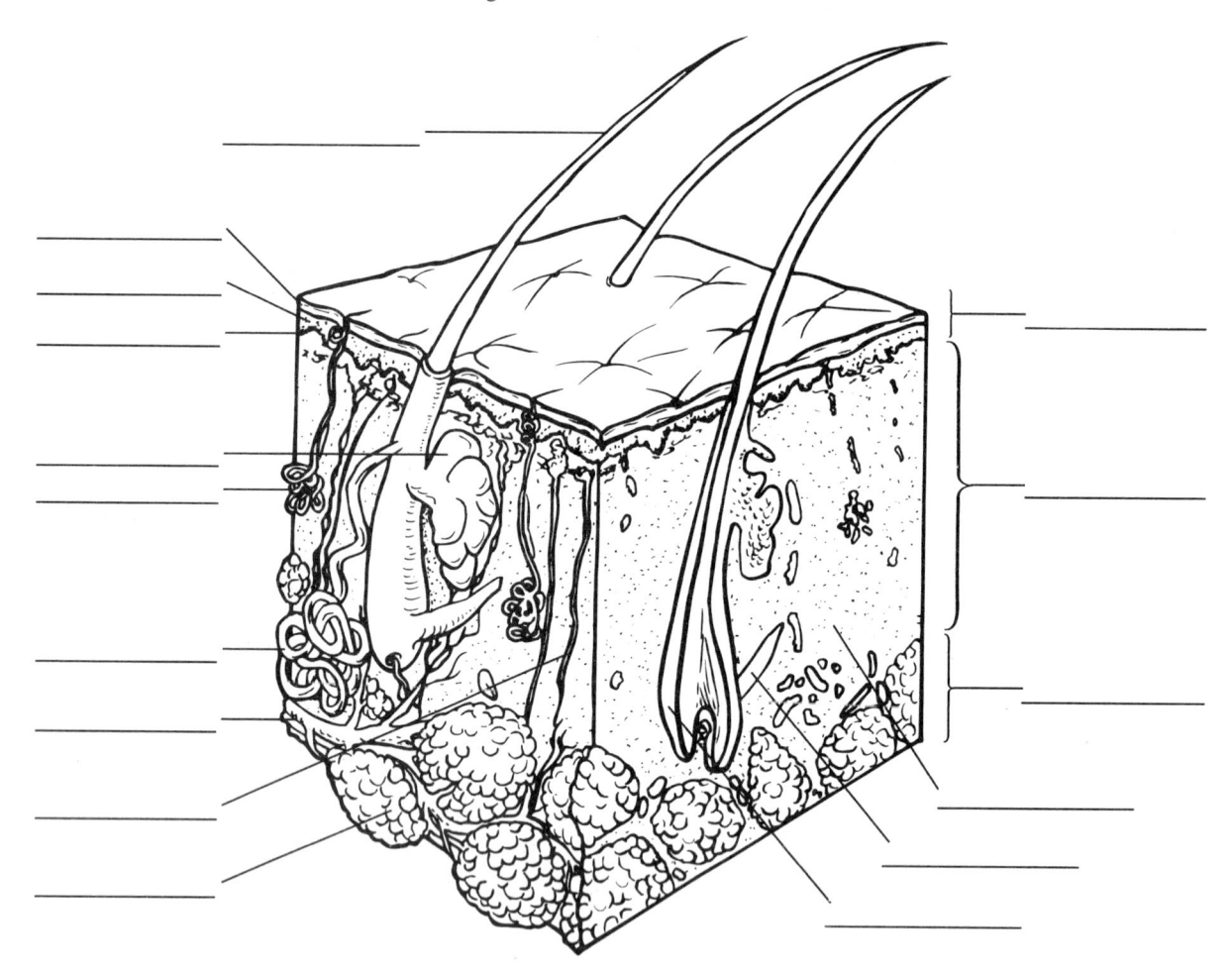

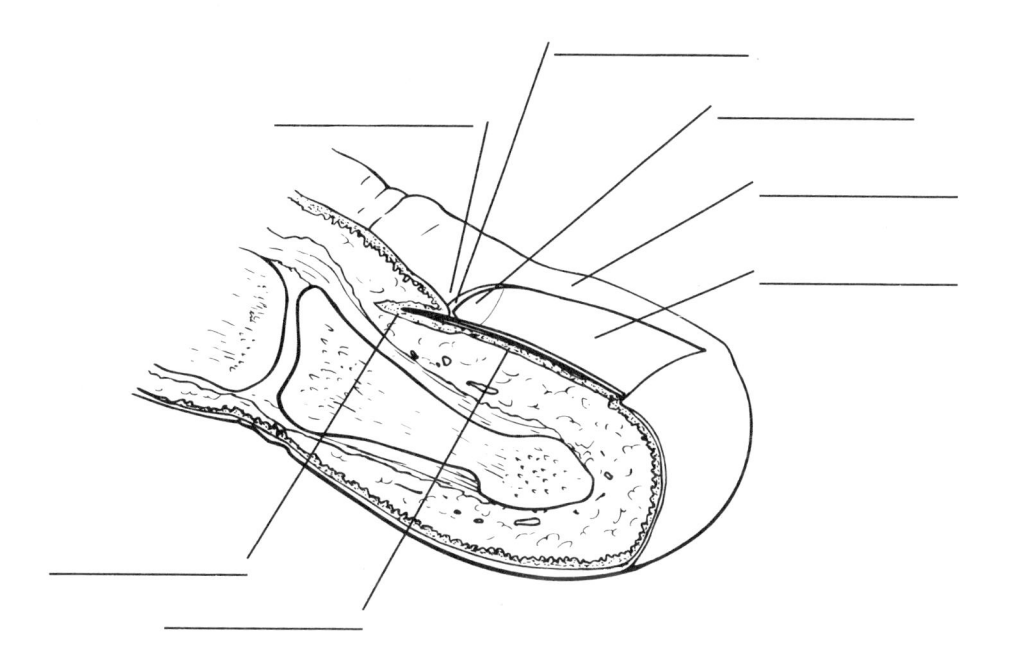

REVIEW AND CLINICAL JUDGEMENT QUESTIONS

This test is for you to check your own mastery of the content. Answers are provided on the text's Evolve site.

1. Select the best description of the secretion of the eccrine glands.
   a. thick, milky
   b. dilute saline solution
   c. protective lipid substance
   d. keratin

2. Nevus is the medical term for
   a. a freckle.
   b. a birthmark.
   c. an infected hair follicle.
   d. a mole.

3. You note a lesion during an examination. Select the description that is most complete.
   a. raised, irregular lesion the size of a quarter, located on dorsum of left hand
   b. open lesion with no drainage or odour approximately 6 mm in diameter
   c. pedunculated lesion below left scapula with consistent red colour, no drainage or odour
   d. dark-brown, raised lesion, with irregular border, on dorsum of right foot, 3 cm in size with no drainage

4. During a routine visit, M.B., age 78 years, asks about small, round, flat, brown macules on the hands. After assessing the area, what is your best response?
   a. "These are the result of sun exposure and do not require treatment."
   b. "These are related to exposure to the sun. They may become cancerous."
   c. "These are the skin tags that occur with aging. No treatment is required."
   d. "I'm glad you brought this to my attention. I will arrange for a biopsy."

5. An area of thin, shiny skin with decreased visibility of normal skin markings is called
   a. lichenification.
   b. plaque.
   c. atrophy.
   d. keloid.

6. Flattening of the angle between the nail and its base is
   a. found in subacute bacterial endocarditis.
   b. a description of spoon-shaped nails.
   c. related to calcium deficiency.
   d. described as clubbing.

7. The configuration for individual lesions arranged in circles or arcs, as occurs with ringworm, is called
   a. linear.
   b. clustered.
   c. annular.
   d. gyrate.

8. The "A" in the ABCDE rule stands for
   a. accuracy.
   b. appearance.
   c. asymmetry.
   d. attenuated.

Match column A to column B. Items in column B may be used more than once.

Column A—Descriptor

9. _____ Basal cell layer
10. _____ Aids protection by cushioning
11. _____ Collagen
12. _____ Adipose tissue
13. _____ Uniformly thin
14. _____ Stratum corneum
15. _____ Elastic tissue

Column B—Skin Layer

a. Epidermis
b. Dermis
c. Subcutaneous layer

Column A—Descriptor

16. _____ Pallor
17. _____ Erythema
18. _____ Cyanosis
19. _____ Jaundice

Column B—Colour Change

a. Intense redness of the skin due to excess blood in the dilated superficial capillaries
b. Bluish, mottled discoloration that signifies decreased perfusion
c. Absence of red-pink tones from the oxygenated hemoglobin in blood
d. Increase in bilirubin in the blood causing a yellow colour in the skin

Column A—Descriptor

20. _____ Tiny punctate red macules and papules on the cheeks, trunk, chest, back, and buttocks
21. _____ Lower half of body turns red, upper half blanches
22. _____ Transient mottling on trunk and extremities
23. _____ Bluish colour around the lips, on the hands and fingernails, and on the feet and toenails
24. _____ Large round or oval patch of light brown usually present at birth
25. _____ Yellowing of skin, sclera, and mucous membranes due to increased numbers of red blood cells hemolyzed following birth
26. _____ Yellow-orange colour in light-skinned people from ingestion of large amounts of foods containing carotene

Column B—Skin Colour Change

a. Harlequin
b. Erythema toxicum
c. Acrocyanosis
d. Physiological jaundice
e. Carotenemia
f. Café au lait
g. Cutis marmorata

27. You are conducting a class for new graduates on skin assessment. Which statement is true regarding the epidermis?
    a. The epidermis consists mostly of connective tissue or collagen.
    b. The epidermis contains the blood vessels.
    c. The epidermal cells are continually lost and replaced with new cells.
    d. A "paper cut" stimulates nerve cells in the epidermis.

28. You are preparing to care for a 63-year-old Black male with a history of heart attack who now presents with heart failure. What is the best technique to assess for cyanosis?
    a. Palpate the skin for increased heat.
    b. Inspect the hard palate of the mouth.
    c. Inspect the feet for an ashen grey look.
    d. Inspect the nail beds for a dusky, pale colour.

29. You are assessing a 57-year-old man's skin during a clinic appointment. Which technique is the best to assess for increased skin temperature?
    a. a grasping with your fingertips of both his hands
    b. laying the palmar surface of your hands on his abdomen
    c. placing the ventral surface of your hands on the person's shins and feet
    d. laying the dorsal surface of your hands on the person's neck

30. You are assessing the general skin colour of a person with dark pigmentation. You would expect which finding?
    a. lighter pigmentation on the palms of the hands
    b. a reddened colour of the lips
    c. patchy pigmentation on the dorsal surface of the hands
    d. small flat macules of browner pigment melanin on the chest

31. You are in the emergency department when a 70-year-old woman is brought by ambulance after falling in her assisted living home and then not found for 14 hours. Vital signs are stable. Imaging shows no broken bones. She is alert and oriented. One of your assessment findings is that the skin on upper chest "tents" after you lift it. This finding is consistent with
    a. edema.
    b. dehydration.
    c. dry skin (xerosis) of aging.
    d. a normal finding for her age and upper chest.

32. A 3-day-old infant has had healthy assessments since birth. On this third day, you notice a yellowing of his skin, sclera, and mucous membranes. You next most appropriate action is
    a. ask the breastfeeding mom to avoid carotene-rich foods.
    b. notify the nurse practitioner or physician that this may be hemolytic disease of the newborn.
    c. record this as physiological jaundice and proceed with the assessment.
    d. perform deep palpation on the abdomen to elicit possible pain associated with biliary tract obstruction.

33. During a sports physical for a 14-year-old female, you observe many papules, pustules, nodules, and "blackheads" covering the cheeks and jaw on the face. Which of these statements would be your most appropriate one?
    a. "Have you heard any other girls say anything about your acne?"
    b. "You have severe acne; it's at its peak and will get better in a year."
    c. "How do you feel about the acne on your face?"
    d. "Would you say your acne has made you feel depressed?"

CRITICAL THINKING EXERCISES

1. Review the article by O'Sullivan et.al. listed at the beginning of this chapter. You encounter an 18-year-old female at your clinic for a sports physical. Compose what you would say in response to her history of using a tanning bed in her gym twice per week. During which part of the examination would you give your response?

2. You are caring for a 78-year-old male of Indigenous descent who has developed Guillain Barré syndrome and has difficulty with mobility. Study the Braden Scale shown in Table 13.1 in your textbook. How would you rate the risk of your patient developing a pressure injury? Review the article by Oozageer Gunowa et.al. listed at the beginning of this chapter. How would differing skin tones impact patient assessment?

SKILLS LABORATORY/CLINICAL SETTING

You are now ready for the clinical component of the integumentary system. Usually the clinical examination of the integumentary system is performed along with the examination of each particular body region. The purpose of practising the steps of this examination separately is so that you begin to think of the skin and its appendages as a separate organ system, and so that you learn the components of skin examination.

Clinical Objectives

1. Inspect and palpate the skin, noting its colour, vascularity, edema, moisture, temperature, texture, thickness, mobility and turgor, and any lesions.

2. Inspect the fingernails, noting colour, shape, and any lesions.

3. Inspect the hair, noting texture, distribution, and any lesions.

4. Record the history and physical examination findings accurately, reach an assessment of the health state, and develop a plan of care.

Instructions

Prepare the examination setting. Wash your hands. Practise the steps of the examination on a peer in the skills laboratory, giving appropriate instructions as you proceed. Choosing a peer from an ethnic background other than your own will further heighten your recognition of the range of normal skin tones. Record your findings using the documentation sheet that follows. The front of the page is intended as a worksheet; the back of the page is intended for your narrative summary recording using the subjective, objective, assessment, plan (SOAP) format.

Note the student competency checklist that follows the documentation sheet. It lists the essential behaviours you should display as an examiner, and it may be used by your clinical instructor to evaluate your clinical teaching of the skin self-examination.

NOTES

DOCUMENTATION—SKIN, HAIR, AND NAILS

Date _____

Examiner _____

Patient _____ Age _____ Gender _____

Occupation _____

I. Health History

	No	Yes, explain
1. Any previous **skin disease**?		
2. Any change in skin colour or **pigmentation**?		
3. Any changes in a **mole**?		
4. Excessive dryness or **moisture**?		
5. Any skin **itching**?		
6. Any excess **bruising**?		
7. Any skin **rash** or **lesions**?		
8. Taking any **medications**?		
9. Any recent hair loss?		
10. Any change in nails?		
11. Any environmental or occupational hazards for skin?		
12. How do you take care of skin? Sunscreen?		

II. Physical Examination

A. Inspect and palpate the skin.

Colour _____

Pigmentation _____

Temperature _____

Moisture _____

Texture _____

Thickness _____

Any edema _____

Mobility and turgor _____

Vascularity and bruising _____

Any lesions (describe) _____

B. Inspect and palpate the hair.

Colour _____

Texture _____

Distribution _____

Any lesions (describe) _____

C. Inspect and palpate the nails.

Shape and contour _____

Consistency _____

Colour _____

Capillary refill _____

D. Teach skin self-examination.

DOCUMENTATION—SKIN, HAIR, AND NAILS _____

Summarize your findings using the SOAP format.

Subjective (Reason for seeking care, health history)

Objective (Physical examination findings)

Record distribution of any rash or lesions below.

Assessment (Assessment of health state or problem, diagnosis)

Plan (Diagnostic evaluation, follow-up care, patient teaching)

STUDENT COMPETENCY CHECKLIST

Teaching Skin Self-Examination (SSE)

	S	U	Comments
I. Cognitive			
A. Explain:			
a) Why skin is examined.			
b) Who should perform skin self-examination.			
c) Frequency of skin examination.			
B. Define the ABCDE rule.			
C. Describe any equipment the patient may need.			
II. Performance			
A. Explains to patient need for SSE.			
B. Instructs patient on technique of SSE by:			
a) Demonstrating the order and body positioning for inspecting skin.			
b) Describing normal skin characteristics.			
c) Describing abnormal findings to look for.			
C. Instructs patient to report unusual findings to nurse or physician at once.			

NOTES

NOTES

14 Head, Face, and Neck, Including Regional Lymphatic System

PURPOSE

This chapter reviews the anatomy and function of structures in the head and neck; the methods of inspection and palpation of these structures; and the accurate recording of the assessment.

READING ASSIGNMENT

Jarvis: *Physical Examination and Health Assessment*, 4th Canadian ed., Chapter 14.

Suggested Readings

Richer, L., Billinghurst, L., Linsdell, M. A., et al. (2016). Medications for the acute treatment of migraine in children and adolescents. *Cochrane Database of Systematic Reviews,* (4). Art. no. CD005220. https://doi.org/10.1002/14651858.CD005220.pub2

Toward Optimized Practice. (2016, September). *Quick reference: Primary care management of headache in adults.* https://actt.albertadoctors.org/CPGs/Lists/CPGDocumentList/Quick-Reference-Headache.pdf

GLOSSARY

Study the following terms after reading the corresponding chapter in the text.

Bruit: a soft blowing, swooshing sound heard through the stethoscope over an area of abnormal blood flow
Dysphagia: difficulty in swallowing
Fontanelles: membrane-covered "soft spots" allow for growth of the brain during the first year
Goitre: an increase in size of the thyroid gland that occurs with hyperthyroidism
Hyoid bone: highest structure in the neck, palpated at the level of the floor of the mouth
Lymph nodes: small, oval clusters of lymphatic tissue that are set at intervals along the lymph vessels, like beads on a string
Lymphadenopathy: enlargement of the lymph nodes (>1 cm) due to infection, allergy, or neoplasm
Macrocephalic: an abnormally large head
Microcephalic: an abnormally small head
Normocephalic: a round, symmetrical skull that is appropriately related to body size
Parotid glands: largest of the salivary glands and located in the cheeks over the mandible, anterior to and below the ear
Thyroid gland: a highly vascular endocrine gland synthesizes and secretes thyroxine (T4) and triiodothyronine (T3), hormones that stimulate the rate of cellular metabolism
Torticollis: a head tilt due to a shortening or spasm of one sternomastoid muscle
Vertigo: an illusory sensation of either the room or one's own body spinning; not the same as dizziness

STUDY GUIDE

After completing the reading assignment, you should be able to answer the following questions in the spaces provided.

1. The major neck muscles are the _____.

2. Name the borders of two regions in the neck: the anterior triangle and the posterior triangle.

3. List the facial structures that should appear symmetrical when inspecting the head.

4. Describe the characteristics of lymph nodes often associated with the following conditions:

   Acute infection _____

   Chronic inflammation _____

   Cancer _____

5. Differentiate *caput succedaneum* from *cephalhematoma* in the newborn infant.

6. Describe the tonic neck reflex in the infant.

7. Describe the characteristics of normal cervical lymph nodes during childhood.

8. List the condition(s) associated with parotid gland enlargement.

9. Describe the facial characteristics that occur with Down syndrome or trisomy 21.

10. Contrast the facial characteristics of hyperthyroidism versus hypothyroidism.

11. Fill in the labels indicated on the following illustrations.

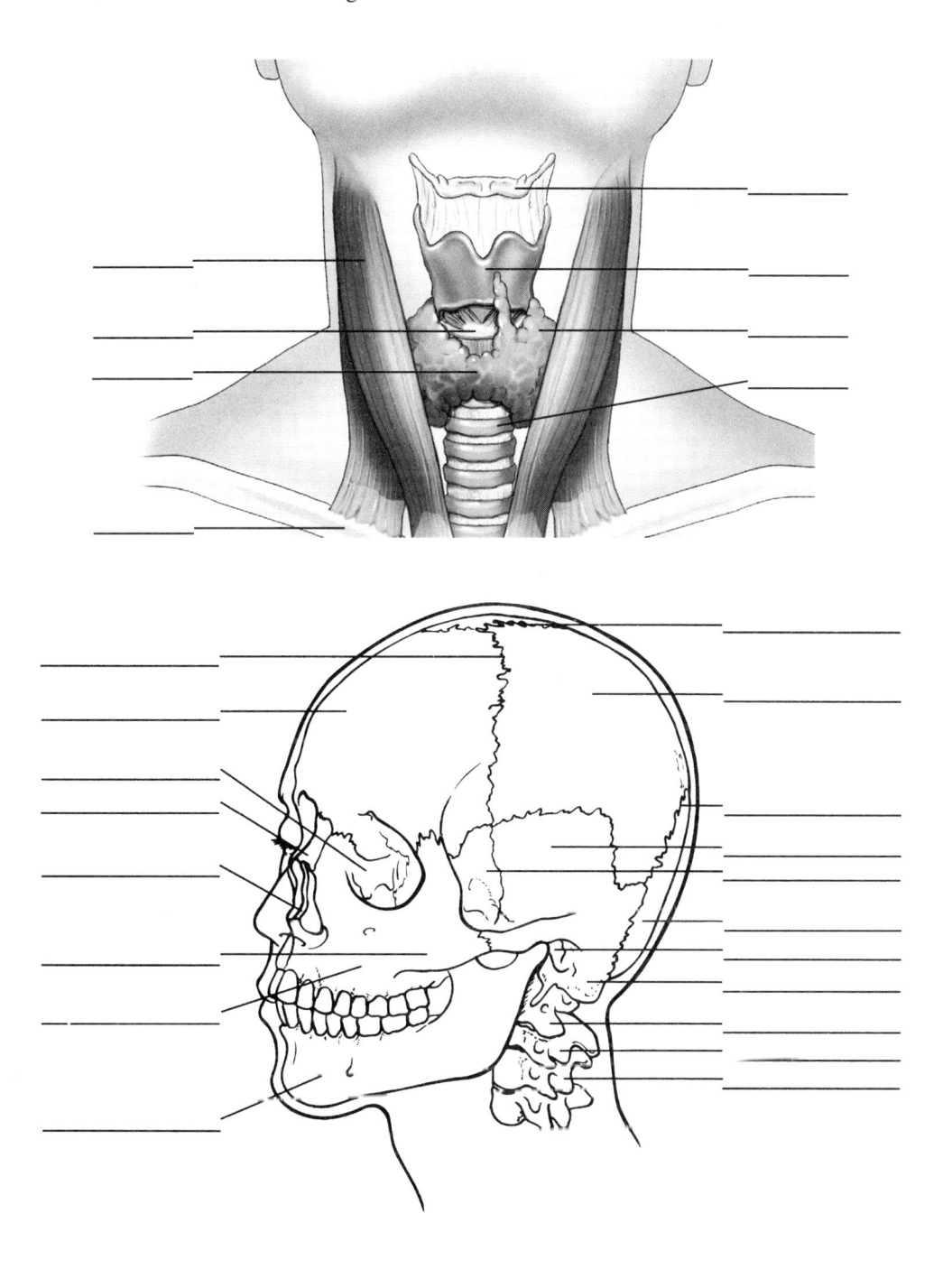

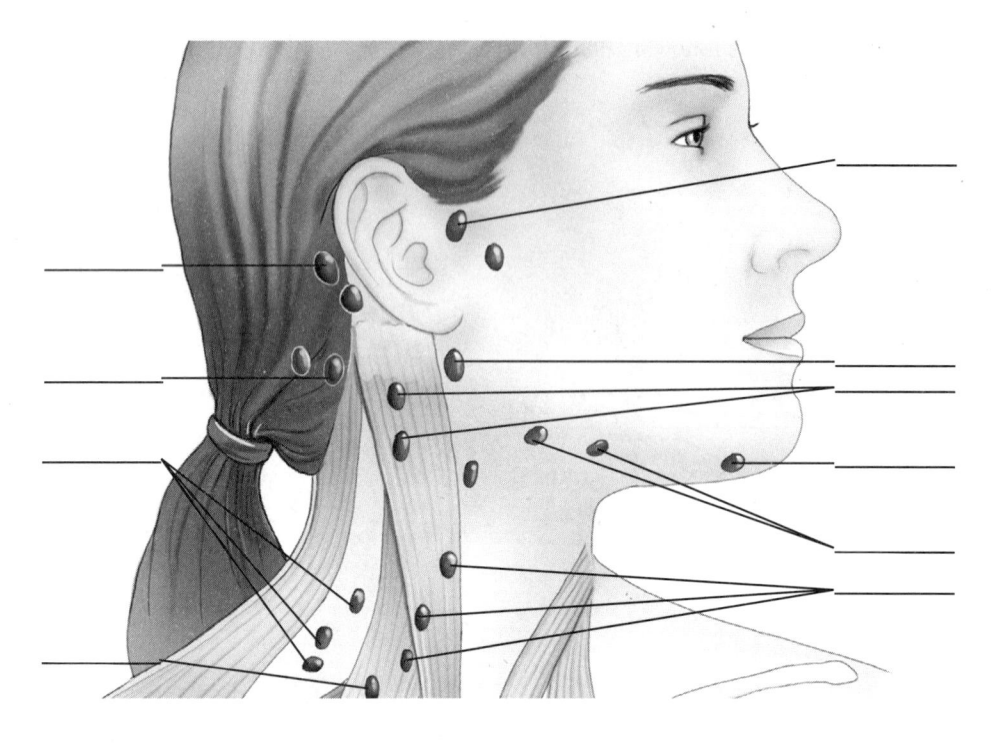

REVIEW AND CLINICAL JUDGEMENT QUESTIONS

This test is for you to check your own mastery of the content. Answers are provided on the text's Evolve site.

1. You are assessing the oral structures in a 58-year-old man with a 40-year history of smoking cigarettes. You will search for the sublingual glands at which location?
   a. in the cheeks, over the mandible, anterior to the ear
   b. beneath the mandible, at the angle of the jaw
   c. in the floor of the mouth, under the side of the tongue
   d. above the temporalis muscle, anterior to the ear

2. Identify the facial bone that articulates at a joint instead of a suture.
   a. zygomatic
   b. maxilla
   c. nasal
   d. mandible

3. During your physical examination, a 30-year-old patient shows you a bulging blood vessel that runs diagonally across the sternomastoid muscle. This vessel is
   a. the temporal artery.
   b. the carotid artery.
   c. the external jugular vein.
   d. the internal jugular vein.

4. You stand behind a 28-year-old pregnant woman to palpate her thyroid gland. You search for the isthmus of the thyroid gland just below
   a. the mandible.
   b. the cricoid cartilage.
   c. the hyoid bone.
   d. the thyroid cartilage.

5. You are taking a health history for a 35-year-old woman who reports that she has had cluster headaches in the past. Which findings would you expect for cluster headaches?
   a. Exacerbated by alcohol, stress, daytime napping, wind or heat exposure.
   b. The usual occurrence is two per month, each lasting 1 to 3 days.
   c. They are described as throbbing.
   d. They tend to be supraorbital, retro-orbital, or frontotemporal.

6. You are testing active range of motion (ROM) in a 79-year-old man. When turning his head to the right and left, you observe he turns more at his shoulders than at his neck. What is your next most appropriate action?
   a. Palpate his shoulders for any pain or tenderness.
   b. Direct him to bend over and touch the toes for complete ROM of spine.
   c. Continue with the examination; this finding is common in an older adult.
   d. Refer him to an orthopedic specialist.

7. A 38-year-old male presents to the clinic with concerns of a headache. While assessing his cranial nerves, you ask the patient to shrug their shoulders while providing resistance. This is a test of the status of which cranial nerve?
   a. II
   b. V
   c. IX
   d. XI

8. L.F. is in the clinic today for a routine 6-month well-baby check. As you palpate the anterior fontanelle on the 6-month-old infant, you note that the fontanelles should feel
   a. tense or bulging.
   b. depressed or sunken.
   c. firm, slightly concave, and well defined.
   d. pulsating.

9. The thyroid gland is enlarged bilaterally in the neck of a 50-year-old woman. Which manoeuvre would be your next most appropriate?
   a. Check for deviation of the trachea.
   b. Continue with the examination; this is an expected finding in a menopausal woman.
   c. Listen for a murmur over the aortic area causing thyroid enlargement.
   d. Listen for a bruit over the thyroid lobes indicating increased blood flow.

10. A 22-year-old adult comes to your clinic for a new patient intake. As you palpate the cervical lymph nodes, which characteristics would be healthy and expected?
    a. mobile, soft, nontender
    b. large, clumped, tender
    c. matted, fixed, hard
    d. one isolated enlargement, fixed, nontender

11. You assess a newborn infant 3 hours after birth and note a soft, fluctuant swelling just over one cranial bone. The parents report a difficult head presentation delivery. What is (are) your next action(s)? (Select all that apply.)
    a. Inform the parents that this is a cephalhematoma and will go away on its own over the next few weeks.
    b. Request an order for blood results to screen for possible jaundice.
    c. Suspect increased intracranial pressure and request a referral.
    d. Inform the parents that this is a caput succedaneum and will go away on its own over the next few weeks.

12. A 20-year-old man suffers a blow to his head from another player's leg during a soccer game. You assess him 6 hours later, and he reports moderate headache and nausea, vomiting one time, and blurred vision while reading his phone screen. He had no loss of consciousness after the injury. There are no further assessment abnormalities. Your most appropriate advice is
    a. physical and cognitive rest for 24 hours—no reading, screen watching, or other brain work activity.
    b. rest with only slow walking for the next 7 days, followed by full return to play.
    c. remain at home for 24 hours, with mild stretching allowed.
    d. no return to game play for 24 hours; otherwise perform usual activity.

13. T.S. presents with a throbbing, unilateral headache associated with nausea, vomiting, and photophobia. These symptoms are characteristic of
    a. a cluster headache.
    b. a subarachnoid hemorrhage.
    c. a migraine headache.
    d. a tension headache.

Match column A to column B.

Column A—Lymph Nodes

14. _____ Preauricular

15. _____ Posterior auricular

16. _____ Occipital

17. _____ Submental

18. _____ Submandibular

19. _____ Jugulodigastric

20. _____ Superficial cervical

21. _____ Deep cervical

22. _____ Posterior cervical

23. _____ Supraclavicular

Column B—Location

a. Above and behind the clavicle
b. Deep under the sternomastoid muscle
c. In front of the ear
d. In the posterior triangle along the edge of the trapezius muscle
e. Superficial to the mastoid process
f. At the base of the skull
g. Halfway between the angle and the tip of the mandible
h. Behind the tip of the mandible
i. Under the angle of the mandible
j. Overlying the sternomastoid muscle

CRITICAL THINKING EXERCISE

Headache (HA) disorders are common neurological disorders, but are often not fully assessed, diagnosed, or treated. Consider your own personal and clinical experience with HA. Review data on headache in Chapter 14 in your textbook and in the articles listed at the beginning of this chapter. Discuss these points:
- List pharmaceutical and nonpharmaceutical interventions for tension-type HA and migraine HA. Discuss your own experiences with these interventions. What evidenced-informed resources can you find to support these interventions?
- List triggers for tension-type, migraine, and cluster HA.
- Discuss lifestyle modifications that may aid in the care of the person with frequent HAs.
- Discuss red-flag HAs that command immediate referral.

SKILLS LABORATORY/CLINICAL SETTING

You are now ready for the clinical component of the head, face, and neck chapter. The purpose of the clinical component is to practise the steps of the head, face, and neck examination on a peer in the skills laboratory and to achieve the following objectives.

Clinical Objectives

1. Collect a health history related to pertinent signs and symptoms of the head and neck.

2. Inspect and palpate the skull, noting size, contour, lumps, or tenderness.

3. Inspect the face, noting facial expression, symmetry, skin characteristics, or lesions.

4. Inspect and palpate the neck for symmetry, range of motion, and integrity of lymph nodes, trachea, and thyroid gland.

5. Record the findings systematically, reach an assessment of the health state, and develop a plan of care.

Instructions

Prepare the examination setting. Wash your hands. Practise the steps of the examination on a peer in the skills laboratory, giving appropriate instructions as you proceed. Record your findings using the documentation sheet that follows. The front of the page is intended as a worksheet; the back of the page is intended for your narrative summary recording using the subjective, objective, assessment, plan (SOAP) format.

DOCUMENTATION—HEAD, FACE, AND NECK

Date _____

Examiner _____

Patient _____ Age _____ Gender _____

Pronouns _____

Occupation _____

I. Health History

	No	Yes, explain
1. Any unusually frequent or unusually severe **headaches**?		
2. Any **head injury**?		
3. Experienced any **dizziness**?		
4. Any neck **pain**?		
5. Any **lumps** or **swelling** in head or neck?		
6. Any surgery on head or neck?		

II. Physical Examination

A. Inspect and palpate the skull.

General size and contour _____

Deformities, lumps, tenderness _____

Temporal artery _____

Temporomandibular joint _____

B. Inspect the face.

Facial expression _____

Symmetry of structures _____

Involuntary movements _____

Edema _____

Masses or lesions _____

Colour and texture of skin _____

C. Inspect the neck.

Symmetry _____

Range of motion, active _____

Test strength of cervical muscles _____

Abnormal pulsations _____

Enlargement of thyroid _____

Enlargement of lymph and salivary glands _____

D. Palpate the lymph nodes.

Exact location _____

Size and shape _____

Presence or absence of tenderness _____

Freely movable, adherent to deeper structures, or matted together _____

Presence of surrounding inflammation _____

Texture (hard, soft, firm) _____

E. Palpate the trachea.

F. Palpate the thyroid gland.

G. Auscultate the thyroid gland (if enlarged).

DOCUMENTATION—HEAD, FACE, AND NECK

Summarize your findings using the SOAP format.

Subjective (Reason for seeking care, health history)

Objective (Physical examination findings)

Assessment (Assessment of health state or problem, diagnosis)

Plan (Diagnostic evaluation, follow-up care, patient teaching)

15 Eyes

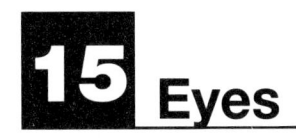

PURPOSE

This chapter reviews the structure and function of the external and internal components of the eyes; the methods of examination of vision, external eye structures, and the ocular fundus; and the accurate recording of the assessment.

READING ASSIGNMENT

Jarvis: *Physical Examination and Health Assessment*, 4th Canadian ed., Chapter 15.

Suggested reading

Carlson, C., Howe, T., Pedersen, C., et al. (2020). Caring for visually impaired patients in the hospital. *The American Journal of Nursing, 120*(5), 48–55.

GLOSSARY

Study the following terms after reading the corresponding chapter in the text.

Accommodation: adaptation of the eye for near vision by increasing the curvature of the lens
Anisocoria: unequal pupil size
Arcus senilis: a grey-white arc or circle around the limbus of the iris that is common with aging
Argyll Robertson pupil: no reaction of pupil to light, but does constrict with accommodation
Arteriovenous crossing: crossing paths of an artery and vein in the ocular fundus
Bitemporal hemianopsia: loss of both temporal visual fields
Blepharitis: inflammation of the glands and eyelash follicles along the margin of the eyelids
Cataract: opacity of the lens of the eye that develops slowly with aging and gradually obstructs vision
Chalazion: an infection or retention cyst of a meibomian gland, showing as a beady nodule on the eyelid
Conjunctivitis: infection of the conjunctiva, "pinkeye"
Cotton wool spots: abnormal soft exudates visible as grey-white areas on the ocular fundus
Cup–disc ratio: ratio of the width of the physiological cup to the width of the optic disc, normally half or less
Dioptre: unit of strength of the lens settings on the ophthalmoscope that changes focus on the eye structures
Diplopia: double vision
Drusen: benign deposits on the ocular fundus that show as round yellow dots and occur commonly with aging
Ectropion: lower eyelid loose and rolling outward
Entropion: lower eyelid rolling inward
Exophthalmos: protruding eyeballs
Fovea centralis: the area of sharpest and keenest vision; it is at the centre of the macula on the ocular fundus
Glaucoma: a group of eye diseases characterized by increased intraocular pressure
Hordeolum: a stye; a red, painful pustule that is a localized infection of the hair follicle at the eyelid margin
Lid lag: the abnormal white rim of sclera visible between the upper eyelid and the iris when a person moves the eyes downward
Macula: a round, darker area of the ocular fundus that mediates vision only from the central visual field
Microaneurysm: abnormal finding of round, punctuate red dots on the ocular fundus that are localized dilations of small vessels
Miosis: constricted pupils
Mydriasis: dilated pupils
Myopia: "nearsightedness"; a refractive error in which near vision is better than far vision
Nystagmus: involuntary, rapid, rhythmic movement of the eyeball
O.D.: oculus dexter, or right eye
Optic atrophy: pallor of the optic disc due to partial or complete death of optic nerve
Optic disc: the area of the ocular fundus in which blood vessels exit and enter
O.S.: oculus sinister, or left eye
Papilledema: stasis of blood flow out of the ocular fundus; sign of increased intracranial pressure

Pingueculae: yellowish elevated nodules caused by a thickening of the bulbar conjunctiva as a result of prolonged exposure to sun, wind, and dust
Presbyopia: the decrease in power of accommodation that occurs with aging
Pterygium: triangular opaque tissue on the nasal side of the conjunctiva that grows toward the centre of the cornea
Ptosis: drooping of upper eyelid over the iris and possibly covering the pupil
Red reflex: the red glow that appears to fill the person's pupil when first visualized through the ophthalmoscope
Strabismus: squint, crossed eye; disparity of the eye axes
Xanthelasma: soft, raised yellow plaques on the eyelids at the inner corners of the eyes

STUDY GUIDE

After completing the reading assignment, you should be able to answer the following questions in the spaces provided.

1. Name the six sets of extraocular muscles and the cranial nerve that innervates each one.

2. Name and describe the three concentric coats of the eyeball.

3. Name the functions of the ciliary body, the pupil, and the iris.

4. Describe the anterior chamber, posterior chamber, and the vitreous body.

5. Describe how an image formed on the retina compares with an object's actual appearance in the outside world.

6. Describe the lacrimal system.

7. Define the pupillary light reflex, fixation, and accommodation.

8. Concerning the pupillary light reflex, describe and contrast a direct light reflex with a consensual light reflex.

9. Identify common age-related changes in the eye.

10. Discuss the most common causes of decreased visual function in the older adult.

11. Explain the statement that normal visual acuity is 20/20.

12. Describe the method of testing for presbyopia.

13. To test for accommodation, the person focuses on a distant object, then shifts the gaze to a near object about 15 cm (6 in.) away. At near distance, you would expect the pupils to _____ (dilate/constrict), and the axes of the eyes to _____.

14. Concerning malalignment of the eye axes, contrast *phoria* with *tropia*.

15. Describe abnormal findings of tissue colour that are possible on the conjunctiva and sclera, and their significance.

16. Describe the method of everting the upper eyelid for examination.

17. Contrast *pingueculae* with *pterygium*.

18. Contrast the use of the negative dioptre (or red lens settings) with the positive dioptre (or black lens settings) on the ophthalmoscope.

19. Explain the rationale for testing for strabismus during early childhood.

20. Describe these findings and explain their significance: epicanthal fold, pseudostrabismus, ophthalmia neonatorum, and Brushfield's spots.

21. Describe the following four types of "red eye," and explain their significance:

    Conjunctivitis _____

    _____

    Subconjunctival hemorrhage _____

    _____

    Iritis _____

    _____

    Acute glaucoma _____

    _____

22. Fill in the labels indicated on the following illustrations.

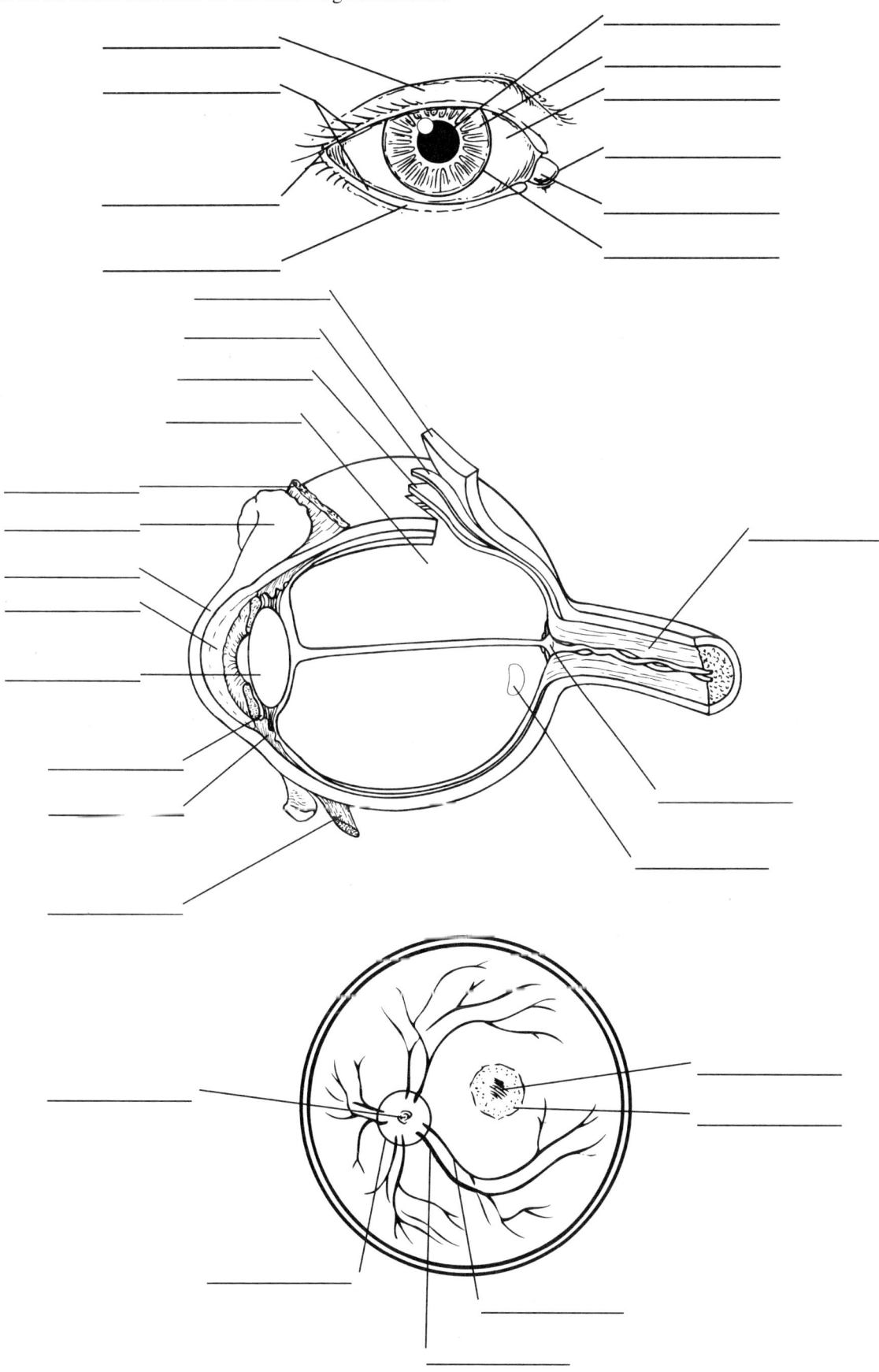

REVIEW AND CLINICAL JUDGEMENT QUESTIONS

This test is for you to check your own mastery of the content. Answers are provided on the text's Evolve site.

1. The palpebral fissure is
   a. the border between the cornea and sclera.
   b. the open space between the eyelids.
   c. the angle where the eyelids meet.
   d. visible on the upper and lower lids at the inner canthus.

2. The corneal reflex is mediated by cranial nerves
   a. II and III.
   b. II and VI.
   c. V and VII.
   d. VI and IV.

3. The retinal structures viewed through the ophthalmoscope are
   a. the optic disc, the retinal vessels, the general background, and the macula.
   b. the cornea, the lens, the choroid, and the ciliary body.
   c. the optic papilla, the sclera, the retina, and the iris.
   d. the pupil, the sclera, the ciliary body, and the macula.

4. The examiner records "positive consensual light reflex." This is
   a. the convergence of the axes of the eyeballs.
   b. the simultaneous constriction of the other pupil when one eye is exposed to bright light.
   c. a reflex direction of the eye toward an object attracting a person's attention.
   d. the adaptation of the eye for near vision.

5. Several changes occur in the eye with the aging process. The thickening and yellowing of the lens is referred to as
   a. presbyopia.
   b. floaters.
   c. macular degeneration.
   d. senile cataract.

6. Be alert to symptoms that may constitute an eye emergency. Identify the symptom(s) that should be referred immediately.
   a. floaters
   b. epiphora
   c. sudden onset of vision change
   d. photophobia

7. Visual acuity is assessed with
   a. the Snellen eye chart.
   b. an ophthalmoscope.
   c. the Hirschberg test.
   d. the confrontation test.

8. The cover–uncover test is used to assess for
   a. nystagmus.
   b. peripheral vision.
   c. muscle weakness.
   d. visual acuity.

9. When using the ophthalmoscope, you would
   a. remove your own glasses and approach the patient's left eye with your left eye.
   b. leave the light on in the examining room and remove glasses from the patient.
   c. remove your glasses, and set the dioptre setting to 0.
   d. use the smaller white light, and instruct the patient to focus on the ophthalmoscope.

10. The six muscles that control eye movement are innervated by cranial nerves
    a. II, III, and V.
    b. IV, VI, and VII.
    c. III, IV, and VI.
    d. II, III, and VI.

11. Conjunctivitis is always associated with
    a. absent red reflex.
    b. reddened conjunctiva.
    c. impairment of vision.
    d. fever.

12. A patient has blurred peripheral vision. You suspect glaucoma and test the visual fields. A person with normal vision would see your moving finger temporally at
    a. 50 degrees.
    b. 60 degrees.
    c. 90 degrees.
    d. 180 degrees.

13. A person is known to be blind in the left eye. What happens to the pupils when the right eye is illuminated by a penlight beam?
    a. No response in both pupils.
    b. Both pupils constrict.
    c. The right pupil constricts, and the left has no response.
    d. The left pupil constricts, and the right has no response.

14. Use of the ophthalmoscope: an interruption of the red reflex occurs when
    a. there is an opacity in the cornea or lens.
    b. the patient has pathology of the optic tract.
    c. the blood vessels are tortuous.
    d. the pupils are constricted.

15. One cause of visual impairment in aging adults is
    a. strabismus.
    b. glaucoma.
    c. amblyopia.
    d. retinoblastoma.

16. You are testing vision using the Snellen eye chart. A 14-year-old girl has a result of 20/40 for the right eye and 20/50−1 for the left eye. You observe her pausing and hesitant about some of the letters. Your next best action would be to
    a. move her 10 ft (3 m) closer to the Snellen eye chart and retest.
    b. assess her near vision using a handheld vision screener.
    c. alert the girl and her parent(s) to the need to refer to an eye specialist.
    d. continue with the examination; this is a common finding during a teenage growth spurt.

17. A 44-year-old male presents to your outpatient clinic for an examination for a bus-driving job. During the diagnostic positions test, you observe a back-and-forth movement of the iris when he looks to the extreme side. Your best action would be to
    a. proceed with the examination, as this is a normal finding.
    b. inquire about the amount of daily alcohol drinking.
    c. ask about dizziness when changing positions, as this eye movement is associated with inflammation of the semicircular canals in the ears.
    d. refer to a physician, as this eye movement is associated with multiple sclerosis.

18. You are inspecting the conjunctiva and sclera of a 53-year-old Black female. Which of the findings below are abnormal and are worthy of referral? (Select all that apply.)
    a. an overall reddening of the blood vessels on the sclera of one eye, but clearer near the iris
    b. a grey-blue or muddy colour of the sclera
    c. an even yellow colour of both sclera, extending up to the iris
    d. a small brown macule on the sclera that the person says has always been there

19. You plan to assess the pupillary light reflex on a hospitalized 20-year-old soccer player suspected of concussion. What would your correct action(s) be? (Select all that apply.)
    a. Ask the person to stare into the distance behind you.
    b. Advance your penlight in from the front to test both pupil responses.
    c. Use a pupil gauge to assess the findings in millimetres.
    d. Refer unequal pupil response to the physician.

20. During a screening examination, you inspect the ocular fundus using the ophthalmoscope on a 21-year-old woman who reports no abnormal symptoms during the history collection. Your best action would be to
    a. remove your own glasses and approach the woman's left eye with your left eye.
    b. leave the light on in the examining room and remove glasses from the woman.
    c. remove your glasses and set the dioptre setting to 0.
    d. use the smaller white light, and instruct the woman to focus on the ophthalmoscope.

21. During the ophthalmoscope examination of a 66-year-old woman, the red reflex is interrupted and appears with a black centre. This finding is associated with
    a. an opacity in the cornea or lens.
    b. a pathological disease in the optic tract.
    c. tortuous and crossing blood vessels in the ocular fundus.
    d. constricted pupils.

22. During the ophthalmoscopic examination, the mechanism causing the red reflex is
    a. petechial hemorrhages in the sclera.
    b. diabetic retinopathy.
    c. light reflecting off the retina.
    d. blood in the vitreous humor.

23. You are assessing infants during screening examinations in a pediatric outpatient clinic. You are alert for the following attending behaviours that suggest the infant can receive visual images and indeed see. (Select all that apply.)
    a. At 2 to 4 weeks of age, the infant can fixate on an object (bright toy).
    b. At 6 weeks of age, the infant can make some visual response to your face.
    c. At 6 to 10 months of age, the infant can fixate on a toy and follow it as you move it in all directions.
    d. At 12 months of age, the infant refuses to reopen eyes for about 20 seconds after exposure to your bright penlight.

24. You are assessing the vision of a 4-year-old child. Which of the following responses are abnormal and indicate referral to an eye specialist? (Select all that apply.)
    a. The child is unable to read letters on the Snellen eye chart.
    b. During the corneal light reflex, the reflected light in the left eye is off centre, but the reflected light in the right eye is centred on the pupil.
    c. During the cover–uncover test, one eye jumps in gaze following removal of the opaque card.
    d. The child has an extra fold of skin at the epicanthus of both eyes.

25. You are assessing the eyes and vision of residents aged 65 years and older at a long-term care facility. Which of the following responses are abnormal and indicate referral to an eye specialist? (Select all that apply.)
    a. The tissue of the upper eyelid is relaxed and rests close to the upper eyelashes.
    b. Bulging exists on the tissue of the lower eyelids.
    c. An opaque wedge-shaped tissue is present on the sclera and continues over the cornea.
    d. A grey-white circle is present around the cornea on the iris.
    e. Yellow papules are present on the upper lids near the inner canthus.
    f. Pupils are small with a resting size of 2 mm.
    g. During the ophthalmoscope examination, a black spot is present in the red reflex.

26. A 19-year-old man presents to the university health centre holding a tissue pressed to his eye. A yellow raised pustule exists at the upper eyelid margin. It has a small red area around it and is extremely painful. The sclera are white and vision is normal. Which of the following is/are your appropriate action(s)?
    a. Inspect the other eye for similar lesion.
    b. Request prescriptions for antibiotic drops/ointment.
    c. Instruct the man that this will resolve on its own and that no treatment is necessary.
    d. Instruct the man to avoid touching both eyes with the same tissue.
    e. Refer the man to the emergency department of the hospital.

27. A 25-year-old woman has been blind in her left eye since birth. What response would you expect in her pupils when the right eye is illuminated by a penlight beam?
    a. No response in both pupils.
    b. Both pupils constrict.
    c. The right pupil constricts, and the left has no response.
    d. The left pupil constricts, and the right has no response.

28. Which of the following eye disorders prompt urgent referral to an emergency department? (Select all that apply.)
    a. sudden acute loss of vision in one eye
    b. obvious trauma to the eyeball
    c. unequal resting pupil size of 1 or 2 mm; both constrict to light
    d. diagnosis of herpes zoster infection (shingles) on the face
    e. one unequal pupil that is dilated, distorted in shape, with redness around the iris

CRITICAL THINKING EXERCISE

Work with a partner in the lab, but try to pair with someone you do not know well. One person is blindfolded. Each person should guide the other on a campus walk with the following requirements:

1. Go through two different sets of doors.

2. Go up *and* down a set of stairs.

3. Drink at a water fountain.

Walk into buildings with which you are less familiar; this highlights a vision deficit in an unfamiliar environment. Be the blindfolded partner for 7 to 10 minutes and then switch roles. Back in the lab, discuss the following:

1. Frustration levels.

2. How did it feel to be led?

3. How did it feel to lead?

4. What worked? What failed to work?

5. What actions developed your trust in the partner who was leading?

6. How did you handle the doorways? The stairs? The water fountain?

7. Did you talk to anyone else on campus? Did you feel self-conscious, as if others were looking at you?

8. What is your takeaway for applying this exercise to your low-vision patients?

SKILLS LABORATORY/CLINICAL SETTING

You are now ready for the clinical component of the eye examination. The purpose of the clinical component is to practise the steps of the examination on a peer in the skills laboratory. Note that the first practice session usually takes a long time because there are so many separate steps. Be aware that success with the use of the ophthalmoscope is hard to achieve during the first practice session. Make sure you are holding the instrument correctly, and practise focusing on various objects about the room before you try to look at a peer's fundus. When you do examine a peer's eye, make sure to offer occasional rest times. It is very tiring for the "patient" to have the ophthalmoscope light shining in the eye. During the first practice session, aim for finding the red reflex and a retinal vessel or two; if you can locate the optic disc, so much the better.

Clinical Objectives

1. Collect a health history related to pertinent signs and symptoms of the eye system.

2. Demonstrate and explain assessment of visual acuity, visual fields, external eye structures, and ocular fundus.

3. Record the history and physical examination findings accurately, reach an assessment of the health state, and develop a plan of care.

Instructions

Prepare the examination setting. Wash your hands. Practise the steps of the examination on a peer in the skills laboratory, giving appropriate instructions as you proceed. Record your findings using the documentation sheet that follows. The front of the page is intended as a worksheet; the back of the page is intended for your narrative summary recording using the subjective, objective, assessment, plan (SOAP) format.

NOTES

DOCUMENTATION—EYES

Date _____

Examiner _____

Patient _____ Age _____ Gender _____

Occupation _____

I. **Health History—Adult**

	No	Yes, explain

1. Any **difficulty seeing** or any blurring?
2. Any eye **pain**?
3. Any history of **crossed eyes**?
4. Any **redness** or **swelling** in eyes?
5. Any **watering** or **tearing**?
6. Any eye conditions, **injury**, or **surgery** to eye?
7. Ever tested for **glaucoma**?
8. Wear **glasses** or **contact lenses**?
9. Ever had vision tested?
10. Anything at home or work that may affect your eyes?
11. Taking any medications?

II. **Physical Examination**

   A. **Test visual acuity.**

   Snellen eye chart _____

   Handheld vision screener for near vision _____ _____

   B. **Test visual fields.**

   Confrontation test _____

   C. **Inspect extraocular muscle function.**

   Corneal light reflex _____ _____

   Cover–uncover test _____

   Diagnostic positions test _____

   D. **Inspect external eye structures.**

   General _____

   Eyebrows _____

   Eyelids and lashes _____

   Eyeballs _____

   Conjunctiva and sclera _____

   Lacrimal gland, puncta _____

E. Inspect anterior eyeball structures.

Cornea _____

Iris _____

Pupil size _____

Pupil direct and consensual light reflex _____

Accommodation _____

F. Inspect ocular fundus.

Optic disc _____

Vessels _____

General background of fundus _____

Macula _____

DOCUMENTATION—EYES

Summarize your findings using the SOAP format.

Subjective (Reason for seeking care, health history)

Objective (Physical examination findings)

Record your findings on the diagram.

R   L

Assessment (Assessment of health state or problem, diagnosis)

Plan (Diagnostic evaluation, follow-up care, patient teaching)

16 Ears

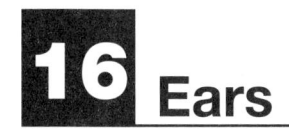

PURPOSE

This chapter reviews the structure and function of the ears; the methods of examination of hearing, external ear structures, and tympanic membrane using the otoscope; and the accurate recording of the assessment.

READING ASSIGNMENT

Jarvis: *Physical Examination and Health Assessment*, 4th Canadian ed., Chapter 16.

Suggested readings

Le Saux, N., & Robinson, J. (2022). *Management of acute otitis media in children six months of age and older.* Canadian Pediatric Society. https://cps.ca/en/documents/position/acute-otitis-media

Tiefel, N.L. (2020). What did you say? A review of the management of sudden sensorineural hearing loss. *The Nurse Practitioner, 45*(12), 43–48.

GLOSSARY

Study the following terms after reading the corresponding chapter in the text.

Annulus: the outer fibrous rim encircling the eardrum
Atresia: congenital absence or closure of the ear canal
Cerumen: a yellow, waxy material that lubricates and protects the ear canal
Cochlea: the inner ear structure containing the central hearing apparatus
Conductive hearing loss: hearing loss caused by fixation of the stapes (bones of the inner ear)
Eustachian tube: an opening that connects the middle ear with the nasopharynx and allows passage of air
Helix: superior, posterior free rim of the pinna
Incus: the middle of the three ossicles of the middle ear
Malleus: the first of the three ossicles of the middle ear
Mastoid process: bony prominence of the skull located just behind the ear
Organ of Corti: the sensory organ of hearing
Otalgia: pain in the ear
Otitis externa: inflammation of the outer ear and ear canal
Otitis media: inflammation of the middle ear and tympanic membrane
Otorrhea: discharge from the ear
Otosclerosis: a gradual hardening that causes the footplate of the stapes to become fixed in the oval window, which impedes the transmission of sound and causes progressive deafness
Pars flaccida: the small, slack, superior section of the tympanic membrane
Pars tensa: the thick, taut, central or inferior section of the tympanic membrane
Pinna: the auricle or outer ear
Presbycusis: gradual sensorineural hearing loss caused by nerve degeneration in the inner ear or auditory nerve, which occurs with aging
Sensorineural hearing loss: also called *perceptive loss*, it signifies pathology of the inner ear, cranial nerve VIII, or the auditory areas of the cerebral cortex
Stapes: the inner of the three ossicles of the middle ear
Tinnitus: ringing in the ears
Tympanic membrane: the eardrum; the thin, translucent, oval membrane that stretches across the ear canal and separates the middle ear from the outer ear
Umbo: the knob of the malleus that shows through the tympanic membrane
Vertigo: a spinning, twirling sensation

STUDY GUIDE

After completing the reading assignment, you should be able to answer the following questions in the spaces provided.

1. List the three functions of the middle ear.

2. Contrast two pathways of hearing.

3. Differentiate among the types of hearing loss, and give examples.

4. Relate the anatomical differences that place the infant at greater risk for middle ear infections.

5. Describe the whispered voice test for hearing acuity.

6. Explain the positioning of normal ear alignment in the child.

7. Define *otosclerosis* and *presbycusis*.

8. Contrast the motions used to straighten the ear canal when using the otoscope with an infant versus an adult.

9. Describe the appearance of the following nodules that could be present on the external ear: Darwin's tubercle; sebaceous cyst; tophi; chondrodermatitis; keloid; and carcinoma.

10. Describe the appearance of the following conditions that could appear in the ear canal: osteoma; exostosis; furuncle; polyp; foreign body.

11. List the disease state suggested by the following descriptions of the appearance of the eardrum:

    Yellow-amber colour _____

    Pearly grey colour _____

    Air/fluid level _____

    Distorted light reflex _____

    Red colour _____

    Dense white patches _____

    Dark oval area _____

    Black or white dots on eardrum or canal _____

    Blue eardrum _____

12. Describe the behaviours that might be demonstrated in a clinical interview by a patient who has hearing loss.

13. Fill in the labels indicated on the following illustrations.

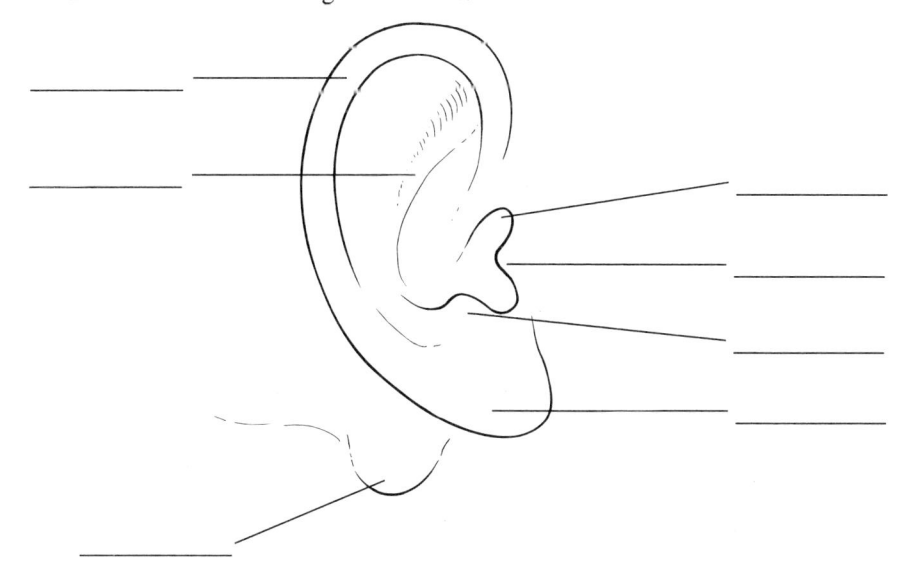

Chapter 16 Ears

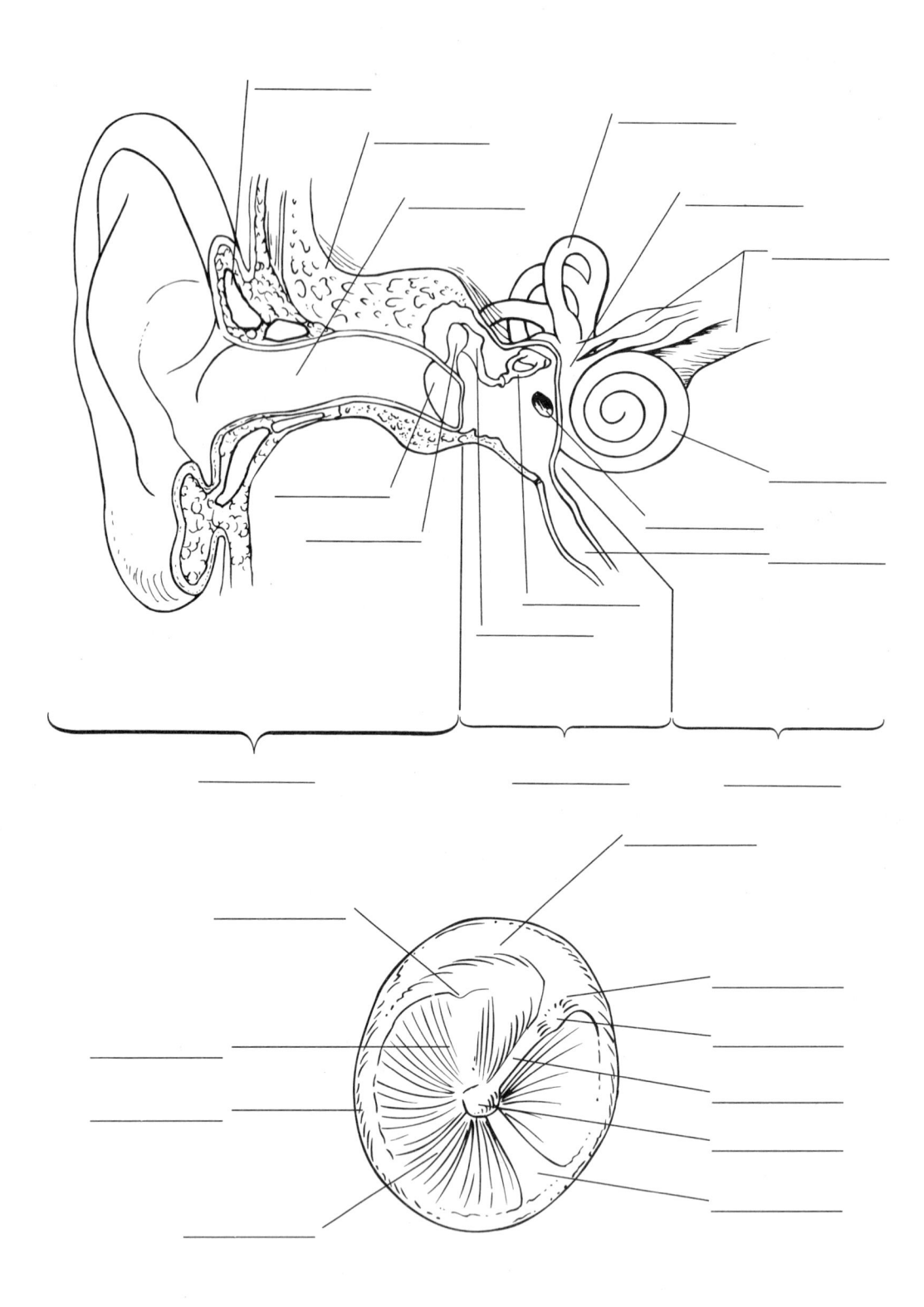

REVIEW AND CLINICAL JUDGEMENT QUESTIONS

This test is for you to check your own mastery of the content. Answers are provided on the text's Evolve site.

1. Using the otoscope, the tympanic membrane is visualized. The colour of a normal membrane is
   a. deep pink.
   b. creamy white.
   c. pearly grey.
   d. dependent upon the ethnicity of the individual.

2. Sensorineural hearing loss may be related to
   a. gradual nerve degeneration.
   b. foreign bodies.
   c. an impacted cerumen.
   d. a perforated tympanic membrane.

3. Before examining the ear with the otoscope, the _____, _____, and _____ should be palpated for tenderness. (Select the three correct structures.)
   a. helix, external auditory meatus, and lobule
   b. mastoid process, tympanic membrane, and malleus
   c. pinna, pars flaccida, and antitragus
   d. pinna, tragus, and mastoid process

4. During the otoscopic examination of a child younger than 3 years of age, the examiner
   a. pulls the pinna up and back.
   b. pulls the pinna down.
   c. holds the pinna gently but firmly in its normal position.
   d. tilts the head slightly toward the examiner.

5. While viewing with the otoscope, the examiner instructs the person to hold the nose and swallow. During this manoeuvre, the eardrum should
   a. flutter.
   b. retract.
   c. bulge.
   d. remain immobile.

6. To differentiate between air conduction and bone conduction hearing loss, the examiner would perform
   a. the Weber test.
   b. the Romberg test.
   c. the Rinne test.
   d. none of the above.

7. In examining the ear of an adult, the canal is straightened by pulling the auricle
   a. down and forward.
   b. down and back.
   c. up and back.
   d. up and forward.

8. Darwin's tubercle is
   a. an overgrowth of scar tissue.
   b. a blocked sebaceous gland.
   c. a sign of gout called tophi.
   d. a congenital, painless nodule at the helix.

9. When the ear is being examined with an otoscope, the patient's head should be
   a. tilted toward the examiner.
   b. tilted away from the examiner.
   c. as vertical as possible.
   d. tilted down.

10. The hearing receptors are located in the
    a. vestibule.
    b. semicircular canals.
    c. middle ear.
    d. cochlea.

11. The sensation of vertigo is the result of
    a. otitis media.
    b. pathology in the semicircular canals.
    c. pathology in the cochlea.
    d. fourth cranial nerve damage.

12. A common cause of a conductive hearing loss is
    a. impacted cerumen.
    b. acute rheumatic fever.
    c. a cerebrovascular accident (CVA).
    d. otitis externa.

13. Upon examination of the tympanic membrane, visualization of which of the following findings indicates acute purulent otitis media infection?
    a. absent light reflex, bluish eardrum, oval dark areas
    b. absent light reflex, reddened eardrum, bulging eardrum
    c. oval dark areas on eardrum
    d. absent light reflex, air/fluid level, or air bubbles behind eardrum
    e. retracted eardrum, very prominent landmarks

14. In examining a young adult woman, you observe that her tympanic membrane is yellow in colour. You suspect that she has
    a. serum in the middle ear.
    b. blood in the middle ear.
    c. infection of the drumhead.
    d. jaundice.

15. Risk reduction for acute otitis media includes
    a. use of pacifiers.
    b. increasing group day care.
    c. avoiding breastfeeding.
    d. eliminating smoking in the house and car.

16. The mother of an 18-month-old is concerned because her son has had three ear infections in the past year. He attends day care and takes a pacifier at bedtime. He has not had a pneumococcal vaccine. What would be your most appropriate response?
    a. "We need to check your son's immune system to see why he is having so many ear infections."
    b. "Ear infections are common in infants and toddlers because they tend to have more cerumen in their external ear."
    c. "At 18 months, the child's eustachian tube is shorter and wider than an adult's, so infections in the throat can extend up to the ear."
    d. "This suggests nerve damage in the inner ear, and we will refer you to a specialist in ear-nose-throat disorders."

17. A 64-year-old woman states that she has no problems hearing and is able to repeat all six numbers/letters presented in the whispered voice test. During otoscopy, her eardrum looks more white and more opaque than you have seen in a younger adult. Your next appropriate response would be to
    a. ask her if she feels "isolated" in family groups.
    b. consider conductive hearing loss and refer her to an audiologist.
    c. proceed with the examination, as this is a common finding in aging.
    d. ask if she has been hit on the side of her head in the past.

18. A 38-year-old woman enters your clinic concerned with roaring and ringing in her ears that is driving her "crazy." What is your best response to this concern?
    a. "How would you say the ringing in your ears affects your ability to do your usual activities?"
    b. "Are you allergic to any medications that you know of?"
    c. "How do you clean your ears?"
    d. "Are you exposed to chronic loud noises in your work or your hobby?"

19. You are assessing hearing acuity using the whispered voice test on a 74-year-old woman. She is able to repeat two of the six numbers/letters you present. Your next action should be to
    a. consider a high-tone hearing sensorineural loss and refer for audiology.
    b. assume that this is an expected response to aging and proceed with the examination.
    c. inspect the ear canal for foreign bodies.
    d. ask the woman whether she experienced recent head trauma.

CRITICAL THINKING EXERCISE

Review the Le Saux and Robinson article listed at the beginning of this chapter. Work with a partner to create and outline a management and an education plan for a 4-year-old female patient and her parents. You encounter the patient at the community primary care clinic, and her parents tell you that the child has complained of right ear pain and has had a fever of 38°C (100.4°F) for 24 hours. On examination, you find a bulging tympanic membrane that is yellowish in colour, with no evidence of perforation or discharge.

SKILLS LABORATORY/CLINICAL SETTING

You are now ready for the clinical component of the ear examination. The purpose of the clinical component is to practise the steps of the ear examination on a peer in the skills laboratory or on a patient in the clinical setting. The use of the otoscope is somewhat easier than the use of the ophthalmoscope; however, you still must be sure you are holding the instrument correctly. Holding the otoscope in an "upside down" position seems awkward at first, but it is important in order to make sure the otoscope tip does not cause pain to the delicate parts of the ear canal. Have someone correct your positioning before you insert the instrument.

Clinical Objectives

1. Collect a health history related to pertinent signs and symptoms of the ear system.
2. Describe the appearance of the normal outer ear and external ear canal.
3. Describe and demonstrate the correct technique of an otoscopic examination.
4. Describe and perform tests for hearing acuity and the vestibular apparatus.
5. Systematically describe the normal tympanic membrane, including position, colour, and landmarks.
6. Record the history and physical examination findings accurately, reach an assessment about the health state, and develop a plan of care.

Instructions

Prepare the examination setting and gather your equipment. Make certain the otoscope light is bright and batteries are freshly charged. Wash your hands. Practise the steps of the examination on a peer in the skills laboratory, giving appropriate instructions as you proceed. Record your findings using the documentation sheet that follows. The front of the page is intended as a worksheet; the back of the page is intended for your narrative summary recording using the subjective, objective, assessment, plan (SOAP) format.

NOTES

DOCUMENTATION—EARS

Date _____

Examiner _____

Patient _____ Age _____ Gender _____

Occupation _____

I. Health History

	No	Yes, explain
1. Any **earache** or ear pain?	_____	_____
2. Any ear infections?	_____	_____
3. Any **discharge** from ears?	_____	_____
4. Any **hearing loss**?	_____	_____
5. Any **loud noises** at home or job?	_____	_____
6. Any **ringing** or **buzzing** in ears?	_____	_____
7. Ever felt **vertigo** (spinning)?	_____	_____
8. How do you clean your ears?	_____	_____

II. Physical Examination

A. Inspect and palpate the external ear.

Size and shape _____

Skin condition _____

Tenderness _____

External auditory meatus _____

B. Inspect using the otoscope.

External canal _____

Tympanic membrane _____

Colour and characteristics _____

Position _____

Integrity of membrane _____

C. Test hearing acuity and the vestibular apparatus.

Whispered voice test _____

Romberg test (Chapter 25, see Fig. 25.18). _____

DOCUMENTATION—EARS

Summarize your findings using the SOAP format.

Subjective (Reason for seeking care, health history)

Objective (Physical examination findings)

Record your findings on the diagram.

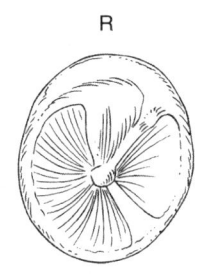

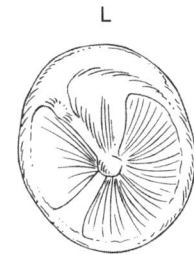

R   L

Assessment (Assessment of health state or problem, diagnosis)

Plan (Diagnostic evaluation, follow-up care, patient teaching)

NOTES

17 Nose, Mouth, and Throat

PURPOSE

This chapter reviews the structure and function of the nose, mouth, and throat; the methods of inspection and palpation of these structures; and the accurate recording of the assessment.

READING ASSIGNMENT

Jarvis: *Physical Examination and Health Assessment*, 4th Canadian ed., Chapter 17.

Suggested readings

RxFiles. (2022). *Pharyngitis: Management considerations.* https://www.rxfiles.ca/rxfiles/uploads/documents/ABX-Pharyngitis.pdf

Sauve, L., Forrester, M., & Top, K. (2021). Group A streptococcal (GAS) pharyngitis: A practical guide to diagnosis and treatment. *Pediatric Child Health, 26*(5), 319. https://cps.ca/en/documents/position/group-a-streptococcal

GLOSSARY

Study the following terms after reading the corresponding chapter in the text.

Aphthous ulcers: small, painful, round ulcers in the oral mucosa of unknown cause; also called *chancre sores*
Buccal: pertaining to the cheek
Candidiasis: moniliasis; a white, cheesy, curdlike patch on the buccal mucosa due to superficial fungal infection
Caries: decay in the teeth
Cheilitis: red, scaling, shallow, painful fissures at the corners of the mouth
Choanal atresia: closure of nasal cavity due to congenital septum between nasal cavity and pharynx
Crypts: indentations on the surface of the tonsils
Epistaxis: nosebleed, usually from the anterior septum
Epulis: nontender, fibrous nodule of the gum
Fordyce's granules: small, isolated, white or yellow papules on the oral mucosa
Frenulum: a midline fold of tissue connecting the tongue to the mouth floor
Gingivitis: red, swollen gum margins that bleed easily
Herpes simplex 1: clear vesicles with red base that evolve into pustules, usually at lip–skin junction
Koplik's spots: small, blue-white spots with irregular red halo scattered over mucosa opposite the molars; they are an early sign of measles
Leukoedema: a bilateral opalescent white appearance on the mucosa that is a variation of the normal anatomy due to cellular changes
Leukoplakia: a chalky-white, thick, raised patch on sides of the tongue, precancerous
Malocclusion: upper or lower dental arches out of alignment
Papillae: rough, bumpy elevations on the dorsal surface of the tongue
Parotid glands: a pair of salivary glands in the cheeks in front of the ears
Pharyngitis: inflammation of the throat
Plaque: soft whitish debris on teeth
Polyp: smooth, pale grey nodules in the nasal cavity due to chronic allergic rhinitis
Rhinitis: red, swollen inflammation of nasal mucosa
Thrush: oral candidiasis in the newborn
Turbinate: one of three bony projections into the nasal cavity
Uvula: the free projection hanging down from the middle of the soft palate

STUDY GUIDE

After completing the reading assignment, you should be able to answer the following questions in the spaces provided.

1. Name the functions of the nose.

2. Describe the size and components of the nasal cavity.

3. List the four sets of paranasal sinuses, and describe their function.

4. List the three pairs of salivary glands, including their location and the locations of their duct openings.

5. Following tooth loss in the middle-aged or older adult, describe the consequences of chewing with the remaining maloccluded teeth.

6. Describe the appearance of a deviated nasal septum and a perforated septum.

7. Describe the appearance of a torus palatinus, and explain its significance.

8. Contrast the physical appearance and clinical significance of leukoedema, candidiasis, leukoplakia, and Fordyce's granules.

9. List the four-point grading scale for the size of tonsils.

10. Describe the appearance and clinical significance of these findings in the infant: sucking tubercle, Epstein pearls, and Bednar aphthae.

11. Contrast the appearance of nasal turbinates versus nasal polyps.

12. Describe the appearance and clinical significance of these findings on the tongue: ankyloglossia, fissured tongue, geographic tongue, black hairy tongue, and macroglossia.

13. In the space below, sketch a cleft palate and a bifid uvula.

14. Describe the appearance of oral Kaposi's sarcoma.

15. Fill in the labels indicated on the following illustrations.

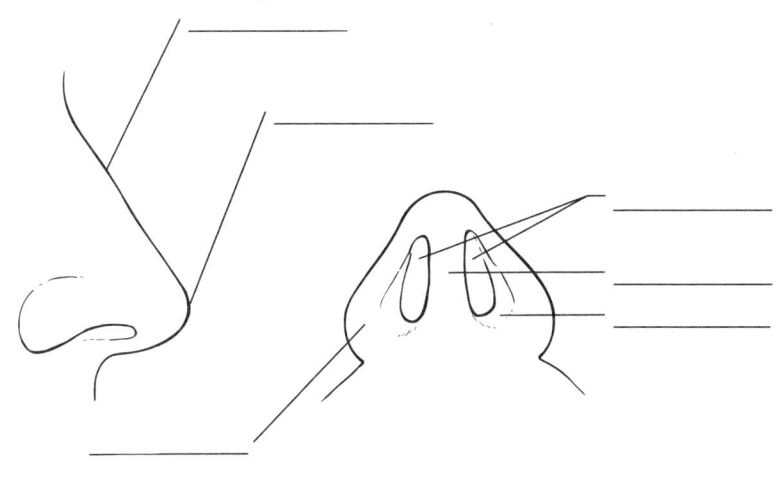

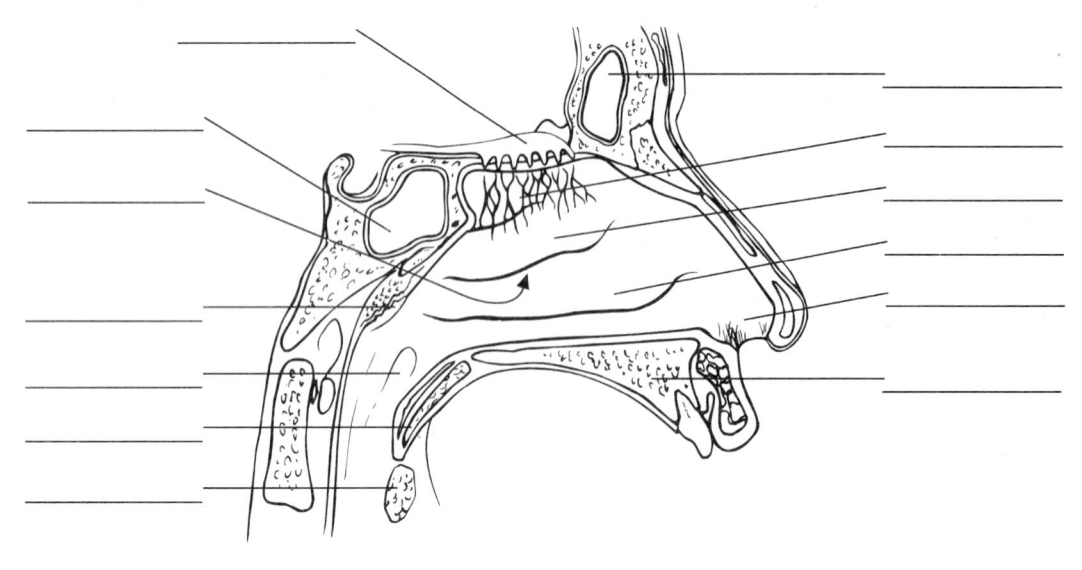

LEFT LATERAL WALL–NASAL CAVITY

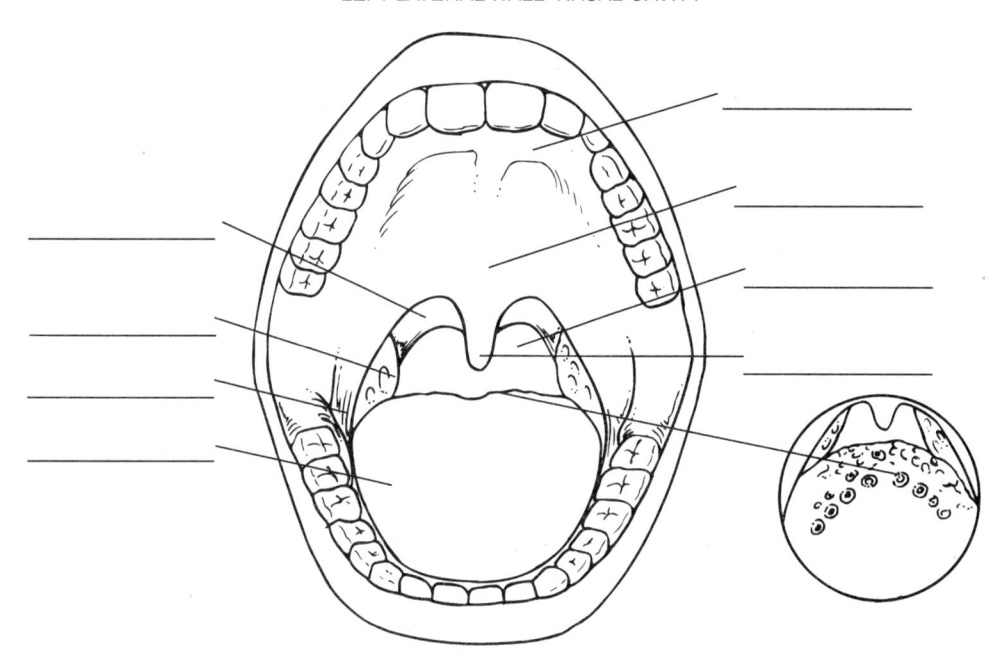

REVIEW AND CLINICAL JUDGEMENT QUESTIONS

This test is for you to check your own mastery of the content. Answers are provided on the text's Evolve site.

1. A 30-year-old man enters your emergency department with profuse bleeding from the nose. He reports no prescription medicine, no street drugs, and no chronic conditions. You proceed with your intervention, knowing that 80 to 90% of nose bleeds occur in which site?
    a. the turbinates.
    b. the columellae.
    c. Kiesselbach's plexus.
    d. the meatus.

2. The sinuses that are accessible to examination are
    a. the ethmoid and sphenoid.
    b. the frontal and ethmoid.
    c. the maxillary and sphenoid.
    d. the frontal and maxillary.

3. The *frenulum* is
   a. the midline fold of tissue that connects the tongue to the floor of the mouth.
   b. the anterior border of the oral cavity.
   c. the arching roof of the mouth.
   d. the free projection hanging down from the middle of the soft palate.

4. The largest salivary gland is located
   a. within the cheeks in front of the ear.
   b. beneath the mandible at the angle of the jaw.
   c. within the floor of the mouth under the tongue.
   d. at the base of the tongue.

5. A 70-year-old woman complains of dry mouth. The most frequent cause of this problem is
   a. the aging process.
   b. related to medications she may be taking.
   c. the use of dentures.
   d. related to a diminished sense of smell.

6. Because of the patient's history of headache, the examiner inspects the nasal cavity. The nasal mucosa in an individual with a chronic allergy would be described as
   a. swollen and bright red.
   b. swollen, boggy, pale, and grey.
   c. pale grey, swollen, and pink.
   d. red with a smooth moist surface.

7. During an inspection of a patient's nares, you observe a deviated septum. The best action is to
   a. request a consultation with an ear, nose, and throat specialist.
   b. document the deviation in the medical record in case the person needs to be suctioned.
   c. teach the person what to do if a nosebleed should occur.
   d. explore further because polyps frequently accompany a deviated septum.

8. A 45-year-old female has a 23-year history of smoking over one pack of cigarettes per day. During the oral examination, you inspect knowing that oral malignancies are most likely to develop
   a. on the soft palate.
   b. on the tongue.
   c. in the buccal cavity.
   d. under the tongue.

9. A 16-year-old has a fever and a sore throat. You grade his tonsils as 3+ because the tonsils are
   a. visible.
   b. halfway between the tonsillar pillars and uvula.
   c. touching the uvula.
   d. touching each other.

10. The function of the nasal turbinates is to
    a. warm the inhaled air.
    b. detect odours.
    c. stimulate tear formation.
    d. lighten the weight of the skull bones.

11. The opening of an adult's parotid gland (Stensen's duct) is opposite
    a. the lower second molar.
    b. the lower incisors.
    c. the upper incisors.
    d. the upper second molar.

12. A nasal polyp can be distinguished from a nasal turbinate by three of the following characteristics. Which characteristic is *false*?
    a. The polyp is highly vascular.
    b. The polyp is movable.
    c. The polyp is pale grey in colour.
    d. The polyp is nontender.

CRITICAL THINKING EXERCISE

Read the Sauve et al. article listed at the beginning of this chapter. Then consider the following scenario. A 6-year-old male patient is brought into your clinic by his dad. He has been experiencing a sore throat for the past 2 days. The patient reports a sore throat that is worse in the morning. It is relieved somewhat with acetaminophen (Tylenol). He has no cough. He believes he has a fever and has been experiencing some chills. On examination, you note that his temperature is 38.1°C (100.5°F). He has large swollen tonsils that are 3+ with purulent exudate. He has tender cervical lymphadenopathy. With this information in mind, consult the RxFiles resource listed at the beginning of this chapter. What is his modified Centor score? Does he require a rapid antigen detecting test or a throat culture? Would you recommend that he receive antibiotics today?

SKILLS LABORATORY/CLINICAL SETTING

You are now ready for the clinical component of the nose, mouth, and throat examination. The purpose of the clinical component is to practise the steps of the examination on a peer in the skills laboratory or on a patient in the clinical setting and to achieve the following.

Clinical Objectives

1. Inspect the external nose.
2. Demonstrate use of the otoscope and nasal attachment to inspect the structures of the nasal cavity.
3. Demonstrate knowledge of infection control practices during inspection and palpation of structures of the mouth and pharynx.
4. Record the history and physical examination findings accurately, reach an assessment of the health state, and develop a plan of care.

Instructions

Prepare the examination setting and gather your equipment. Wash your hands. Practise the steps of the examination on a peer in the skills laboratory, giving appropriate instructions as you proceed. Record your findings using the documentation sheet that follows. The front of the page is intended as a worksheet; the back of the page is intended for your narrative summary recording using the subjective, objective, assessment, plan (SOAP) format.

NOTES

DOCUMENTATION—NOSE, MOUTH, AND THROAT

Date _____

Examiner _____

Patient _____ Age _____ Gender _____

Occupation _____

I. Health History

	No	Yes, explain

A. Nose

1. Any nasal **discharge**?
2. Unusually frequent or severe colds?
3. Any **sinus pain** or sinusitis?
4. Any **trauma** or injury to nose?
5. Any **nosebleeds**? How often?
6. Any **allergies** or hay fever?
7. Any change in sense of smell?

B. Mouth and throat

1. Any **sores** in mouth, tongue?
2. Any **sore throat**? How often?
3. Any **bleeding gums**?
4. Any **toothache**?
5. Any **hoarseness**, voice change?
6. Any difficulty **swallowing**?
7. Any change in sense of taste?
8. Do you smoke? How much each day?
9. Tell me about usual dental care.

II. Physical Examination

A. Inspect and palpate the nose.

Symmetry _____

Deformity, asymmetry, inflammation _____

Test patency of each nostril _____

Using a nasal speculum, note:

  Colour of nasal mucosa _____

  Discharge, foreign body _____

  Septum: deviation, perforation, bleeding _____

  Turbinates: colour, swelling, exudates, polyps _____

B. Palpate the sinus area.

Frontal _____

Maxillary _____

C. Inspect the mouth.

Lips _____

Teeth and gums _____

Buccal mucosa _____

Palate and uvula _____

Tonsils (grade) _____

Tongue _____

D. Inspect the throat.

Tonsils: condition and grade _____

Pharyngeal wall _____

Any breath odour _____

DOCUMENTATION—NOSE, MOUTH, AND THROAT

Summarize your findings using the SOAP format.

Subjective (Reason for seeking care, health history)

Objective (Physical examination findings)

Record your findings on the diagram.

Assessment (Assessment of health state or problem, diagnosis)

Plan (Diagnostic evaluation, follow-up care, patient teaching)

18 Breasts and Regional Lymphatic System

PURPOSE

This chapter reviews the structure and function of the breast and regional lymphatic system; the rationale for and methods of breast examination; and the accurate recording of the assessment. It also discusses how to determine, according to current evidence-informed guidelines, when it is appropriate to conduct a clinical breast examination and when it is appropriate to teach people to do breast self-examination (BSE).

READING ASSIGNMENT

Jarvis: *Physical Examination and Health Assessment*, 4th Canadian ed., Chapter 18.

Suggested readings

Canadian Task Force on Preventive Health Care. (2020). *Breast cancer update—1000 person tool.* https://canadiantaskforce.ca/tools-resources/breast-cancer-update/1000-person-tool/

Freudenheim, J. L. (2020). Alcohol's effects on breast cancer in women. *Alcohol Research: Current Reviews, 40*(2), 1–12. https://doi.org/10.35946/arcr.v40.2.11

Klarenbach, S., Sims-Jones, N., Lewin, G., et al. (2018). Recommendations on screening for breast cancer in women aged 40–74 years who are not at increased risk for breast cancer. *Canadian Medical Association Journal, 190*(49), E1441–E1451. https://doi.org/10.1503/cmaj.180463

GLOSSARY

Study the following terms after reading the corresponding chapter in the text.

Alveoli: the smallest structures of the mammary gland; they produce milk

Areola: darkened area surrounding the nipple

Colostrum: a thick, yellow fluid that is the precursor of milk; it is secreted during later stages of pregnancy and for a few days after delivery

Cooper's ligaments: suspensory ligaments; they are fibrous bands that extend from the inner breast surface to the chest wall muscles

Fibroadenoma: benign breast mass

Galactorrhea: milky-white breast discharge in a woman who is not pregnant and not breastfeeding; may also occur in men

Gynecomastia: excessive breast development in the male

Inframammary ridge: a firm, transverse ridge of compressed tissue in the lower quadrants of the breast, especially noticeable when palpating large breasts

Intraductal papilloma: a small, usually benign lesion that grows in the lactiferous ducts, associated with serous or serosanguineous nipple discharge

Inverted: nipples that are depressed or invaginated

Lactiferous: conveying milk

Mastalgia: breast pain; it may be cyclical (i.e., occurring with the menstrual cycle) or noncyclical

Mastitis: inflammation of the breast; often associated with breastfeeding

Menarche: the onset of menstruation; it usually occurs during stage 3 or 4 of breast development

Montgomery's glands: small, elevated sebaceous glands in the areola that secrete protective lipid during lactation; also called *tubercles of Montgomery*

Paget's disease: intraductal carcinoma in the breast

Peau d'orange: orange-peel appearance of breast due to edema; it is produced by lymphatic obstruction

Retraction: dimpling or puckering on the skin; it usually results from fibrosis in the breast tissue and may be related to a growing neoplasm

Striae: atrophic pink, purple, or white linear streaks on the breasts; they are associated with pregnancy, excessive weight gain, or rapid growth during adolescence

Supernumerary nipple: a minute extra nipple along the embryonic milk line

Tail of Spence: superior lateral corner of breast tissue that extends into the axilla

Tanner staging: classic system for describing and rating sexual maturity

Thelarche: the beginning of breast development; it usually precedes menarche by about 2 years

STUDY GUIDE

After completing the reading assignment, you should be able to answer the following questions in the spaces provided.

1. Identify appropriate history questions to ask regarding the breast examination.

2. Describe the anatomy of the breast.

3. Correlate changes in the female breast with normal developmental stages.

4. Describe the components of the breast examination.

5. List points to include when advising patients about breast self-examination (BSE).

6. Explain the significance of a supernumerary nipple.

7. Differentiate between the female, male, and transgendered person's breast examination procedure and findings.

8. Discuss the following pathological changes that may occur in the breast:

    Benign breast disease

Abscess

Acute mastitis

Fibroadenoma

Cancer

Paget's disease

9. List and describe the characteristics to consider when a mass is noted in the breast.

10. Define *gynecomastia*.

11. Describe the Canadian Task Force on Preventive Health Care (2020) breast screening recommendations for routine mammography, BSE, and clinical breast examination for diagnosis of breast lesions.

12. List the modifiable and unmodifiable factors that increase the usual risk for breast cancer.

13. Fill in the labels on the following diagrams.

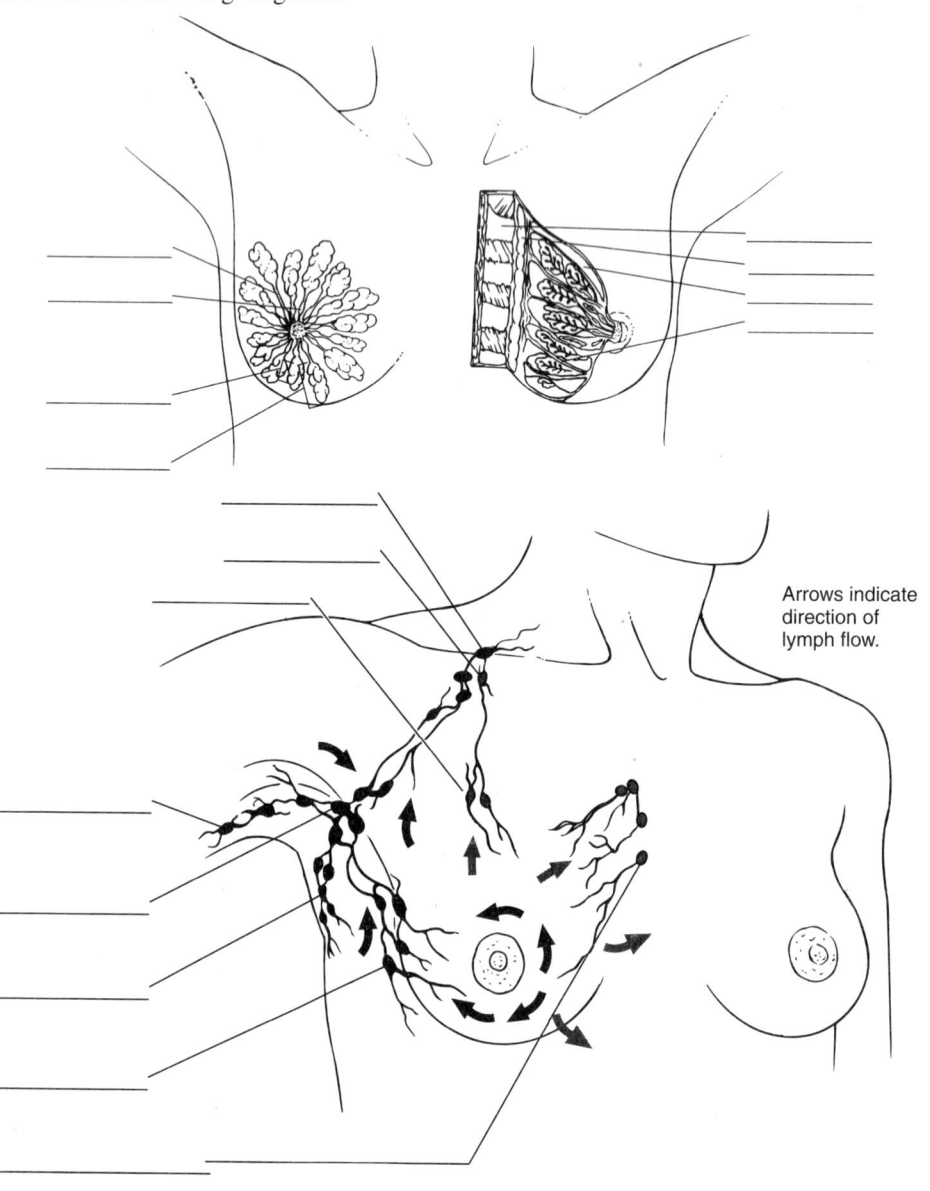

Arrows indicate direction of lymph flow.

REVIEW AND CLINICAL JUDGEMENT QUESTIONS

This test is for you to check your own mastery of the content. Answers are provided on the text's Evolve site.

1. You are presenting the internal anatomy of the breast to a community health care clinic. Which of the following are accurate points to include? (Select all that apply.)
   a. The bulk of the breast is mainly pectoralis muscle tissue.
   b. The fibrous connective tissue extends from inside the breast skin surface toward the chest wall muscles.
   c. The breast tissue slopes upward into the axilla.
   d. Most lymphatic drainage of the breast flows inward to deeper chest lymph ducts.

2. You are performing a clinical breast examination on a 52-year-old female who is concerned about a lump in her right breast. While performing the examination, you reflect that the most common site of breast tumours is
   a. the upper inner quadrant.
   b. the upper outer quadrant.
   c. the lower inner quadrant.
   d. the lower outer quadrant.

3. A 13-year-old female presents to your clinic for a HEADSS assessment. She asks you why her breasts "don't match" in size. What is your best response?
   a. "One breast temporarily may grow faster than the other during development."
   b. "In these cases, I usually ask another examiner to come in and double-check."
   c. "It's a sign you will have small cystic lumps on one side; these are common."
   d. "This may show a temporary hormonal imbalance. We will check again in 6 months."

4. When teaching BSE, you would inform patients that
   a. all patients at risk for breast cancer should perform BSE routinely.
   b. there are no risks associated with doing BSE.
   c. the decision to do BSE is not routinely recommended and is an individual decision, based on personal risk factors and patient preference.
   d. BSE is the best way to assess a patient's risk for breast cancer.

5. You are providing health promotion for a 56-year-old female at your clinic. According to the Canadian Task Force on Preventive Health Care (2020), what is the current recommendation for breast cancer screening mammography for your patient?
   a. every year for patients aged 50 to 69 years.
   b. every 2 to 3 years for patients aged 50 to 69 years.
   c. twice a year for all patients.
   d. only the baseline examination is needed unless the patient has symptoms.

6. You are inspecting an adult woman's breasts for retraction signs. Her best position is
   a. lying supine with arms at the sides.
   b. leaning forward with hands outstretched.
   c. sitting with hands pushing onto hips.
   d. lying supine with one arm elevated over her head.

7. You are teaching a learner how to perform a clinical breast examination. The preferred palpation technique for the clinical breast examination is
   a. spokes-on-a-wheel pattern.
   b. concentric circles pattern.
   c. vertical strip pattern.
   d. bimanual technique.

8. During the examination of a 70-year-old man, you note gynecomastia. You next best action is to
   a. refer for a biopsy.
   b. refer for a mammogram.
   c. review his medications for agents that have gynecomastia as a side effect.
   d. proceed with the examination. This is a normal part of the aging process.

9. A 57-year-old female presents to your clinic for a health checkup, having deferred any health care visits for 1.5 years. During a breast examination, you palpate a 2-cm firm mass with irregular edges. What is your next best action?
   a. Request a breast biopsy.
   b. Request a mammogram.
   c. Review her medication list for drugs that cause breast lumps.
   d. Proceed with the examination; this is a common finding in a menopausal woman.

10. You are teaching a 34-year-old patient who is 2 months pregnant what common breast changes to expect. What would you include? (Select all that apply.)
    a. The areolae become darker brown.
    b. Nipples may retract.
    c. The ability to express breast milk can be expected after 2 months.
    d. A blue vascular pattern may appear over both breasts.

11. You have examined the following female patients during your shift. Which one(s) should you refer for further evaluation? (Select all that apply.)
    a. a 28-year-old with multiple distinct nodules palpated in each breast
    b. a 48-year-old who has a 6-month history of a reddened and sore left nipple and areolar area
    c. a 22-year-old with asymmetric breasts and inversion of nipples since adolescence
    d. a 64-year-old with an ulcerated area at the tip of the right nipple; no masses, tenderness, or enlarged lymph nodes present

12. You are examining a 10-year-old female who has been brought in by her mom for concerns about scoliosis and a general health check. Which is the first physical change associated with puberty in girls? (Select all that apply.)
    a. Breasts enlarge and areolae enlarge over breasts.
    b. A small mound of breast tissue develops under the nipple.
    c. A height spurt occurs.
    d. Pubic hair develops.

13. During the examination of a 30-year-old patient with preferred pronouns "they" and "them," they ask about "the large mole" below their left breast/chest. After inspecting a 1-cm circular brown area with a central bump, what is your best response?
    a. "I think you should be examined by a dermatologist."
    b. "This is a common finding of an extra, undeveloped nipple."
    c. "These are Montgomery glands, which are common."
    d. "This is a common finding occurring with Paget's disease of the breast."

14. You visit the home of a 35-year-old mother with her first baby. She is 4 days postpartum. She has a tender thickening in one breast with the overlying skin reddened and tender. She has fatigue but no fever. What teaching would you give? (Select all that apply.)
    a. "Nurse the baby on the affected side first at each nursing."
    b. "Nurse the baby frequently to keep the breast as empty as possible."
    c. "This condition is common when you and the baby are both learning to nurse."
    d. "I will request an antibiotic for you that will not harm the baby."

15. A 12-year-old male patient presents to your clinic with his caregiver due to concerns regarding recent unilateral breast enlargement. Your best response is as follows:
    a. "This requires regular monitoring every 6 weeks."
    b. "This is normal, common, and temporary, and will eventually go away as you continue to grow."
    c. "This could be an early sign of male breast cancer."
    d. "This is a normal condition that will persist into early adulthood."

CRITICAL THINKING EXERCISE

A.G. is a healthy 39-year-old female who is attending your primary care clinic for her annual flu shot. While discussing health promotion with her, she tells you that she is very concerned about breast cancer as one of her friends was recently diagnosed with it. She has never been diagnosed with breast cancer herself and has no family members who have been diagnosed with it. She has started doing a BSE monthly, while showering. However, she feels guilty about forgetting to do it routinely.

- Review the Canadian Task Force on Preventive Health Care resource listed at the beginning of this chapter. What information would you give A.G. about breast cancer screening?
- Are BSEs indicated for A.G. currently?
- When should A.G. receive her first mammogram?
- Why is family history important when determining breast cancer risk?

SKILLS LABORATORY/CLINICAL SETTING

You are now ready for the clinical component of the breast assessment. The purpose of the clinical component is to practise the steps of the assessment on a peer in the skills laboratory and to achieve the following.

Clinical Objectives

1. Demonstrate knowledge of the symptoms related to the breasts and axillae by obtaining a health history.
2. Perform inspection and palpation of the breasts, with the patient in sitting and supine positions, using proper technique and providing appropriate draping.
3. List the points to include in advising a patient about BSE.
4. Record the history and physical examination findings accurately, reach an assessment of the health state, and develop a plan of care.

Instructions

Practise the steps of the breast examination on your school's breast simulation equipment, or under the supervision and with the guidance of your instructor, in the clinical area. It is not appropriate to practice this sensitive exam with your peer. Record your findings on the documentation sheet that follows. The front of the page is intended as a worksheet; the back of the page is intended for your narrative summary recording using the subjective, objective, assessment, plan (SOAP) format.

Note the student competency checklist that follows the documentation sheet. It lists the essential behaviours you should display as an examiner, and it may be used by your clinical instructor to evaluate your clinical performance of clinical breast examination.

NOTES

NOTES

DOCUMENTATION—BREASTS AND AXILLAE

Date _____

Examiner _____

Patient _____ Age _____ Gender _____

Occupation _____

I. Health History

	No	Yes, explain
1. Any **pain** or tenderness in breasts?	_____	_____
2. Any **lump** or thickening in breasts?	_____	_____
3. Any **discharge** from nipples?	_____	_____
4. Any **rash** on breasts?	_____	_____
5. Any **swelling** in breasts?	_____	_____
6. Any **traum**a or injury to breasts?	_____	_____
7. Any **history** of breast disease?	_____	_____
8. Ever had **surgery** on breasts?	_____	_____
9. Ever been taught BSE?	_____	_____
10. Ever had mammography?	_____	_____

II. Physical Examination
  A. Inspection
    1. Breasts _____

      Symmetry _____

      Skin colour and condition _____

      Texture _____

      Lesions _____

    2. Areolae and nipples

      Shape _____

      Direction _____

      Surface characteristics _____

      Discharge _____

    3. Response to arm movement _____

    4. Axillae _____

  B. Palpation
    1. Breasts

      Texture _____

      Masses _____

      Tenderness _____

2. Areolae and nipples

   Masses _____

   Discharge _____

3. Axillae and lymph nodes

   Size _____

   Shape _____

   Consistency _____

   Mobility _____

   Discrete or matted _____

   Tenderness _____

C. **Discuss the risks and benefits of BSE, and teach BSE if requested.**

DOCUMENTATION—BREASTS AND AXILLAE

Summarize your findings using the SOAP format.

Subjective (Reason for seeking care, health history)

Objective (Physical examination findings)

Record your findings on the diagram.

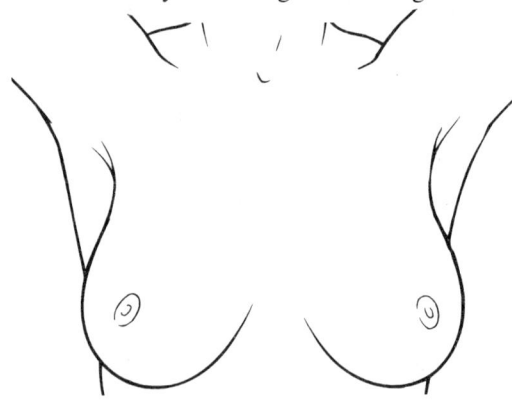

Assessment (Assessment of health state or problem, diagnosis)

Plan (Diagnostic evaluation, follow-up care, patient teaching)

STUDENT COMPETENCY CHECKLIST

Counselling and Teaching Women about Breast Self-Examination (BSE)

	S	U	Comments
I. Cognitive			
A. Explain:			
a) Who should do BSE, according to the Canadian Task Force on Preventive Health Care (2020) recommendations.			
b) Why breasts are examined.			
(1) In the shower.			
(2) Before a mirror.			
(3) Supine with pillow under side of breast being examined.			
c) Frequency of breast examination.			
B. State the area of breast where most lumps are found.			
C. Give two reasons a person may not report significant findings to a health care provider.			
II. Performance			
A. Explain to woman the risks and benefits of BSE.			
B. Instruct woman on technique of BSE by:			
a) Inspecting and bilaterally comparing breasts in front of mirror.			
b) Noting new or unusual rash or redness on skin and areola.			
c) Palpating breast in a systemic manner, using pads of three fingers and with woman's arm raised overhead.			
d) Palpating tail of Spence and axilla.			
e) Gently compressing nipples.			
C. Instruct woman to report unusual findings to a health care provider at once.			
D. Ask woman to do return demonstration.			

NOTES

NOTES

19 Thorax and Lungs

PURPOSE

This chapter reviews the structure and function of the thorax and lungs; the methods of examination of the respiratory system; normal lung sounds; the characteristics of adventitious lung sounds; and the accurate recording of the assessment. At the end of this chapter, you will be able to perform a complete physical examination of the respiratory system.

READING ASSIGNMENT

Jarvis: *Physical Examination and Health Assessment*, 4th Canadian ed., Chapter 19.

Suggested Readings

CASCADES. (2022). *Environmentally sustainable opportunities for health systems metered dose inhalers (MDIs)*. https://cascadescanada.ca/wp-content/uploads/2022/07/June-2022-Inhalers-Infographic-Updated.pdf

Cook, L. K., & Wulf, J. A. (2020). Community-acquired pneumonia: A review of current diagnostic criteria and management. *American Journal of Nursing, 120*(12), 34–42.

GLOSSARY

Study the following terms after reading the corresponding chapter in the text.

Alveoli: functional units of the lung; the thin-walled chambers surrounded by networks of capillaries that are the site of respiratory exchange of carbon dioxide and oxygen

Angle of Louis: manubriosternal angle; the articulation of the manubrium and body of the sternum; it is continuous with the second rib

Apnea: cessation of breathing

Asthma: an abnormal respiratory condition associated with allergic hypersensitivity to certain inhaled allergens, characterized by bronchospasm, wheezing, and dyspnea

Atelectasis: an abnormal respiratory condition characterized by collapsed, shrunken, deflated section of alveoli

Bradypnea: slow breathing, fewer than 10 breaths/min, regular rate

Bronchiole: one of the smaller respiratory passageways into which the segmental bronchi divide

Bronchitis: inflammation of the bronchi with partial obstruction of bronchi due to excessive mucus secretion

Bronchophony: the spoken voice sound heard through the stethoscope, which sounds soft, muffled, and indistinct over normal lung tissue

Bronchovesicular: the normal breath sound heard over major bronchi, characterized by moderate pitch and an equal duration of inspiration and expiration

Chronic obstructive pulmonary disease (COPD): a functional category of abnormal respiratory conditions characterized by airflow obstruction; for example, emphysema and chronic bronchitis

Cilia: millions of hairlike cells lining the tracheobronchial tree

Consolidation: the solidification of portions of lung tissue as it fills up with infectious exudate, as in pneumonia

Crackles: rales; abnormal, discontinuous, adventitious lung sounds heard on inspiration

Crepitus: a coarse, crackling sensation palpable over the skin when air abnormally escapes from the lung and enters the subcutaneous tissue

Dead space: passageways that transport air but are not available for gaseous exchange; for example, trachea and bronchi

Dyspnea: difficult, laboured breathing

Egophony: the voice sound of "eeeeee" heard through the stethoscope

Emphysema: the COPD characterized by enlargement of alveoli distal to terminal bronchioles

Fissure: the narrow crack dividing the lobes of the lungs

Fremitus: a palpable vibration from the spoken voice felt over the chest wall

Friction rub: a coarse, grating, adventitious lung sound heard when the pleurae are inflamed

Hypercapnia: hypercarbia; an increased level of carbon dioxide in the blood

Hyperventilation: an increased rate and depth of breathing

Hypoxemia: a decreased level of oxygen in the blood

Intercostal space: space between the ribs

Kussmaul's respirations: a type of hyperventilation that occurs with diabetic ketoacidosis
Orthopnea: the ability to breathe easily only in an upright position
Paroxysmal nocturnal dyspnea: a sudden awakening from sleeping with shortness of breath
Percussion: striking over the chest wall with short sharp blows of the fingers in order to determine the size and density of the underlying organ
Pleural effusion: abnormal fluid between the layers of the pleura
Rhonchi: low-pitched, musical, snoring, adventitious lung sounds caused by airflow obstruction from secretions
Tachypnea: rapid, shallow breathing, more than 24 breaths/min
Vesicular: the soft, low-pitched, normal breath sounds heard over peripheral lung fields
Vital capacity: the amount of air, following maximal inspiration, that can be exhaled
Wheeze: a high-pitched, musical, squeaking, adventitious lung sound
Whispered pectoriloquy: a whispered phrase heard through the stethoscope that sounds faint and inaudible over normal lung tissue
Xiphoid process: the sword-shaped lower tip of the sternum

STUDY GUIDE

After completing the reading assignment, you should be able to answer the following questions in the spaces provided.

1. Describe the pertinent health history information for the respiratory system.

2. Describe the pleura and its function.

3. List the structures that compose the respiratory dead space.

4. Summarize the mechanics of respiration.

5. List the elements included in the inspection of the respiratory system.

6. Discuss the significance of a "barrel chest."

7. List and describe common thoracic deformities.

8. List and describe three types of normal breath sounds.

9. Define two types of adventitious breath sounds.

10. The manubriosternal angle is also called the _____.
    Why is it a useful landmark?

11. How many degrees is the normal costal angle?

12. When comparing the anteroposterior diameter of the chest to the transverse diameter, what is the expected ratio?

    What is the significance of this?

13. What is the tripod position?

14. List three factors that affect the normal intensity of tactile fremitus.

    a.

    b.

    c.

15. During percussion, which sound would you expect to predominate over normal lung tissue?

16. Normal findings for symmetrical chest expansion are

17. List five factors that can cause extraneous noise during auscultation.

    a.

    b.

    c.

    d.

    e.

18. Describe the three types of normal breath sounds:

Name	Location	Description

19. Fill in the labels indicated on the following illustrations.

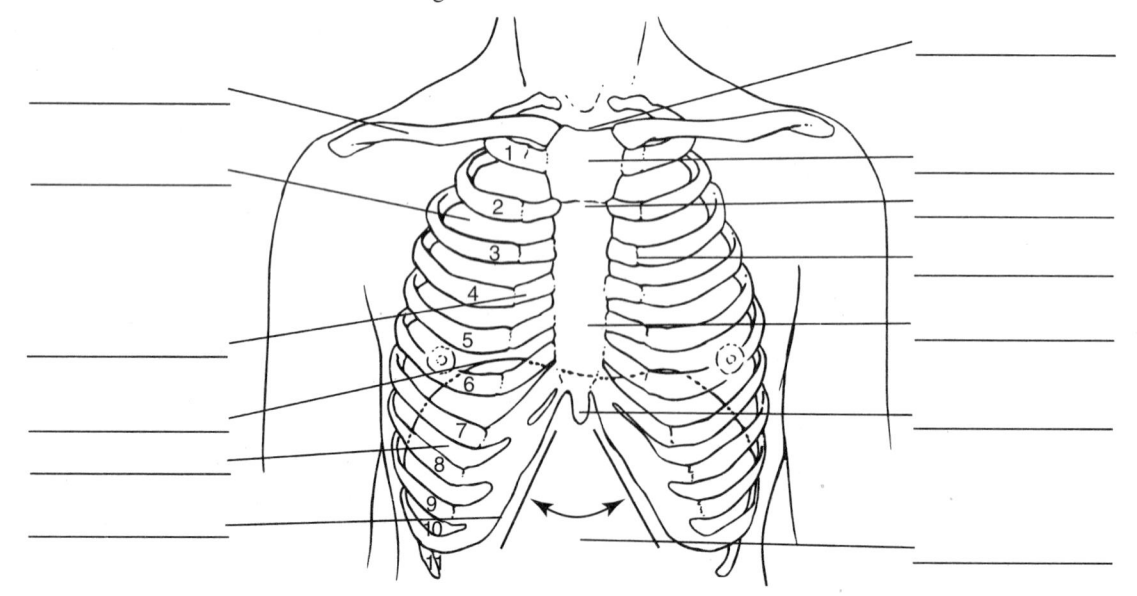

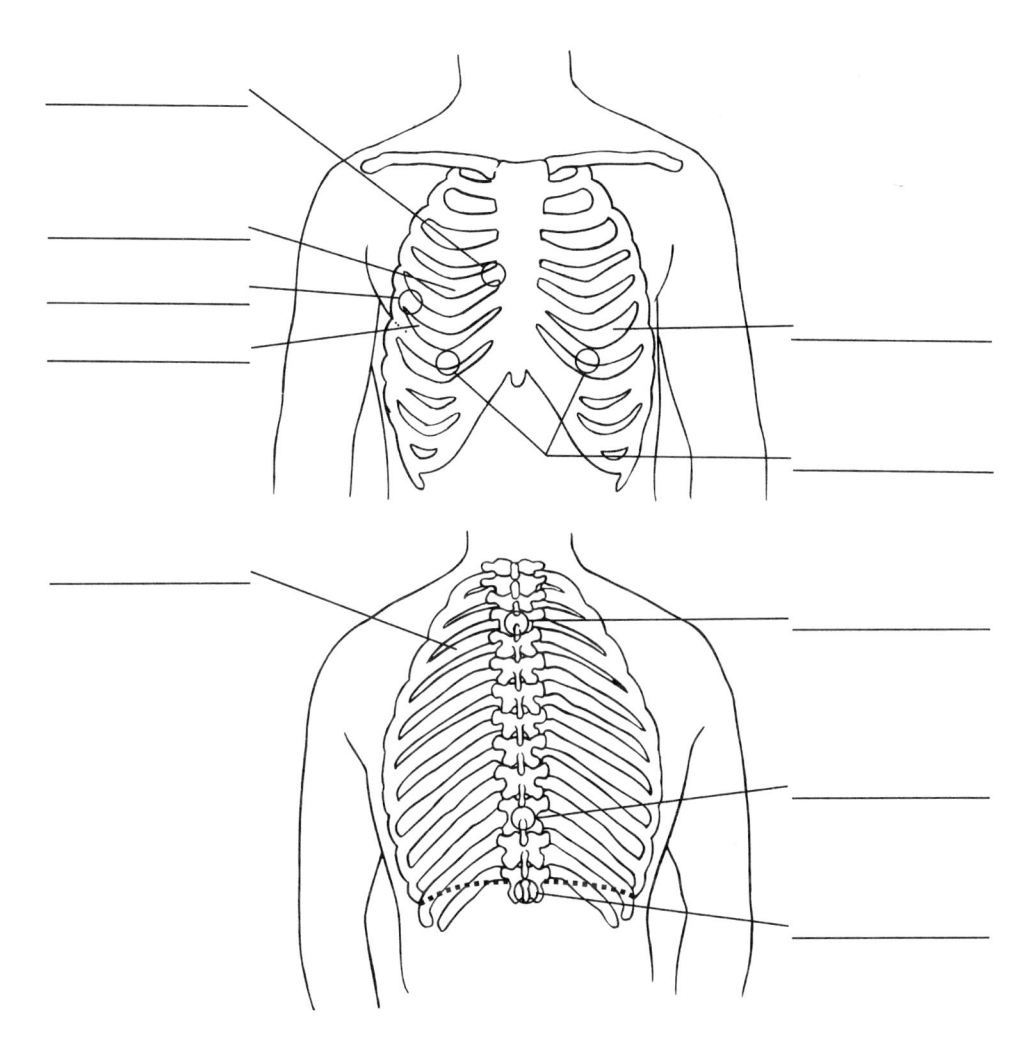

REVIEW AND CLINICAL JUDGEMENT QUESTIONS

This test is for you to check your own mastery of the content. Answers are provided on the text's Evolve site.

1. You are examining a hospitalized woman who is on bed rest and has difficulty turning. Which is your best approach to complete the inspection, palpation, and auscultation of the thorax?
   a. Inspect, palpate, and auscultate the anterior and lateral thorax only, omitting the posterior thorax to optimize patient comfort.
   b. Find an assistant to help you turn the woman side to side, and perform the complete assessment while comparing bilaterally as much as possible.
   c. Have the woman turn as best as she can, omitting assessment of areas of the thorax that are not accessible.
   d. Omit inspection of the posterior thorax, and push down the mattress to move your hand and stethoscope endpiece under the woman while palpating and auscultating.

2. You are taking a health history on a 44-year-old man who reports use of cigarettes. You calculate a 24-year history of smoking 1.5 packs per day and learn that he has never attempted to quit before. What is your best statement to facilitate a discussion of quitting smoking?
   a. "Smoking is deadly; you really need to stop as soon as possible."
   b. "Do you have any family members who have died because of smoking-related illnesses?"
   c. "Here is a list of resources for when you are ready to quit smoking."
   d. "Are you interested in exploring options to help you quit smoking?"

3. Select the correct description of the left lung.
   a. narrower than the right lung with three lobes
   b. narrower than the right with two lobes
   c. wider than the right lung with two lobes
   d. shorter than the right with three lobes

4. You are seeing a 71-year-old patient who describes a cough with characteristic timing that you suspect may be due to chronic bronchitis. The cough associated with chronic bronchitis is best described as
    a. continuous throughout the day.
    b. a productive cough for at least 3 months of the year for 2 years in a row.
    c. occurring in the afternoon or evening because of exposure to irritants at work.
    d. occurring in the early morning.

5. Symmetrical chest expansion is best confirmed by
    a. placing the hands on the posterolateral chest wall with thumbs at the level of T9 or T10.
    b. inspection of the shape and configuration of the chest wall.
    c. placing the palmar surface of the fingers of one hand against the chest and having the person repeat the words "ninety-nine."
    d. percussion of the posterior chest.

6. A 19-year-old man is noted to have a left-sided pneumothorax. Which assessment findings are expected? (Select all that apply.)
    a. dullness to percussion on the left side
    b. decreased breath sounds on the left side
    c. decreased tactile fremitus on the left side
    d. lag in expansion on the left side

7. You are auscultating breath sounds on a 70-year-old man who states he feels dizzy. Which is your next best action?
    a. Quickly move through the remaining auscultatory points.
    b. Stop the examination and record that the patient could not tolerate auscultation portion.
    c. Ask the patient to hold his breath for 10 seconds, then continue with auscultation.
    d. Allow the patient to take a break, then resume auscultation while monitoring for any worsening dizziness.

8. Select the best description of bronchovesicular breath sounds.
    a. high-pitched, of longer duration on inspiration than expiration
    b. moderate pitch, inspiration equal to expiration
    c. low-pitched, inspiration greater than expiration
    d. rustling sound, like the wind in the trees

9. After examining a patient, you make the following notation: Increased respiratory rate, chest expansion decreased on left side, dull to percussion over left lower lobe, breath sounds louder with fine crackles over left lower lobe. These findings are consistent with a diagnosis of
    a. bronchitis.
    b. asthma.
    c. pleural effusion.
    d. lobar pneumonia.

10. Upon examining a patient's anterior chest, you note cutaneous angiomas on the upper chest wall. These findings are consistent with
    a. adult respiratory distress syndrome.
    b. tuberculosis.
    c. chronic, congenital heart disease, and COPD.
    d. liver disease or portal hypertension.

11. Upon examination of a patient, you note a coarse, low-pitched sound during both inspiration and expiration on auscultation. This patient reports pain with breathing. These findings are consistent with
    a. fine crackles.
    b. wheezes.
    c. atelectatic crackles.
    d. pleural friction rub.

12. You are examining a patient with decreased air entry to their right middle lobe and right lower lobe. You decide to perform an egophony. In order to use the technique of egophony, ask the patient to
    a. take several deep breaths, then hold for 5 seconds.
    b. say "eeeeee" each time the stethoscope is moved.
    c. repeat the phrase "ninety-nine" each time the stethoscope is moved.
    d. whisper a phrase as auscultation is performed.

13. You are working at triage in an emergency department. A patient presents with shortness of breath. As you are gathering their vital signs, you note the pulse oximeter reads 92%. The pulse oximeter measures
    a. arterial oxygen saturation.
    b. venous oxygen saturation.
    c. combined saturation of arterial and venous blood.
    d. carboxyhemoglobin levels.

Match column A to column B.

Column A—Lung Borders

14. _____ Apex
15. _____ Base
16. _____ Lateral left
17. _____ Lateral right
18. _____ Posterior apex

Column B—Location

a. Rests on the diaphragm
b. C7
c. Sixth rib, midclavicular line
d. Fifth intercostal
e. 3 to 4 cm above the inner third of the clavicles

Match column A to column B.

Column A—Configurations of the Thorax

19. _____ Normal chest
20. _____ Barrel chest
21. _____ Pectus excavatum
22. _____ Pectus carinatum
23. _____ Scoliosis
24. _____ Kyphosis

Column B—Description

a. Anteroposterior diameter equal to transverse diameter
b. Exaggerated posterior curvature of thoracic spine
c. Lateral, S-shaped curvature of the thoracic and lumbar spine
d. Sunken sternum and adjacent cartilages
e. Elliptical shape with an anteroposterior to transverse diameter in the ratio of 1:2
f. Forward protrusion of the sternum with ribs sloping back at either side

CRITICAL THINKING EXERCISE

Climate change affects Canadians daily. Unfortunately, the health care system contributes to climate change by producing a large quantity of greenhouse gas emissions. Metered dose inhalers (MDIs), used in the treatment of asthma and COPD, contribute significantly to these emissions. Review the CASCADES resource on MDIs listed at the beginning of this chapter. As a health care provider, how can you help create a sustainable health care system?

SKILLS LABORATORY/CLINICAL SETTING

You are now ready for the clinical component of the respiratory system. The purpose of the clinical component is to practise the examination on a peer in the skills laboratory or on a patient in the clinical setting and to achieve the following.

Clinical Objectives

1. Demonstrate knowledge of the symptoms related to the respiratory system by obtaining a health history from a peer.
2. Correctly locate anatomical landmarks on the thorax of a peer.
3. Using a grease pencil, and with the peer's permission, draw lobes of the lungs on a peer's thorax.
4. Demonstrate correct techniques for inspection, palpation, percussion, and auscultation of the respiratory system.
5. Record the history and physical examination findings accurately, reach an assessment of the health state, and develop a plan of care.

Instructions

Gather your equipment. Wash your hands. Clean the stethoscope endpiece with an alcohol wipe. Practise the steps of the examination of the thorax and lungs on a peer or on a patient in the clinical area. Record your findings using the documentation sheet that follows. The front of the page is intended as a worksheet; the back of the page is intended for your narrative summary using the subjective, objective, assessment, plan (SOAP) format.

NOTES

DOCUMENTATION—THORAX AND LUNGS

Date _____

Examiner _____

Patient _____ Age _____ Gender _____

Occupation _____

I. Health History

	No	Yes, explain
1. Do you have a **cough**?	_____	_____
2. Any shortness of **breath**?	_____	_____
3. Any **chest pain** with breathing?	_____	_____
4. Any **past history** of lung disease?	_____	_____
5. Ever **smoke** cigarettes? Vape? How many/much each day?	_____	_____
6. Any living or work conditions that affect your breathing?	_____	_____
7. Last tuberculin skin test, chest X-ray, examination, flu vaccine, COVID-19 vaccine?	_____	_____

II. Physical Examination

A. Inspection

1. Thoracic cage _____

2. Respiratory rate and pattern _____

3. Skin _____

4. Person's position _____

5. Person's facial expression _____

6. Level of consciousness _____

B. Palpation

1. Confirm symmetrical chest expansion _____

2. Tactile fremitus _____

3. Detect any lumps, masses, tenderness _____

4. Trachea _____

C. Percussion

1. Determine percussion note that predominates over lung fields _____

2. Symmetrical chest expansion _____

D. Auscultation
1. Listen: posterior

   a. Any abnormal breath sounds? _____

   b. Any adventitious breath sounds? _____

2. Listen: lateral

   a. Any abnormal breath sounds? _____

   b. Any adventitious breath sounds? _____

3. Listen: anterior

   a. Any abnormal breath sounds? _____

   b. Any adventitious breath sounds? _____

DOCUMENTATION—THORAX AND LUNGS

Summarize your findings using the SOAP format.

Subjective (Reason for seeking care, health history)

Objective (Physical examination findings)

Record your findings on the diagram.

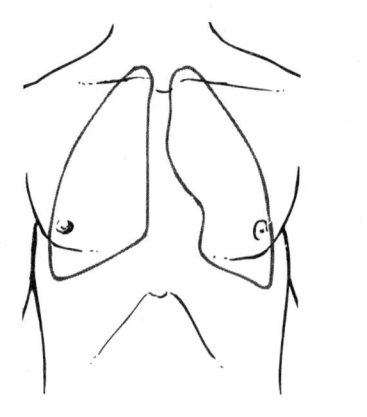

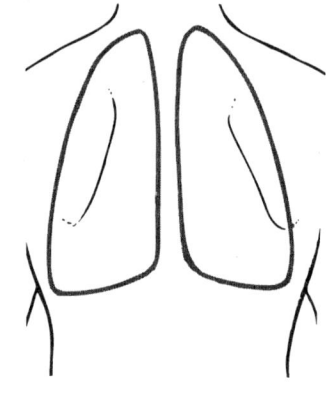

Assessment (Assessment of health state or problem, diagnosis)

Plan (Diagnostic evaluation, follow-up care, patient teaching)

20 Heart and Neck Vessels

PURPOSE

This chapter reviews the structure and function of the heart, valves, and great vessels; the cardiac cycle; heart sounds; the rationale for and methods of examination of the heart; and the accurate recording of the assessment. At the end of this chapter, you will be able to perform a complete assessment of the heart and neck vessels.

READING ASSIGNMENT

Jarvis: *Physical Examination and Health Assessment*, 4th Canadian ed., Chapter 20.

Suggested Readings

Leung, A. A., Bell, A., Tsuyuki, R. T., et al. (2021). Refocusing on hypertension control in Canada. *Canadian Medical Association Journal, 193*(23), E854–E855. https://doi.org/10.1503/cmaj.210140

McCormack, J., & Pfiffner, P. (2017). *The absolute CVD risk/benefit calculator.* https://cvdcalculator.com

GLOSSARY

Study the following terms after reading the corresponding chapter in the text.

Afterload: the opposing pressure that the ventricle must generate to open the aortic valve against the higher aortic pressure

Angina pectoris: acute chest pain that occurs when myocardial demand exceeds its oxygen supply

Aortic regurgitation: aortic insufficiency; incompetent aortic valve that allows backward flow of blood into the left ventricle during diastole

Aortic stenosis: calcification of aortic valve cusps that restricts forward flow of blood during systole

Aortic valve: the left semilunar valve separating the left ventricle and the aorta

Apex of the heart: tip of the heart pointing down toward the fifth left intercostal space

Apical impulse: point of maximal impulse (PMI); pulsation created as the left ventricle rotates against the chest wall during systole, normally at the fifth left intercostal space in the midclavicular line

Base of the heart: the broader area of the heart's outline located superior and medially to the apex

Bell (of the stethoscope): cup-shaped endpiece used for soft, low-pitched heart sounds

Bradycardia: slow heart rate, less than 50 beats/min in the adult

Clubbing: a bulbous enlargement of distal phalanges of fingers and toes that occurs with chronic cyanotic heart and lung conditions

Coarctation of the aorta: a severe narrowing of the descending aorta; a congenital heart defect

Cyanosis: a dusky-blue mottling of the skin and mucous membranes due to an excessive amount of reduced hemoglobin in the blood

Diaphragm (of the stethoscope): flat endpiece of the stethoscope used for hearing relatively high-pitched heart sounds

Diastole: the heart's filling phase

Dyspnea: difficult, laboured breathing

Edema: swelling of the legs or a dependent body part due to increased interstitial fluid

First heart sound (S_1): it occurs with closure of the atrioventricular (AV) valves, signalling the beginning of systole

Fourth heart sound (S_4): it occurs in late diastole, at presystole, when the ventricle is resistant to filling; the atria contract and push blood into a noncompliant ventricle

Gallop rhythm: the addition of a third or a fourth heart sound, making the rhythm sound like the cadence of a galloping horse

Left ventricular hypertrophy (LVH): an increase in thickness of the myocardial wall; it occurs when the heart pumps against chronic outflow obstruction (e.g., aortic stenosis)

Midclavicular line (MCL): imaginary vertical line bisecting the middle of the clavicle in each hemithorax

Mitral regurgitation: mitral insufficiency; incompetent mitral valve allows regurgitation of blood back into left atrium during systole

Mitral stenosis: calcified mitral valve impedes forward flow of blood into left ventricle during diastole

Mitral valve: the left AV valve separating the left atria and ventricle

Palpitation: uncomfortable awareness of rapid or irregular heart rate

Paradoxical split: the opposite of a normal split S_2 so that the split is heard in expiration, and in inspiration the sounds fuse to one sound
Pericardial friction rub: a high-pitched scratchy extracardiac sound heard when the precordium is inflamed
Physiological splitting: a normal variation in S_2 heard as two separate components during inspiration
Precordium: the area of the chest wall overlying the heart and great vessels
Preload: the venous return that builds during diastole
Pulmonic regurgitation: pulmonic insufficiency; backflow of blood through incompetent pulmonic valve into the right ventricle
Pulmonic stenosis: calcification of pulmonic valve that restricts forward flow of blood during systole
Pulmonic valve: the right semilunar valve separating the right ventricle and pulmonary artery
Second heart sound (S_2): it occurs with closure of the semilunar valves, aortic and pulmonic, and signals the end of systole
Syncope: fainting; temporary loss of consciousness due to decreased cerebral blood flow, caused by ventricular asystole, pronounced bradycardia, or ventricular fibrillation
Systole: the heart's pumping phase
Tachycardia: rapid heart rate, faster than 100 bpm in the adult
Third heart sound (S_3): the soft, low-pitched, ventricular filling sound that occurs in early diastole (S_3 gallop) and may be an early sign of heart failure
Thrill: a palpable vibration on the chest wall accompanying severe heart murmur
Tricuspid valve: the right AV valve separating the right atria and ventricle

STUDY GUIDE

After completing the reading assignment, you should be able to answer the following questions in the spaces provided.

1. Define the *apical impulse* and describe its normal location, size, amplitude, and duration.

    Which *normal* variations may affect the location of the apical impulse?

    Which *abnormal* conditions may affect the location of the apical impulse?

2. Explain the mechanism producing normal first and second heart sounds.

3. Describe the effect of respiration on the heart sounds.

4. Describe the characteristics of the first heart sound and its intensity at the apex of the heart and at the base.

    Which conditions *increase* the intensity of S_1?

Which conditions *decrease* the intensity of S_1?

5. Describe the characteristics of the second heart sound and its intensity at the apex of the heart and at the base.

   Which conditions accentuate the intensity of S_2?

   Which conditions diminish the intensity of S_2?

6. Explain the physiological mechanism for normal splitting of S_2 in the pulmonic valve area.

7. Define the *third heart sound*. When in the cardiac cycle does it occur? Describe its intensity, quality, location in which it is heard, and method of auscultation.

8. Differentiate a physiological S_3 from a pathological S_3.

9. Define the fourth heart sound. When in the cardiac cycle does it occur? Describe its intensity, quality, location in which it is heard, and method of auscultation.

10. Explain the position of the valves during each phase of the cardiac cycle.

11. Define *venous pressure* and *jugular venous pulse*.

12. Differentiate between the carotid artery pulsation and the jugular vein pulsation.

13. List the areas of questioning to address during the health history for the cardiovascular system.

14. Define *bruit*, and discuss what it indicates.

15. Define *heave* or *lift*, and discuss what it indicates.

16. State four guidelines to distinguish S_1 from S_2.
    a.
    b.
    c.
    d.

17. Define *pulse deficit*, and discuss what it indicates.

18. Define *preload* and *afterload*.

19. List the characteristics to explore when you hear a murmur, including the "grades" of murmurs.

20. Discuss the characteristics of an innocent or functional murmur.

21. Fill in the labels indicated on the following illustrations.

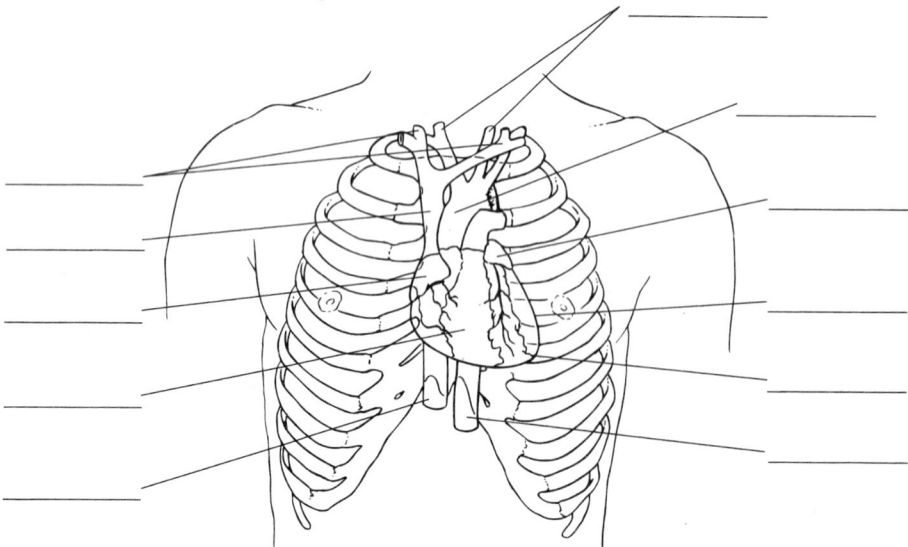

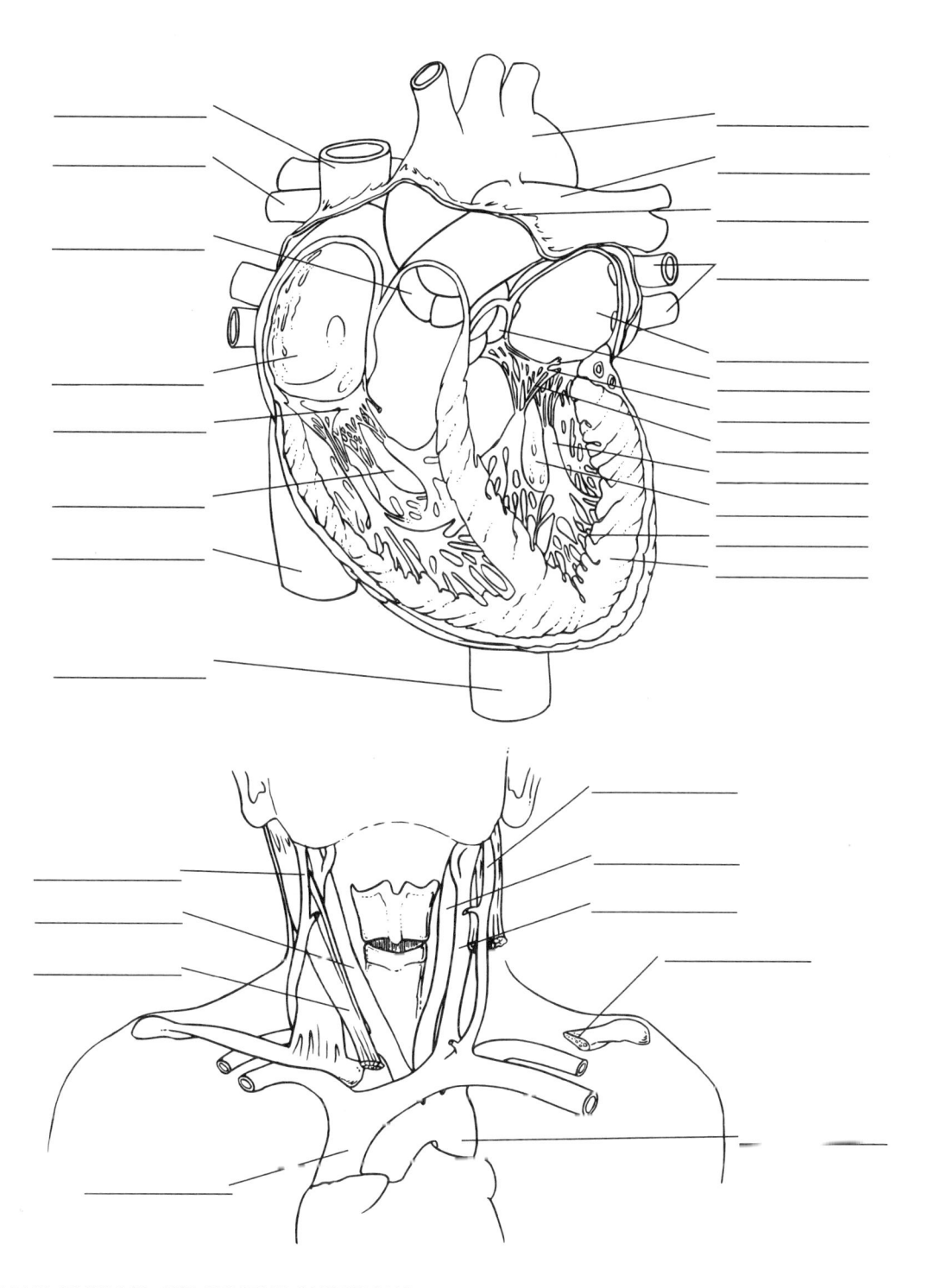

REVIEW AND CLINICAL JUDGEMENT QUESTIONS

This test is for you to check your own mastery of the content. Answers are provided on the text's Evolve site.

1. The *precordium* is
   a. a synonym for the mediastinum.
   b. the area on the chest where the apical impulse is felt.
   c. the area on the anterior chest overlying the heart and great vessels.
   d. a synonym for the area where the superior and inferior venae cavae return unoxygenated venous blood to the right side of the heart.

2. Select the best description of the tricuspid valve.
   a. left semilunar valve
   b. right atrioventricular (AV) valve
   c. left atrioventricular (AV) valve
   d. right semilunar valve

3. The function of the pulmonic valve is to
   a. divide the left atrium and left ventricle.
   b. guard the opening between the right atrium and right ventricle.
   c. protect the orifice between the right ventricle and the pulmonary artery.
   d. guard the entrance to the aorta from the left ventricle.

4. For a patient experiencing orthopnea, which physical assessment findings would be most relevant? (Select all that apply.)
   a. right-sided carotid bruit
   b. elevated jugular venous pressure
   c. presence of a split S_2 toward the end of every expiration
   d. presence of an S_3 heart sounds in both supine and sitting positions

5. The second heart sound is the result of
   a. opening of the mitral and tricuspid valves.
   b. closing of the mitral and tricuspid valves.
   c. opening of the aortic and pulmonic valves.
   d. closing of the aortic and pulmonic valves.

6. You are conducting a focused cardiac examination on a 63-year-old patient with heart failure. As you palpate the apical pulse, you note that the normal size of this impulse is
   a. less than 1 cm.
   b. about 2 cm.
   c. 3 cm.
   d. variable, depending on the size of the person.

7. The examiner wishes to listen in the pulmonic valve area. To do this, the stethoscope would be placed at the
   a. second right interspace.
   b. second left interspace.
   c. left lower sternal border.
   d. fifth interspace, left midclavicular line.

8. You are assessing a patient and suspect that you hear a pericardial friction rub. Select the best method of auscultation.
   a. Listen with the diaphragm, with the patient sitting up and leaning forward, breath held in expiration.
   b. Listen using the bell with the patient leaning forward.
   c. Listen at the base during normal respiration.
   d. Listen with the diaphragm, with the patient turned to the left side.

9. It is your first day working as a student nurse on the pediatric unit. You are assigned a patient who has a history of congenital heart disease. When auscultating the heart, your first step is to
   a. identify S_1 and S_2.
   b. listen for S_3 and S_4.
   c. listen for murmurs.
   d. identify all four sounds on the first round.

10. You are assessing a 14-year-old athlete. As you auscultate the heart, you believe that you hear a split S_2. You will hear a split S_2 most clearly in what area?
    a. apical
    b. pulmonic
    c. tricuspid
    d. aortic

11. The stethoscope bell should be pressed lightly against the skin so that
    a. chest hair does not simulate crackles.
    b. high-pitched sounds can be heard better.
    c. it does not act as a diaphragm.
    d. it does not interfere with amplification of heart sounds.

12. A murmur heard after S_1 and before S_2 is classified as
    a. diastolic (possibly benign).
    b. diastolic (always pathological).
    c. systolic (possibly benign).
    d. systolic (always pathological).

13. While auscultating a patient's heart rate and rhythm, you note that it sounds irregular. What additional assessments would help you determine the cause? (Select all that apply.)
    a. Note if there is any pattern to the irregularity.
    b. Note if the rate varies with inspiration and expiration.
    c. Carefully listen to the bilateral carotid arteries.
    d. Auscultate the apical beat while palpating the radial pulse, and note any difference in rate.

14. A 62-year-old man complains of chest pain. You ask him to describe the chest pain. Which statement would cause you to consider an ischemic cardiovascular cause?
    a. "The pain is much worse when I take a deep breath, and I keep coughing too."
    b. "It feels sharp and stabbing, but it's a bit better when I lean forward."
    c. "This pain is burning; I notice it more after I eat and my mouth tastes terrible."
    d. "My chest feels tight and heavy, but it does go away when I rest a few minutes."

15. A 74-year-old woman with a history of coronary artery disease describes a history of orthopnea for the last 2 months. She is now sleeping on three pillows because "it's easier to breathe." You are concerned that the woman may have
    a. heart failure.
    b. pneumonia.
    c. acute coronary syndrome.
    d. gastroesophageal reflux.

Match column A to column B.

Column A—Definition

16. _____ Tough, fibrous, double-walled sac that surrounds and protects the heart

17. _____ Thin layer of endothelial tissue that lines the inner surface of the heart chambers and valves

18. _____ Reservoir for holding blood

19. _____ Ensures smooth, friction-free movement of the heart muscle

20. _____ Muscular pumping chamber

21. _____ Muscular wall of the heart

Column B—Cardiovascular Terminology

a. Pericardial fluid
b. Ventricle
c. Endocardium
d. Myocardium
e. Pericardium
f. Atrium

22. Fill in the blanks.

S_1 is best heard at the _____ of the heart, whereas S_2 is loudest at the _____ of the heart.

CRITICAL THINKING EXERCISE

The Absolute CVD Risk/Benefit Calculator (https://cvdcalculator.com) is a valuable clinical tool used to help determine a person's absolute estimate (%) of having a cardiovascular event over a specific period of time. Using the Absolute CVD Risk/Benefit Calculator, calculate your own cardiovascular risk. After determining your risk, interview an older asymptomatic adult without a clinical history of cardiovascular disease and calculate their absolute risk. Obtain a global risk score, and then develop a teaching plan individualized to the risk score of your interviewee.

SKILLS LABORATORY/CLINICAL SETTING

You are now ready for the clinical component of the cardiovascular system. The purpose of the clinical component is to practise the cardiovascular examination on a peer in the skills laboratory or a patient in the clinical setting, and to achieve the following.

Clinical Objectives

1. Demonstrate knowledge of the symptoms related to the cardiovascular system by obtaining a health history from a peer or patient.
2. Correctly locate anatomical landmarks on the chest wall of a peer.
3. Using a grease pencil, and with the peer's permission, outline the borders of the heart, and label the auscultatory areas on a peer's chest wall.
4. Demonstrate correct techniques for inspection, auscultation, and palpation of the neck vessels.
5. Demonstrate correct techniques for inspection, palpation, and auscultation of the precordium.
6. Record the history and physical examination findings accurately, reach an assessment of the health state, and develop a plan of care.

Instructions

Gather your equipment. Wash your hands. Clean the stethoscope endpiece with an alcohol wipe. Practise the steps of the examination of the cardiovascular system on a peer or on a patient in the clinical area. Record your findings using the documentation sheet that follows. The front of the page is intended as a worksheet; the back of the page is intended for your narrative recording using the subjective, objective, assessment, plan (SOAP) format.

NOTES

DOCUMENTATION—CARDIOVASCULAR SYSTEM

Date _____

Examiner _____

Patient _____ Age _____ Gender _____

Occupation _____

I. Health History

	No	Yes, explain
1. Any **chest pain** or tightness?		
2. Any **shortness of breath**?		
3. Use more than one pillow to sleep?		
4. Do you have a **cough**?		
5. Do you seem to **tire easily**?		
6. Facial skin ever turn blue or ashen?		
7. Any **swelling** of feet or legs?		
8. Awaken at night to urinate?		
9. Any past history of heart disease?		
10. Any family history of heart disease?		
11. Assess cardiac risk factors.		

II. Physical Examination

A. Carotid arteries
   Inspect and palpate:

   Grade: R _____ L _____
   (0 = absent, 1+ weak, 2+ normal, 3+ increased, 4+ bounding)

B. Jugular venous system

   External jugular veins (circle one):
   - collapsed supine
   - meniscus visible at _____ bed elevated not visible

   Internal jugular venous pulsations (circle one):
   - visible at _____ bed elevated

C. Precordium
   Inspect and palpate:

   1. Skin colour and condition _____

   2. Chest wall pulsations _____

   3. Heave or lift _____

   4. Apical impulse in the _____ at _____

      Size _____ Amplitude _____

D. **Auscultation**

1. Identify anatomical areas where you will listen.

2. Note the rate and rhythm: _____

3. Identify S_1 and S_2 in the diagram at right and note any variation: _____

   S_1_____S_2_____S_1_____S_2_____

   S1 _____

   S2 _____

4. Listen in systole and diastole:

   Extra heart sounds _____

   Systolic murmur _____

   Diastolic murmur _____

DOCUMENTATION—CARDIOVASCULAR SYSTEM

Summarize your findings using the SOAP format.

Subjective (Reason for seeking care, health history)

Objective (Physical examination findings)

Record your findings on the diagram.

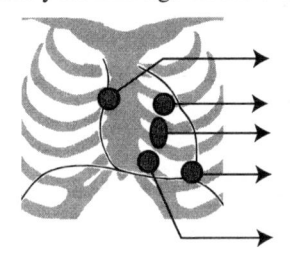

Assessment (Assessment of health state or problem, diagnosis)

Plan (Diagnostic evaluation, follow-up care, patient teaching)

21 Peripheral Vascular System and Lymphatic System

PURPOSE

This chapter reviews the structure and function of the peripheral vascular system and the lymphatic system; the peripheral pulse sites; the methods of examination of the peripheral vascular and lymphatic systems; and the accurate recording of the assessment. At the end of this chapter, you will be able to perform a complete assessment of the peripheral vascular and lymphatic systems.

READING ASSIGNMENT

Jarvis: *Physical Examination and Health Assessment*, 4th Canadian ed., Chapter 21.

Suggested Readings

Embil, J., Albalawi, Z., Bowering, K., et al. (2018). *Foot care*. Diabetes Canada. https://www.diabetes.ca/health-care-providers/clinical-practice-guidelines/chapter-32#panel-tab_FullText

Kohlman-Trigoboff, D. (2021). Healthcare inequity in PAD. *Journal of Vascular Nursing, 39*(3), 54–56.

GLOSSARY

Study the following terms after reading the corresponding chapter in the text.

Aneurysm: a defect or sac formed by dilation in the artery wall due to atherosclerosis, trauma, or congenital defect
Arteriosclerosis: a thickening and loss of elasticity of the arterial walls
Atherosclerosis: plaques of fatty deposits formed in the inner layer (intima) of the arteries
Bradycardia: a slow heart rate; less than 50 bpm in the adult
Bruit: a soft blowing, swooshing sound heard through a stethoscope when an artery is partially occluded
Cyanosis: a dusky-blue mottling of the skin and mucous membranes due to excessive amount of reduced hemoglobin in the blood
Diastole: the heart's filling phase
Ischemia: a deficiency of arterial blood to a body part, due to constriction or obstruction of a blood vessel
Lymph nodes: small oval clumps of lymphatic tissue located at grouped intervals along lymphatic vessels
Lymphedema: the swelling of an extremity due to obstructed lymph channel; nonpitting
Pitting edema: the indentation left after the examiner depresses the skin over swollen edematous tissue
Profile sign: viewing the finger from the side to detect early clubbing
Pulse: the pressure wave created by each heartbeat, palpable at body sites where the artery lies close to the skin and over a bone
Pulsus alternans: a regular rhythm, but the force of the pulse varies with alternating beats of large and small amplitude
Pulsus bigeminus: an irregular rhythm in which every other beat is premature; premature beats have weakened amplitude
Pulsus bisferiens: an abnormal rhythm in which two strong systolic peaks occur, with a dip in between each pulse
Pulsus paradoxus: beats have a weaker amplitude with respiratory inspiration, stronger with expiration
Systole: the heart's pumping phase
Tachycardia: a rapid heart rate; more than 100 bpm in the adult
Thrombophlebitis: inflammation of a vein associated with thrombus formation
Ulcer: an open skin lesion extending into the dermis with sloughing of necrotic inflammatory tissue
Varicose vein: dilated tortuous veins with incompetent valves

STUDY GUIDE

After completing the reading assignment, you should be able to answer the following questions in the spaces provided.

1. Describe the structure and function of arteries and veins.

2. List the pulse sites accessible to examination.

3. Describe three mechanisms that help return venous blood to the heart.

4. Define the term *capacitance vessels*, and explain its significance.

5. List the risk factors for venous stasis.

6. Describe the function of the lymphatic system.

7. Describe the function of the lymph nodes.

8. Name the related organs in the lymphatic system.

9. List the symptom areas to address during history-taking relating to the peripheral vascular system.

10. Fill in the grading scale for assessing the force of an arterial pulse: 0 = _____; 1+ = _____; 2+ = _____; 3+ = _____

11. Differentiate between mild, moderate, and severe lymphedema.

12. List the skin characteristics expected with arterial insufficiency to the lower legs.

13. Compare the characteristics of leg ulcers associated with arterial insufficiency to ulcers with venous insufficiency.

14. Fill in the description of the grading scale for pitting edema:

    1+ = _____

    2+ = _____

    3+ = _____

    4+ = _____

15. Describe the technique for using the Doppler ultrasonic stethoscope to detect peripheral pulses.

16. Raynaud's phenomenon has associated progressive tricolour changes of the skin from _____ to _____ and then to _____. State the mechanism for each of these colour changes.

17. Fill in the labels indicated on the following arteries and pulse sites.

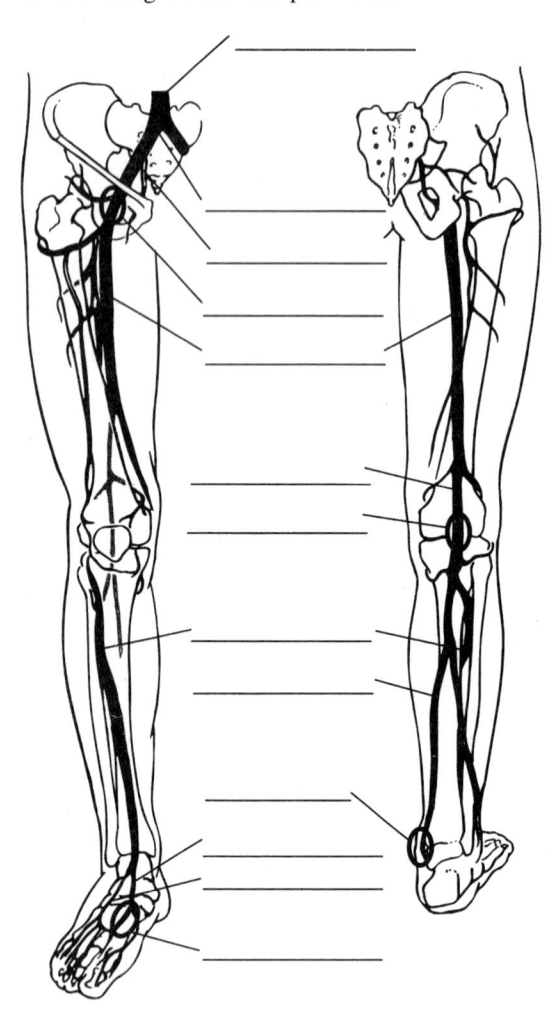

REVIEW AND CLINICAL JUDGEMENT QUESTIONS

This test is for you to check your own mastery of the content. Answers are provided on the text's Evolve site.

1. A function of the venous system is
    a. to hold more blood when blood volume increases.
    b. to conserve fluid and plasma proteins that leak out of the capillaries.
    c. to form a major part of the immune system that defends the body against disease.
    d. to absorb lipids from the intestinal tract.

2. The organs that aid the lymphatic system are
    a. the liver, lymph nodes, and stomach.
    b. the pancreas, small intestine, and thymus.
    c. the spleen, tonsils, and thymus.
    d. the pancreas, spleen, and tonsils.

3. Ms. T. has come for a prenatal visit. She reports dependent edema, varicosities in the legs, and hemorrhoids. The best response is
    a. "If these symptoms persist, we will perform an amniocentesis."
    b. "If these symptoms persist, we will discuss having you hospitalized."
    c. "These symptoms are caused by the pressure of the growing uterus on the veins and are common during pregnancy."
    d. "At this time, the symptoms are a minor inconvenience. You should learn to accept them."

4. You are assessing a patient on the surgical unit and note that the patient has a pulse with an amplitude of 3+. What condition(s) can contribute to a bounding 3+ pulse? (Select all that apply.)
   a. hyperthyroidism
   b. shock
   c. fever
   d. anxiety

5. Inspection of a person's right hand reveals a red, swollen area. To further assess for infection, you would palpate the
   a. cervical node.
   b. axillary node.
   c. epitrochlear node.
   d. inguinal node.

6. What are known risk factors for venous ulcer development? (Select all that apply.)
   a. obesity
   b. multiple pregnancies
   c. a history of hypertension
   d. daily Aspirin therapy

7. During an examination of the lower extremities, you are unable to palpate the popliteal pulse. Your next best action is to
   a. proceed with the examination. It is often impossible to palpate this pulse.
   b. refer the patient to a vascular surgeon for further evaluation.
   c. schedule the patient for a venogram.
   d. schedule the patient for an arteriogram.

8. While reviewing the nursing assessment from the shift before, you note a notation of 4+ edema of the right leg. The best description of this type of edema is
   a. mild pitting, no perceptible swelling of the leg.
   b. moderate pitting, indentation subsides rapidly.
   c. deep pitting, leg looks swollen.
   d. very deep pitting, indentation lasts a long time.

9. After raising a patient's legs 30 cm off the table for 30 seconds and then having the person sit up and dangle the legs, you note the colour returned to both legs in 30 seconds. What should be your next action?
   a. Notify the provider of a potential acute arterial occlusion.
   b. Assess pulse amplitude and ask the patient about symptoms of claudication.
   c. Order a lower extremity venous ultrasound test.
   d. Proceed with the examination, as this is a normal finding.

10. A 54-year-old woman with five children has varicose veins of the lower extremities. Her most characteristic sign is
    a. reduced arterial circulation.
    b. blanching, deathlike appearance of the extremities on elevation.
    c. loss of hair on feet and toes.
    d. dilated, tortuous, superficial bluish vessels.

11. Atrophic skin changes that occur with peripheral arterial insufficiency include
    a. thin, shiny skin with loss of hair.
    b. brown discoloration.
    c. thick, leathery skin.
    d. slow-healing blisters on the skin.

12. During a diabetes clinic, a 76-year-old patient informs you that they have done some research on their symptoms and believe they have intermittent claudication. Intermittent claudication is
    a. muscular pain relieved by exercise.
    b. neurological pain relieved by exercise.
    c. muscular pain brought on by exercise.
    d. neurological pain brought on by exercise.

13. You are assessing a woman with a history of breast cancer. She underwent a right mastectomy 2 months ago and is getting radiation therapy. She is concerned because her right arm is swollen, and she thinks she may have a blood clot. Your examination reveals firm, nonpitting edema. Her arm pulses are 2+ bilaterally. Her skin is warm, and there are no areas of redness or tenderness.

    Underline the cues from the patient's history and physical examination that suggest lymphedema as the likely cause of the arm swelling.

14. You are caring for a patient who presented to the emergency department with right leg pain. She reports an acute, sudden onset of very severe pain. Your physical examination reveals pallor, coolness, and pulselessness in the right leg. You suspect the patient has acute arterial insufficiency and your next action is to
    a. contact the provider immediately.
    b. document your findings carefully.
    c. teach the patient to avoid prolonged sitting.
    d. apply compression stockings.

15. A 62-year-old man reports pain in his left calf in multiple positions. You examine his legs and note unilateral swelling and warmth. You are concerned that he may be experiencing
    a. peripheral artery disease.
    b. chronic venous insufficiency.
    c. acute deep vein thrombosis.
    d. cellulitis.

16. Match the finding to the most likely condition in each row.

Finding	Peripheral Artery Disease	Chronic Venous Insufficiency	Acute Deep Vein Thrombosis
Thin, shiny, trophic skin			
Thick skin with brown discoloration (hemosiderin staining)			
Unilateral erythema, and skin warm to touch			
Hair loss			
Bilateral diminished pulses			
Varicose veins			
Unilateral edema with cyanotic toes			
Ulcers occur at toes, metatarsal heads, heels, and lateral ankle and are characterized by pale ischemic base, well-defined edges, and no bleeding			
Ulcers occur at medial malleolus and are characterized by bleeding and uneven edges			

CRITICAL THINKING EXERCISE

You are working in a wound care clinic and your patient, M.S., reports a tender, swollen calf. Your patient is a 48-year-old female who was in an ebike accident last month. She underwent general anaesthesia for a splenectomy (due to internal bleeding), and her left foot through mid-calf is in a cast due to an ankle fracture. She is reporting that the cast has become tight in the last day. Her left upper calf is tender to palpation along the venous system; the skin is of similar colour and temperature to the right, and there are no dilated vessels. While there is no visible swelling of the entire left leg, you measure a calf circumference of 33 cm on the right leg and 35 cm on the left leg; the left lower leg also has 1+ pitting edema, while the right lower leg has none. She has no other past medical history including no active cancer and

no history of deep vein thrombosis (DVT). Based on your assessment, you are immediately concerned that she may have developed DVT.
- Calculate the Wells score for DVT for this patient. (See Jarvis: *Physical Examination and Health Assessment*, 4th ed., p. 566, or https://www.mdcalc.com/calc/362/wells-criteria-dvt.)
- Based on her Wells criteria, what are your next steps?
- What are the risks of missing a DVT diagnosis?
- What education would you provide to M.S. regarding DVTs and prevention?

SKILLS LABORATORY/CLINICAL SETTING

You are now ready for the clinical component of the peripheral vascular system. The purpose of the clinical component is to practise the components of the peripheral vascular examination on a peer in the skills laboratory or a patient in the clinical setting and to achieve the following.

Clinical Objectives

1. Demonstrate knowledge of the symptoms related to the peripheral vascular system by obtaining a health history from a peer or patient.
2. Demonstrate palpation of peripheral arterial pulses (brachial, radial, femoral, popliteal, posterior tibial, dorsalis pedis) by assessing amplitude and symmetry, noting any signs of arterial insufficiency.
3. Demonstrate inspection and palpation of peripheral veins by noting any signs of venous insufficiency.
4. Demonstrate palpation of the lymphatic system by identifying enlargement, clumping, or abnormal firmness of regional lymph nodes.
5. Record the history and physical examination findings accurately, reach an assessment of the health state, and develop a plan of care.

Instructions

Gather your equipment. Wash your hands. Practise the steps of the examination of the peripheral vascular system on a peer. Record your findings using the documentation sheets that follow. The first part is intended as a worksheet; the last page is intended for your narrative summary recording using the subjective, objective, assessment, plan (SOAP) format. Note that the peripheral examination and cardiovascular examination usually are practised together.

NOTES

DOCUMENTATION—PERIPHERAL VASCULAR SYSTEM

Date _____

Examiner _____

Patient _____ Age _____ Gender _____

Occupation _____

I. **Health History**

	No	Yes, explain
1. Any leg **pain** (cramps)? Where?		
2. Any **skin changes** in arms or legs?		
3. Any sores or **lesions** in arms and legs?		
4. Any **swelling** in the legs?		
5. Any **swollen glands**? Where?		
6. What medications are you taking?		

II. **Physical Examination**

  A. **Inspection**

   1. The arms
      Inspect:

      Colour of skin and nail beds _____

      Symmetry _____

      Lesions _____

      Edema _____

      Clubbing _____

      Palpate:

      Temperature _____

      Texture _____

      Capillary refill _____

      Locate and grade pulses (record on back) _____

      Check epitrochlear lymph node _____

   2. The legs
      Inspect:

      Colour _____

      Hair distribution _____

      Venous pattern and varicosities _____

      Size _____

         Swelling and edema _____

         Atrophy _____

         If so, measure calf circumference in cm   R _____   L _____

      Skin lesions or ulcers _____

Palpate:

Temperature _____

Tenderness _____

Inguinal lymph nodes _____

Locate and grade pulses (record on back) _____

Check pretibial edema (grade if present) _____

Auscultate for bruit (if indicated) _____

	Brachial	Radial	Femoral	Popliteal	D. pedis	P. tibial
R						
L						

0 = absent, 1+ = weak, 2+ = normal, 3+ = increased, bounding

3. Manual compression test _____

Check colour change: elevate legs, then dangle; colour returns in _____ seconds.

NOTES

DOCUMENTATION—PERIPHERAL VASCULAR SYSTEM

Summarize your findings using the SOAP format.

Subjective (Reason for seeking care, health history)

Objective (Physical examination findings)

Record your findings on the diagram.

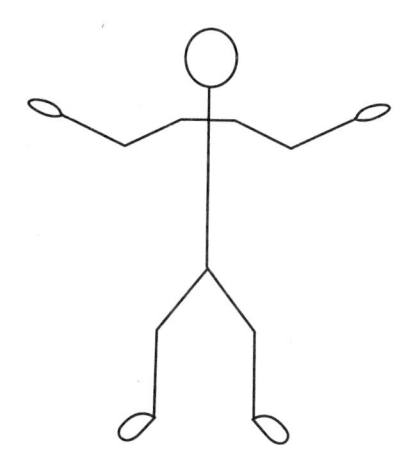

Assessment (Assessment of health state or problem, diagnosis)

Plan (Diagnostic evaluation, follow-up care, patient teaching)

NOTES

22 The Abdomen

PURPOSE

This chapter reviews the structure and function of the abdominal organs; the location of the abdominal organs; bowel sounds; the rationale for and methods of examination of the abdomen; and the accurate recording of the assessment. At the end of this chapter, you will be able to perform a complete assessment of the abdomen.

READING ASSIGNMENT

Jarvis: *Physical Examination and Health Assessment*, 4th Canadian ed., Chapter 22.

Suggested Readings

Chaudhari, H., Schneeweiss, M., Rebinsky, R., et al. (2021). An advanced nursing directive for children with suspected appendicitis: Protocol for a quality improvement feasibility study. *Journal of Medical Internet Research Research Protocols, 10*(10), e33158. doi:10.2196/33158.

Rogers, J., & Schallmo, M. (2021). Understanding the most commonly billed diagnoses in primary care: Abdominal pain. *The Nurse Practitioner, 46*(1), 13–20.

GLOSSARY

Study the following terms after reading the corresponding chapter in the text.

Abdominal adhesions: scar tissue in the abdomen; inflammatory bands that connect opposite sides of serous surfaces after trauma or surgery

Aneurysm: a defect or sac formed by dilation in the artery wall due to atherosclerosis, trauma, or congenital defect

Anorexia: a loss of appetite for food

Ascites: the abnormal accumulation of serous fluid within the peritoneal cavity; it is associated with heart failure, cirrhosis, cancer, or portal hypertension

Borborygmi: loud, gurgling bowel sounds signalling increased motility or hyperperistalsis; they occur with early bowel obstruction, gastroenteritis, diarrhea, laxative use, and subsiding paralytic ileus

Bruit: a soft blowing, swooshing sound heard through a stethoscope when an artery is partially occluded; it indicates turbulent blood flow

Celiac disease: an inherited autoimmune condition in which intestinal tissue is damaged in response to eating gluten, which prevents nutrients from being properly absorbed

Cholecystitis: inflammation of the gallbladder, resulting in biliary colic

Costal margin: lower border of the rib margin formed by the medial edges of the eighth, ninth, and tenth ribs

Costovertebral angle (CVA): an angle formed by the twelfth rib and the vertebral column on the posterior thorax, overlying the kidney

Diastasis recti: a midline longitudinal ridge in the abdomen that is a separation of the abdominal rectus muscles

Dysphagia: difficulty swallowing

Epigastrium: name of the abdominal region between the costal margins

Familial adenomatous polyposis (FAP): a condition caused by a genetic mutation that can be inherited; a risk factor for colon cancer

Hematemesis: bloody vomitus; it occurs with stomach or duodenal ulcers and esophageal varices

Hepatomegaly: the abnormal enlargement of the liver

Hernia: the protrusion of abdominal viscera through an abnormal opening in the muscle wall; depending on location, it is described as inguinal, umbilical, epigastric, or incisional

Lactose intolerance: a condition affecting certain individuals who have lower levels of lactase, the intestinal enzyme that digests lactose found in milk, and causing intolerance to milk and other dairy products

Linea alba: a midline tendinous seam joining the abdominal muscles

Paralytic ileus: a complete absence of peristaltic movement that may follow abdominal surgery or complete bowel obstruction

Peritoneal friction rub: a rough, grating sound heard through the stethoscope over the site of peritoneal inflammation

Peritonitis: inflammation of the peritoneum
Pyloric stenosis: a congenital narrowing of the pyloric sphincter, forming outflow obstruction of the stomach; it is usually seen in newborns within the first weeks of life
Pyrosis: heartburn; a burning sensation in the upper abdomen, due to reflux of gastric acid
Rectus abdominis muscle: a midline abdominal muscle extending from the rib cage to the pubic bone; its edge is often palpable
Scaphoid: an abnormally sunken abdominal wall; one with a "caved in" appearance, as with malnutrition or underweight
Splenomegaly: the abnormal enlargement of the spleen
Striae: linea albicantes; a silvery-white or pink scar tissue formed by stretching of the abdominal skin, as with pregnancy or obesity
Suprapubic: name of the abdominal region just superior to the pubic bone; also sometimes referred to as the *hypogastric area*
Tympany: a high-pitched, musical, drumlike percussion note heard when percussing over the stomach and intestine
Umbilicus: depression on the abdomen marking site of entry of the umbilical cord; umbilical refers to the area surrounding the umbilicus
Viscera: internal organs contained within the abdominal cavity; referred to as either *solid viscera* or *hollow viscera*, depending on organ characteristics

STUDY GUIDE

After completing the reading assignment, you should be able to answer the following questions in the spaces provided.

1. Draw a picture of the borders of the abdomen. Draw in the organs.

2. Name the organs that are normally palpable on abdominal examination.

3. Describe the proper positioning and preparation of the patient for abdominal examination.

4. State the rationale for performing auscultation of the abdomen before palpation or percussion.

5. Discuss inspection of the abdomen, including normal findings.

6. Describe the procedure for auscultation of bowel sounds.

7. Differentiate the following abdominal sounds: normal, hyperactive, and hypoactive bowel sounds; succussion splash; and bruit.

8. Identify and give the rationale for each of the percussion notes heard over the abdomen.

    a. List four conditions that may alter normal percussion notes.

9. Differentiate between light and deep palpation, and explain the purpose of each.

    a. List two abnormalities that may be detected by light palpation and two detected by deep palpation.

10. Contrast involuntary rigidity with voluntary guarding.

11. Contrast visceral pain and somatic (parietal) pain.

12. Describe rebound tenderness.

13. Describe palpation of the liver, spleen, and kidney.

14. List the eight characteristics the examiner should note when a mass is palpated.

15. Describe the expected examination findings of the abdomen in each of the following conditions:

    Obesity _____

    Gaseous distension _____

    Tumour _____

    Pregnancy _____

    Ascites _____

    Enlarged liver _____

    Enlarged spleen _____

    Appendicitis _____

16. Fill in the labels indicated on the following illustrations.

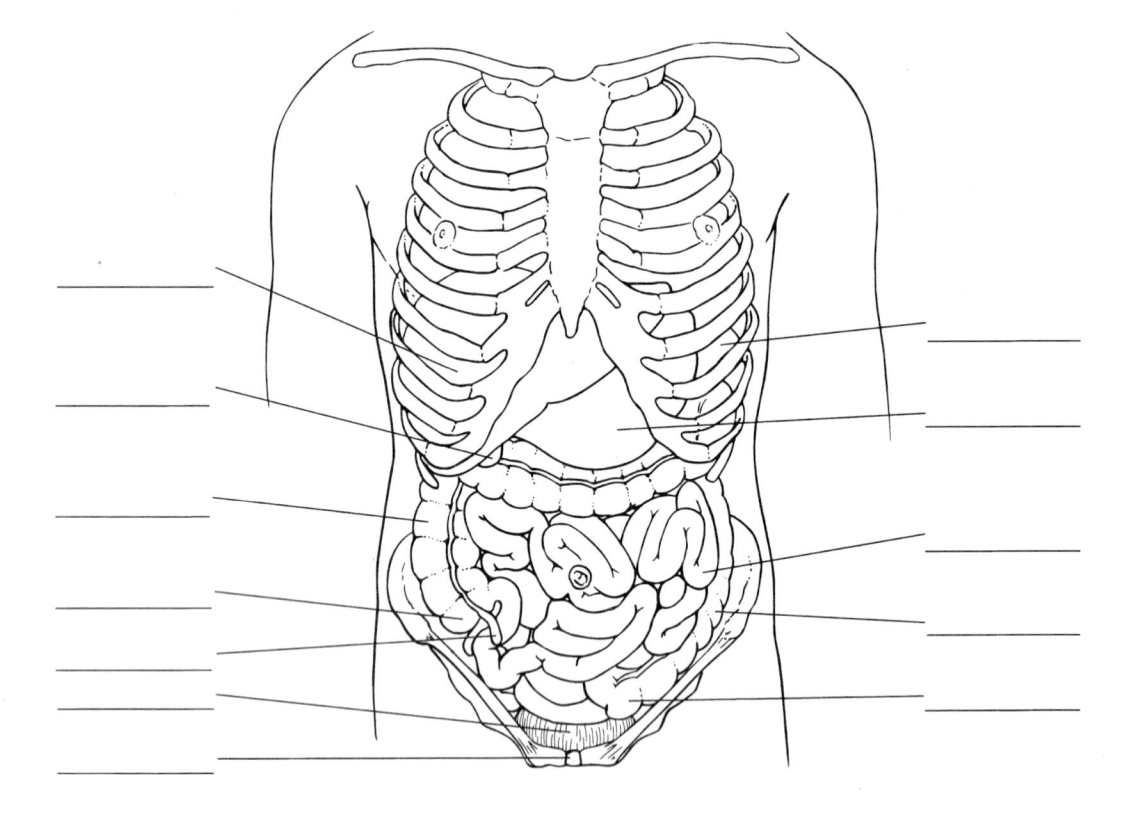

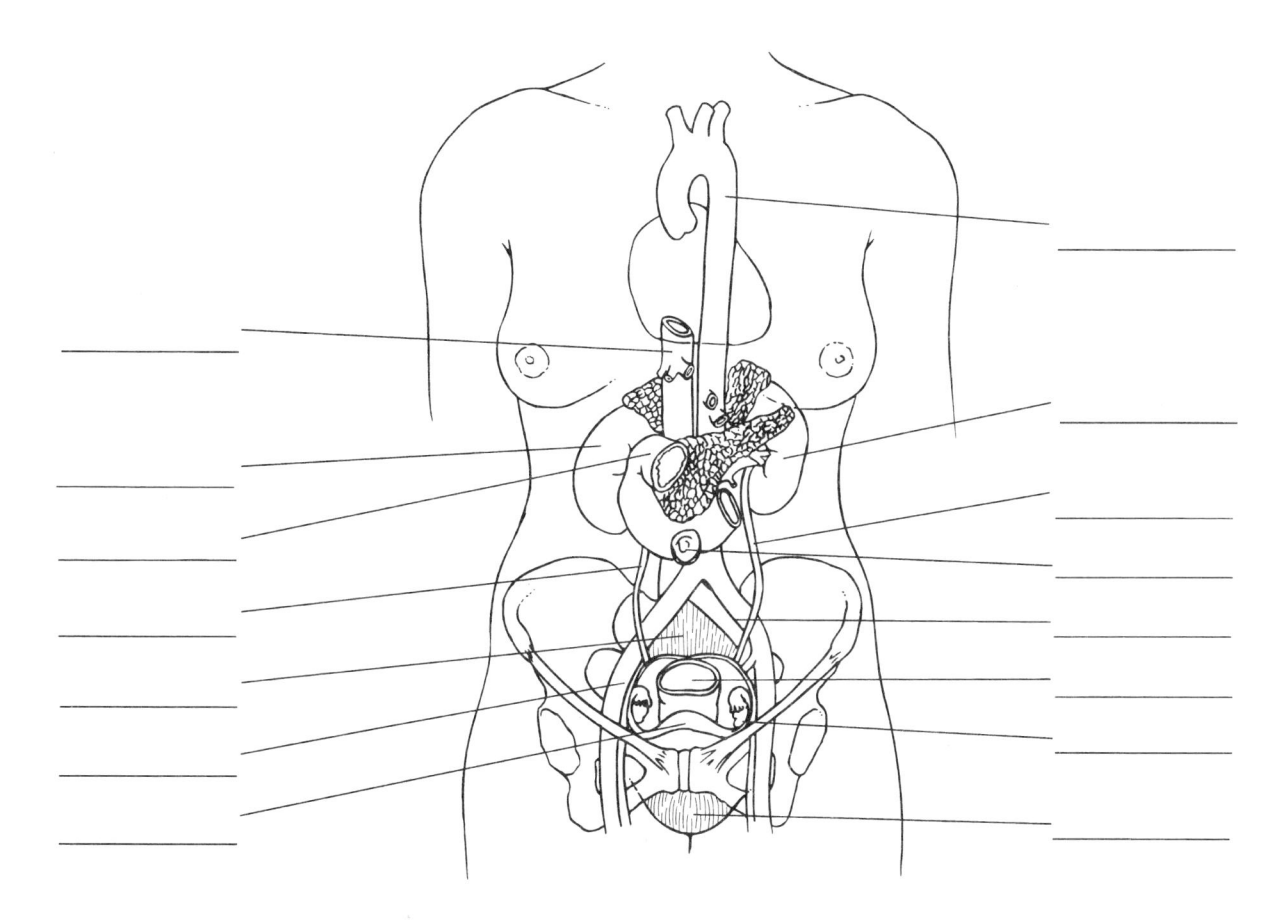

REVIEW AND CLINICAL JUDGEMENT QUESTIONS

This test is for you to check your own mastery of the content. Answers are provided on the text's Evolve site.

1. Select the sequence of techniques used during an examination of the abdomen.
    a. percussion, inspection, palpation, auscultation
    b. inspection, palpation, percussion, auscultation
    c. inspection, auscultation, percussion, palpation
    d. auscultation, inspection, palpation, percussion

2. You are auscultating a patient's abdomen and hear a soft, high-pitched, irregular gurgling sound over the right lower quadrant. What is the next best action?
    a. Move on to percussion of the abdomen, as this is a normal finding.
    b. Continue auscultating the abdomen in all four quadrants, moving clockwise.
    c. Contact the nurse practitioner or physician, as the patient may have a bowel obstruction.
    d. Continue listening to the right lower quadrant for a full 5 minutes.

3. Right upper quadrant tenderness may indicate pathology in
    a. the liver, pancreas, or gallbladder.
    b. the liver and stomach.
    c. the sigmoid colon, spleen, or rectum.
    d. the appendix or ileocecal valve.

4. You are palpating the left lower quadrant, and the patient grimaces slightly and states that the area is tender. What is your next best action?
    a. Contact the nurse practitioner or physician; the patient may have appendicitis.
    b. Document the finding, which is normal, and move on with the examination.
    c. Explain to the patient that this is probably constipation.
    d. Contact the nurse practitioner or physician; the patient may have cholecystitis.

5. The absence of bowel sounds is established after listening for
   a. 1 full minute.
   b. 3 full minutes.
   c. 5 full minutes.
   d. none of the above.

6. Auscultation of the abdomen may reveal bruits of which arteries?
   a. aortic, renal, iliac, and femoral
   b. jugular, aortic, carotid, and femoral
   c. pulmonic, aortic, and portal
   d. renal, iliac, internal jugular, and basilic

7. You are conducting a focused abdominal examination on a patient whom you suspect has hepatitis. As you percuss the liver margins, you note that the range of normal liver span in the right midclavicular line in the adult is
   a. 2–6 cm.
   b. 4–8 cm.
   c. 8–14 cm.
   d. 6–12 cm.

8. The left upper quadrant (LUQ) contains
   a. the liver.
   b. the appendix.
   c. the left ovary.
   d. the spleen.

9. While assessing a 36-year-old female patient, you note striae on her abdomen. What additional questions could you ask? (Select all that apply.)
   a. When was your last menstrual period?
   b. Have you gained any weight recently?
   c. Have you recently been or are you currently pregnant?
   d. What caused these scars on your abdomen?

10. Auscultation of the abdomen is begun in the right lower quadrant (RLQ) because
    a. bowel sounds are always normally present here.
    b. peristalsis through the descending colon is usually active.
    c. this is the location of the pyloric sphincter.
    d. vascular sounds are best heard in this area.

11. A patient reports a burning abdominal pain that occurs after meals, and you suspect gastroesophageal reflux disease (GERD). What is your best statement to the patient?
    a. "You probably should avoid all dairy products. Have you ever tried nondairy milks as an alternative?"
    b. "Consider taking ibuprofen (Advil) to help manage these symptoms"
    c. "You may be experiencing heartburn. While waiting to see your primary care provider, avoid foods that trigger it and consider taking an over-the-counter antacid."
    d. "I think you should try low-fat foods and probiotics for a while and see how your symptoms are affected."

12. You note abdominal distension in a patient with a history of cirrhosis. The shape of the abdomen is protuberant with a single, uniform curve, and the skin appears shiny and taut. What condition is most likely causing the abdominal distension?
    a. enlarged liver
    b. ascites
    c. bowel obstruction
    d. obesity

13. Tenderness during abdominal palpation is expected when palpating
    a. the liver edge.
    b. the spleen.
    c. the sigmoid colon.
    d. the kidneys.

14. Murphy's sign is best described as
    a. the pain felt when the hand of the examiner is rapidly removed from an inflamed appendix.
    b. a sharp pain felt when taking a deep breath when the examiner's fingers are on the approximate location of the inflamed gallbladder, leading the patient to abruptly stop inspiration midway.
    c. a sharp pain felt by the patient when one hand of the examiner is used to thump the other at the costovertebral angle.
    d. an invalid examination technique.

15. You are assessing a 16-year-old athlete who has mononucleosis. You are able to palpate the spleen in the lower quadrants. What is your best next action?
    a. Thoroughly palpate the borders to document a detailed description of its size and location.
    b. Proceed with the examination; this is a normal finding.
    c. Push into the spleen firmly while observing the facial expression for any signs of tenderness.
    d. Stop palpating the spleen and contact the nurse practitioner or physician of possible enlarged spleen.

CRITICAL THINKING EXERCISE

You are working in the emergency department, and a 4-year-old patient, S.L., presents with right-sided abdominal pain. S.L.'s dad reports that the pain started yesterday and has increased today. Dad also reports that S.L. has a decreased appetite, lethargy, and limited activity today. Dad gave S.L. acetaminophen (Tylenol) 2 hours ago because he thought S.L. had a slight fever. He reports that S.L. has had no vomiting. You suspect this patient may have appendicitis. On assessment, S.L. indicates increased abdominal pain with movement and with percussion. Upon palpation, you note tenderness over the right iliac fossa. Review the Chaudhari et al. article listed at the beginning of this chapter. According to the advanced nursing directive (AND), would this patient qualify for the advanced nursing directive order set? What blood work is included in the AND order set? From your clinical and personal experiences, do you feel ANDs are beneficial for Canada's health care system?

SKILLS LABORATORY/CLINICAL SETTING

You are now ready for the clinical component of the abdominal system. The purpose of the clinical component is to practise the regional examination on a peer in the skills laboratory or on a patient in the clinical setting and to achieve the following.

Clinical Objectives

1. Demonstrate knowledge of the symptoms related to the abdominal system by obtaining a focused health history from a peer or patient.
2. Demonstrate inspection of the abdomen by assessing skin condition, symmetry, contour, pulsation, umbilicus, and nutritional state.
3. Demonstrate auscultation of the abdomen by assessing characteristics of bowel sounds and by screening for bruits.
4. Demonstrate percussion of the abdomen by identifying the predominant percussion note, determining liver span, and noting borders of spleen.
5. Demonstrate light palpation by assessing muscular resistance, tenderness, and any masses.
6. Demonstrate deep palpation by assessing for any masses; assessing the liver, spleen, kidneys, and aorta; and assessing any CVA or rebound tenderness.
7. Demonstrate the correct technique of performing the following additional tests when indicated: inspiratory arrest (Murphy's sign); iliopsoas muscle test; obturator test; and rebound tenderness.
8. Record the history and physical examination findings accurately, reach an assessment of the health state, and develop a plan of care.

Instructions

Gather your equipment. Wash your hands. Assess the patient's comfort before starting. Practise the steps of the examination on a peer or a patient in the clinical setting, giving appropriate instructions as you proceed.

Record your findings using the documentation sheets that follow. The first part is intended as a worksheet; the last page is intended for your narrative summary recording using the subjective, objective, assessment, plan (SOAP) format.

NOTES

DOCUMENTATION—THE ABDOMEN

Date _____

Examiner _____

Patient _____ **Age** _____ **Gender** _____

Occupation _____

I. **Health History**

	No	Yes, explain
1. Any change in **appetite**? Loss?		
2. Any difficulty **swallowing**?		
3. Any foods you **cannot tolerate**?		
4. Any **abdominal pain**?		
5. Any **nausea or vomiting**?		
6. How often are **bowel movements**?		
7. Any past history of **gastro-intestinal disease**?		
8. What **medications** are you taking?		

9. Tell me all the food you ate in the last **24 hours**:

   Breakfast   Snack   Lunch   Snack   Dinner   Snack

II. **Physical Examination**

   A. **Inspection**

      Contour of abdomen _____

      General symmetry _____

      Skin colour and condition _____

      Pulsation or movement _____

      Umbilicus _____

      Hair distribution _____

      State of hydration and nutrition _____

      Person's facial expression and position in bed _____

   B. **Auscultation**

      Bowel sounds _____

      Note any vascular sounds _____

   C. **Percussion**

      Percuss in all four quadrants _____

      Percuss borders of liver span in R MCL _____ cm _____

      Percuss spleen _____

_____

D. Palpation

Light palpation in all four quadrants:

Muscle wall _____

Tenderness _____

Enlarged organs _____

Masses _____

Deep palpation in all four quadrants:

Masses _____

Contour of liver _____

Spleen _____

Kidneys _____

Aorta _____

Rebound tenderness _____

CVA tenderness _____

E. Additional tests, if indicated

NOTES

DOCUMENTATION—THE ABDOMEN

Summarize your findings using the SOAP format.

Subjective (Reason for seeking care, health history)

Objective (Physical examination findings)

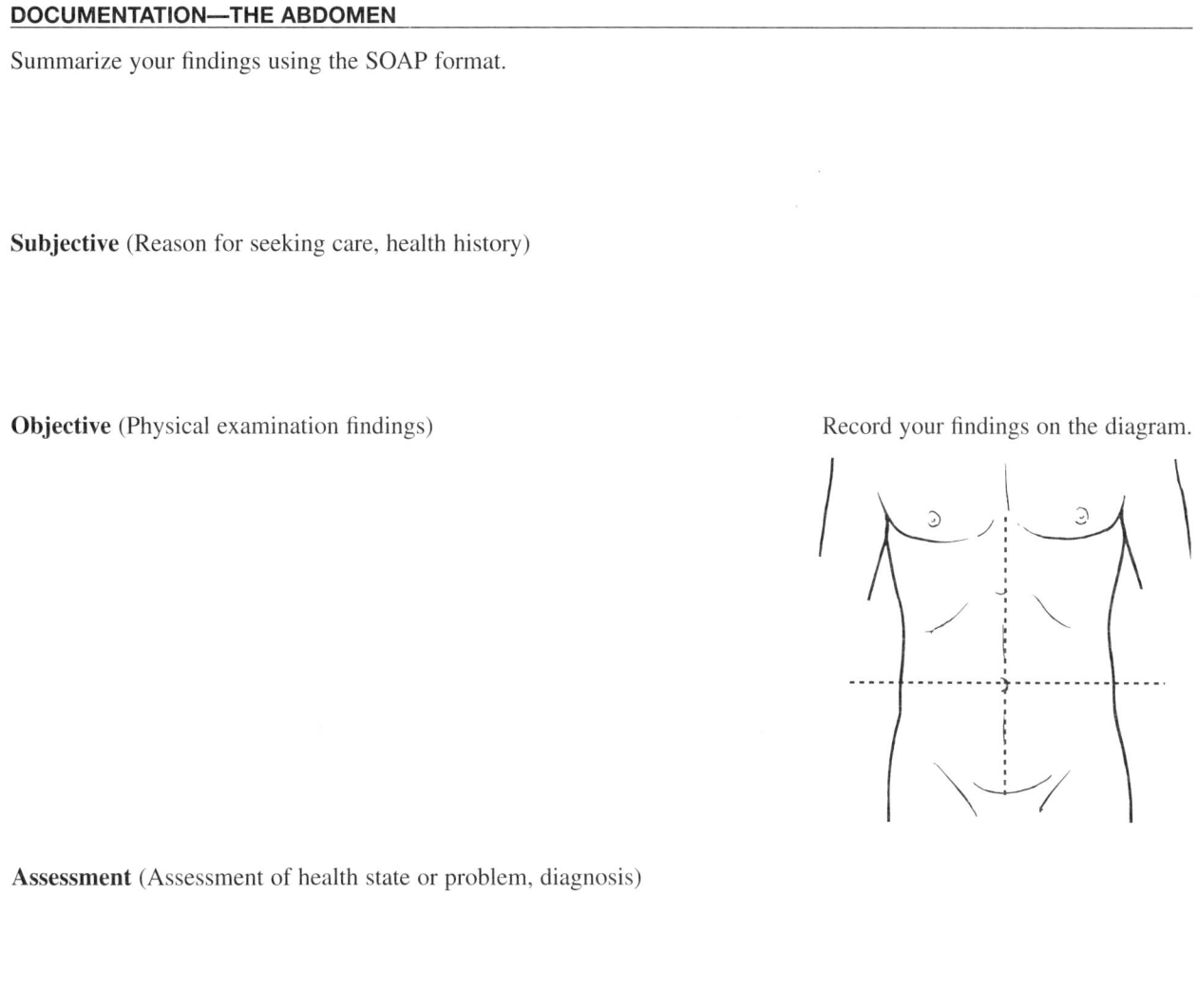

Record your findings on the diagram.

Assessment (Assessment of health state or problem, diagnosis)

Plan (Diagnostic evaluation, follow-up care, patient teaching)

NOTES

23 Anus, Rectum, and Prostate

PURPOSE

This chapter reviews the structure and function of the anus and rectum, and the male prostate gland; the methods of inspection and palpation of these structures; and the accurate recording of the assessment.

READING ASSIGNMENT

Jarvis: *Physical Examination and Health Assessment*, 4th Canadian ed., Chapter 23.

Suggested Readings

Bell, N., Connor Gorber, S., Shane, A., et al. (2014). Recommendations on screening for prostate cancer with the prostate-specific antigen test. *Canadian Medical Association Journal, 186*(16), 1225–1234. https://doi.org/10.1503/cmaj.140703

Dunlap, J. J., & Dunlap, B. S. (2021). Constipation. *Gastroenterology Nursing, 44*(5), 361–364, https://doi.org/10.1097/sga.0000000000000632

GLOSSARY

Study the following terms after reading the corresponding chapter in the text.

Anorectal fistula: an abnormal passage from inner anus or rectum out to skin surrounding anus, created by chronic inflammation in the gastro-intestinal tract; it usually originates from a local abscess

Constipation: a decrease in frequency of bowel movements, defined as three or fewer stools per week, with difficult passing of hard, dry stools

Dyschezia: pain with defecation

Encopresis: persistent involuntary passing of stools into clothing (fecal incontinence) by a child older than age 4 years

Fissure: a painful longitudinal tear in tissue; for example, in the superficial mucosa at the anal margin

Hemorrhoid: flabby papules of skin or mucous membrane in the anal region caused by a varicose vein of the hemorrhoidal plexus

Melena: black or bloody stools

Pruritus: an itching or a burning sensation in the skin

Steatorrhea: excessive fat in the stool, as occurs in malabsorption of fat

Valves of Houston: one of three semilunar transverse folds that cross half the circumference of the rectal lumen

STUDY GUIDE

After completing the reading assignment, you should be able to answer the following questions in the spaces provided.

1. State the length of the anal canal and the rectum in the adult, and describe the location of these structures in the lower abdomen.

2. Describe the size, shape, and location of the male prostate gland.

3. List a few examples of high-fibre foods of the soluble type and of the insoluble type. What advantages do these foods have for the body?

4. List screening measures that are recommended for early detection of colon or rectal cancer, and identify the factors that may indicate a patient is at a higher-than-average risk for colon or rectal cancer.

5. Describe the normal physical characteristics of the prostate gland that would be assessed by palpation, and discuss screening measures recommended for early detection of prostate cancer.

Size _____

Shape _____

Surface _____

Consistency _____

Mobility _____

Sensitivity _____

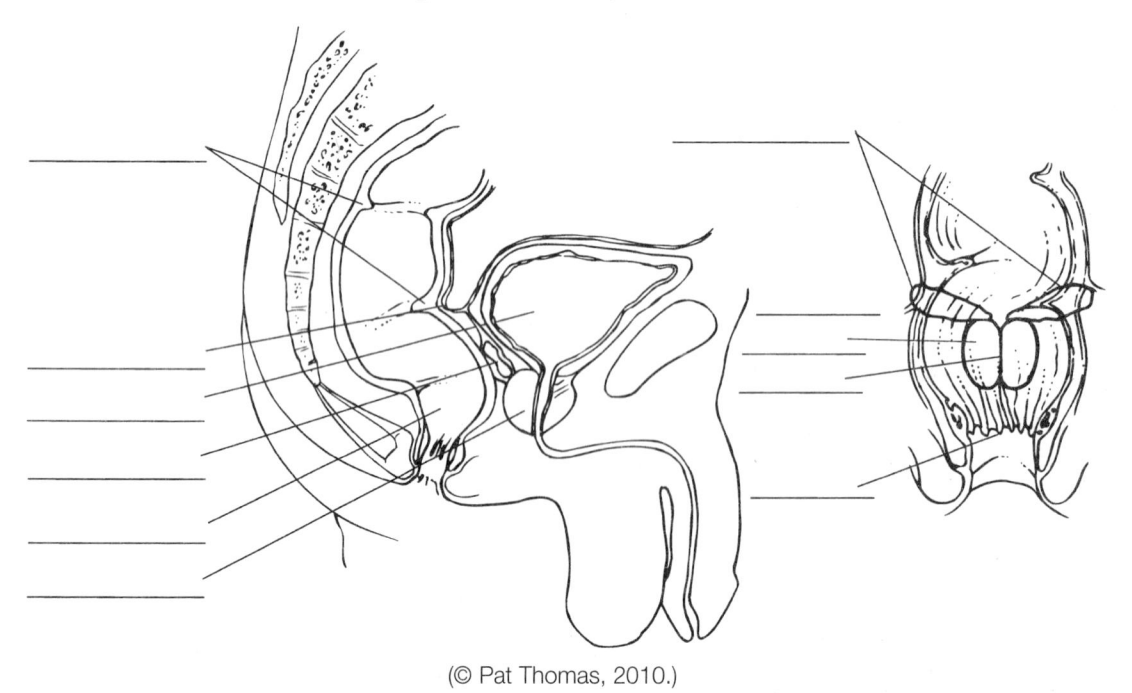

6. Describe the physical appearance and clinical significance of a pilonidal cyst and an anorectal fistula.

7. Define *benign prostatic hypertrophy (BPH)*, list the usual symptoms that a man experiences with this condition, and describe the physical characteristics.

8. Fill in the labels indicated on the following illustration.

(© Pat Thomas, 2010.)

REVIEW AND CLINICAL JUDGEMENT QUESTIONS

This test is for you to check your own mastery of the content. Answers are provided on the text's Evolve site.

1. The gastrocolic reflex is
    a. a peristaltic wave.
    b. the passage of meconium in the newborn.
    c. another term for *borborygmi*.
    d. reverse peristalsis.

2. The incidence of BPH
    a. is highest among males aged 40 to 60 years.
    b. increases with age.
    c. decreases with age.
    d. is not related to age.

3. Select the best description of the anal canal.
    a. a 12-cm-long portion of the large intestine
    b. under involuntary control of the parasympathetic nervous system
    c. a 3.8-cm-long outlet of the gastro-intestinal tract
    d. an S-shaped portion of the colon

4. While good nutrition is important for everyone, foods believed to help reduce the risk for colon cancer are
    a. high in fibre.
    b. low in fat.
    c. high in protein.
    d. high in carbohydrate.

5. Which finding in the prostate gland suggests prostate cancer?
    a. a symmetrical smooth enlargement
    b. extreme tenderness to palpation
    c. a boggy soft enlargement
    d. diffuse hardness

6. The bulbourethral gland
    a. is assessed during an examination of a female patient.
    b. is assessed during an examination of both male and female patients.
    c. is assessed during an examination of a male patient.
    d. cannot be assessed with a rectal examination.

7. Inspection of stool is an important part of the rectal examination. Normal stool is
    a. black in colour and tarry in consistency.
    b. brown in colour and soft in consistency.
    c. clay-coloured and dry in consistency.
    d. variable depending on the individual's diet.

8. Which symptoms suggest BPH?
    a. weight loss and bone pain
    b. fever, chills, urinary frequency, and urgency
    c. difficulty initiating urination and a weak stream
    d. dark, tarry stools

9. A false positive may occur on fecal occult blood tests of the stool if the person has ingested significant amounts of
    a. red meat.
    b. candies with red dye #2.
    c. cranberry juice.
    d. red beets.

10. During history collection, a 66-year-old man tells you that he has trouble urinating, and his provider says his prostate gland is enlarged. He says, "Why do I even have a prostate gland?" Which is your best response?
    a. "It makes a thin, milky fluid to help the sperm stay alive during intercourse."
    b. "The prostate gland often shrinks as you grow older, so your urine troubles can get better."
    c. "The prostate gland secretes mucus into the rectum to help you pass stool."
    d. "The prostate gland passes a substance into the urine to make it more acidic and less likely to get infected."

11. Write a narrative account of a rectal assessment with normal findings.

CRITICAL THINKING EXERCISES

Communication is a crucial component of every patient encounter.

1. Read the Dunlap and Dunlap article listed at the beginning of this chapter. In a small discussion group during your laboratory, address these topics in the article:
   - Compare the causes of primary (functional) constipation and secondary constipation.
   - What further assessment tests are needed when constipation is present?
   - List nonpharmacological interventions to employ with constipation.
   - Many older adults experience constipation. Some discuss it freely; others do not discuss it unless pressed. Think about the older adults with whom you have had experience. How did you react to their discussions of constipation?
2. Read the Bell et al. article listed at the beginning of this chapter. Work with a partner to practise how you would counsel and educate a 53-year-old gentleman with no family history of prostate cancer who, after seeing a "Movember" ad on television, requests a routine prostate-specific antigen (PSA) test.

SKILLS LABORATORY/CLINICAL SETTING

You are now ready for the clinical component of the rectal examination. This regional examination usually is combined with the examination of the male genitalia or with examination of the female genitalia.

Clinical Objectives
1. Demonstrate knowledge of the signs and symptoms related to the rectal area by obtaining a pertinent health history.
2. Inspect and palpate the perianal region.
3. Test any stool specimen for occult blood.
4. Record the history and physical examination findings accurately.

Instructions
Prepare the examination setting, and gather your equipment. Wash your hands; wear gloves during the examination and wash your hands again after removing the gloves. Practise the steps of the examination on a patient in the clinical setting, giving appropriate instructions as you proceed, and assisting the patient as necessary to assume the preferred position. Record your findings using the documentation sheet that follows. Note that only the worksheet is included in this chapter. Your narrative summary recording using the subjective, objective, assessment, plan (SOAP) format can be included with the narrative summary of the genitalia.

NOTES

DOCUMENTATION—ANUS, RECTUM, AND PROSTATE

Date _____

Examiner _____

Patient _____ **Age** _____ **Gender** _____

Occupation _____

I. Health History

	No	Yes, explain
1. Describe usual bowel routine and stools: (regularity, frequency, colour, consistency, straining, pain, incomplete emptying, fecal incontinence)	___	___
2. Describe any **change** in usual bowel habits.	___	___
3. Describe any occurrence of **black or bloody stool, clay-coloured stool, mucus or pu**s in stool, **frothy** stool, or **excessive flatus**.	___	___
4. List relevant **medications** (laxatives, stool softeners, suppositories, enemas, hemorrhoid preparations, iron supplements).	___	___
5. Describe any **rectal conditions** (itching, pain, fissures, fistulae, fecal incontinence, **or hemorrhoids**).	___	___
6. Describe any family history of **colon or rectal polyps, or cancer**.	___	___
7. Describe self-care behaviours (high-fibre foods, most recent examinations, screening, investigations).	___	___

II. Physical Examination

A. Inspect the perianal area.

Skin condition _____

Sacrococcygeal area _____

Note skin integrity while patient performs Valsalva manoeuvre.

B. Palpate the anus, rectum, and surrounding structures.

Anal sphincter _____

Anal canal _____

Rectal wall _____

Prostate gland (for males)

    Size _____

    Shape _____

    Surface _____

    Consistency _____

    Mobility _____

    Any tenderness _____

Cervix through anterior rectal wall (for females) _____

C. Examine stool.

Visual inspection _____

Test for occult blood _____

NOTES

24 Musculo-Skeletal System

PURPOSE

This chapter reviews the structure, function, and normal range of motion of various joints in the body. It also indicates how to position the patient comfortably during the examination. As well, it reviews the rationale for and methods of examination of the musculo-skeletal system; the assessment of functional ability; and the accurate recording of the assessment. At the end of this chapter, you will be able to perform a complete assessment of the musculo-skeletal system.

READING ASSIGNMENT

Jarvis: *Physical Examination and Health Assessment*, 4th Canadian ed., Chapter 24.

Suggested Readings

Korownyk, C. S., Montgomery, L., Young, J., et al. (2022). PEER simplified chronic pain guideline: Management of chronic low back, osteoarthritic, and neuropathic pain in primary care. *Canadian Family Physician, 68*(3), 179–190. https://doi.org/10.46747/cfp.6803179

Niu, S., & Lim, F. (2020). The effects of smoking on bone health and healing. *American Journal of Nursing, 120*(7), 40–46.

GLOSSARY

Study the following terms after reading the corresponding chapter in the text.

Abduction: moving a limb away from the midline of the body

Adduction: moving a limb toward the midline of the body

Ankylosis: immobility, consolidation, and fixation of a joint because of disease, injury, or surgery; it is most often due to chronic rheumatoid arthritis

Bursa: an enclosed sac filled with viscous fluid located in joint areas of potential friction

Circumduction: moving the arm in a circle around the shoulder

Crepitation: a dry, crackling sound or sensation due to grating of the ends of damaged bone

Dorsal: directed toward or located on the surface

Dupuytren's contracture: flexion contractures of the fingers due to chronic hyperplasia of the palmar fascia

Eversion: moving the sole of the foot outward at the ankle

Extension: straightening a limb at a joint

Flexion: bending a limb at a joint

Ganglion cyst: a round, cystic, nontender nodule overlying a tendon sheath or joint capsule, usually on the dorsum of the wrist

Hallux valgus: lateral or outward deviation of the great toe

Inversion: moving the sole of the foot inward at the ankle

Kyphosis: an outward or a convex curvature of the thoracic spine; hunchback

Ligaments: fibrous bands running directly from one bone to another bone that strengthen the joint

Lordosis: inward or concave curvature of the lumbar spine

Nucleus pulposus: the centre of the intervertebral disc

Olecranon process: a bony projection of the ulna at the elbow

Osteoporosis: a loss of bone density

Patella: kneecap

Plantar: surface of the sole of the foot

Pronation: turning the forearm so that the palm is down

Protraction: moving a body part forward and parallel to the ground
Range of motion (ROM): extent of movement of a joint
Retraction: moving a body part backward and parallel to the ground
Rheumatoid arthritis: a chronic systemic inflammatory disease of the joints and surrounding connective tissue
Sciatica: nerve pain along the course of the sciatic nerve that travels down from the back or thigh through the leg and into the foot
Scoliosis: an S-shaped curvature of the thoracic spine
Supination: turning the forearm so that the palm is up
Talipes equinovarus: clubfoot; congenital deformity of the foot in which it is plantar flexed and inverted
Tendon: a strong, fibrous cord that attaches a skeletal muscle to a bone

STUDY GUIDE

After completing the reading assignment, you should be able to answer the following questions in the spaces provided.

1. List four signs that suggest acute inflammation in a joint.

2. Differentiate the following:

    Dislocation

    Subluxation

    Contracture

    Ankylosis

3. Describe the condition of osteoporosis.

    Which bones are most affected?

    Who is at highest risk?

4. Differentiate testing of active range of motion (ROM) versus passive ROM.

5. State the expected range of degrees of flexion and extension of the following joints:

   Elbow

   Wrist

   Fingers (at metacarpophalangeal joints)

6. State the expected range of degrees of flexion and extension of the following joints:

   Hip

   Knee

   Ankle

7. Explain the method for measuring leg length.

8. Describe the Ortolani manoeuvre for checking an infant's hips.

9. State four landmarks to note when checking an adolescent for scoliosis.

10. When performing a functional assessment for an older adult, state the common adaptations the aging person makes when attempting these manoeuvres:
    Walking _____
    Climbing up stairs _____
    Walking down stairs _____
    Picking up an object on the floor _____
    Rising up from sitting in a chair _____
    Rising up from lying in bed _____

11. Describe the symptoms and signs in carpal tunnel syndrome.

    Name and describe two techniques of examination for the syndrome.

12. Draw and describe swan-neck deformity and boutonnière deformity.

13. Contrast Bouchard's nodes with Heberden's nodes.

14. Contrast syndactyly and polydactyly.

15. Fill in the labels indicated on the following illustrations.

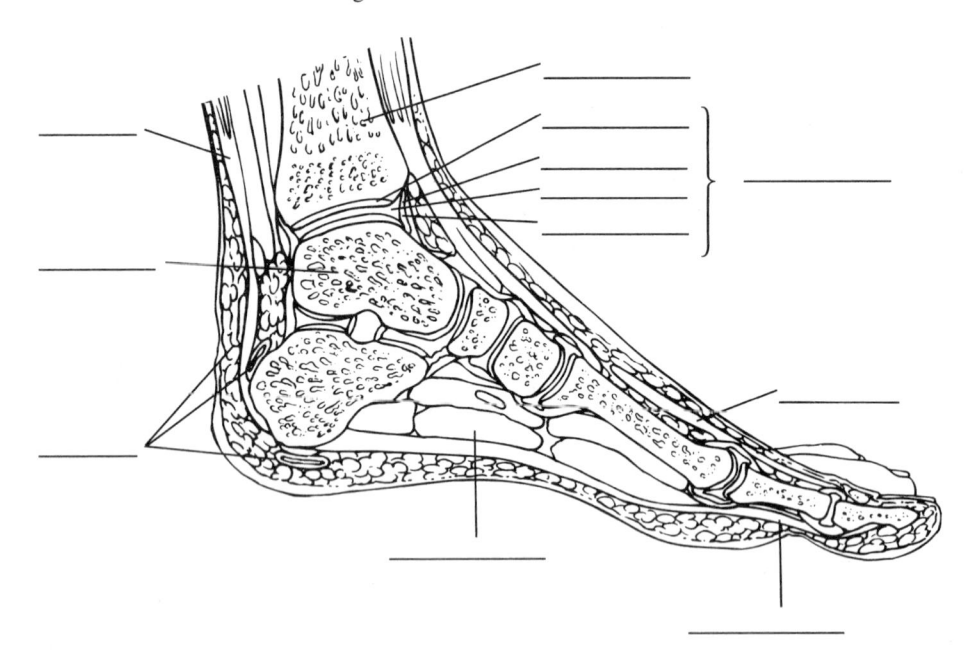

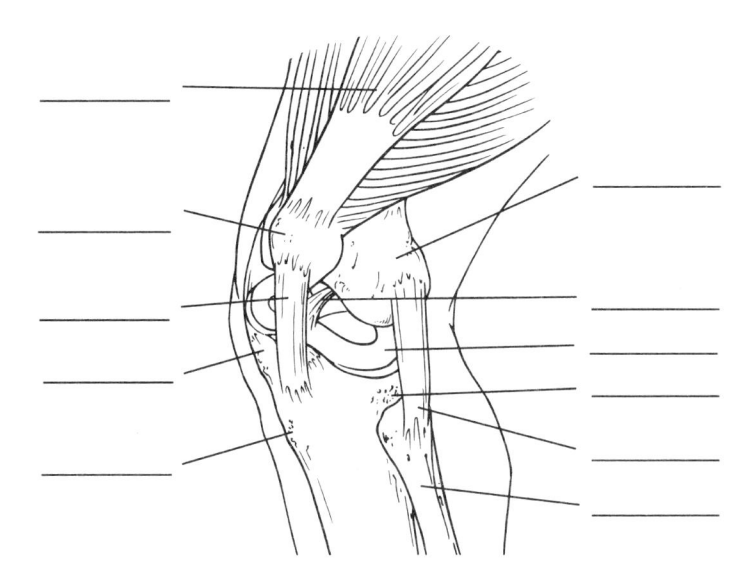

REVIEW AND CLINICAL JUDGEMENT QUESTIONS

This test is for you to check your own mastery of the content. Answers are provided on the text's Evolve site.

1. During an assessment of the spine, the patient would be asked to
   a. adduct and extend.
   b. supinate, evert, and retract.
   c. extend, adduct, invert, and rotate.
   d. flex, extend, abduct, and rotate.

2. Pronation and supination of the hand and forearm are the result of the articulation of
   a. the scapula and clavicle.
   b. the radius and ulna.
   c. the patella and condyle of fibula.
   d. the femur and acetabulum.

3. Anterior and posterior stability is provided to the knee joint by
   a. the medial and lateral menisci.
   b. the patellar tendon and ligament.
   c. the medial collateral ligament and quadriceps muscle.
   d. the anterior and posterior cruciate ligaments.

4. A 70-year-old woman has come for a health examination. As you complete the assessment, you notice several changes in the musculo-skeletal system. Please mark each change as expected or not expected with normal healthy aging.

	Expected	Not Expected
Boggy metacarpophalangeal joints		
Kyphosis		
Lordosis		
Flexion of the hips		
Flexion of the knees		
Osteoarthritis		

5. The timing of joint pain may assist the examiner in determining the cause. The joint pain associated with rheumatic fever would
   a. be worse in the morning.
   b. be worse later in the day.
   c. be worse in the morning but improve during the day.
   d. occur 10 to 14 days after an untreated sore throat.

6. Examination of the shoulder includes
   a. forward flexion, internal rotation, abduction, and external rotation.
   b. abduction, adduction, pronation, and supination.
   c. circumduction, inversion, eversion, and rotation.
   d. elevation, retraction, protraction, and circumduction.

7. The bulge sign is a test for
   a. swelling in the suprapatellar pouch.
   b. carpal tunnel syndrome.
   c. Heberden's nodes.
   d. olecranon bursa inflammation.

8. The examiner is going to measure the patient's legs for length discrepancy. The normal finding would be
   a. no difference in measurements.
   b. a 0.5–cm difference.
   c. within 1 cm of each other.
   d. a 2-cm difference.

9. A 2-year-old child has been brought to the clinic for a health examination. A common finding would be
   a. kyphosis.
   b. lordosis.
   c. scoliosis.
   d. no deviation is normal.

10. Briefly describe the functions of the musculo-skeletal system.

11. Identify which assessment findings are expected in each group. Some findings may be expected in multiple groups.

	Infant	Toddler	Preschool/School Age	Pregnant Woman
Lordosis				
Varus position of feet/legs (flexible)				
Valgus position of feet/legs (flexible)				
Cervical flexion				

12. You are caring for a 52-year-old woman with a 5-year history of rheumatoid arthritis. As you complete the musculo-skeletal assessment, you identify the following assessment and history findings that are expected deviations with rheumatoid arthritis. (Select all that apply.)
    a. symmetrical joint involvement
    b. unilateral joint involvement
    c. lymphadenopathy
    d. increased appetite
    e. weight gain
    f. fatigue
    g. hard, bony protuberances
    h. ulnar drift
    i. bone spur
    j. anorexia

13. You are providing osteoporosis education to a 67-year-old female who is at your clinic for her annual check-up. She has no chronic medical conditions, and her last bone mineral density (BMD) test was normal. The following is the most appropriate teaching for this patient.
    a. "It is recommended that you have a dual-energy X-ray absorptiometry (DEXA) scan to check for osteoporosis every 2 to 5 years. You'll want to continue to eat a healthy diet, exercise at least twice a week, and drink no more than one standard drink per day."
    b. "It is recommended that you have a DEXA scan at least every 5 years. You should continue to 'eat the rainbow' and maintain a healthy weight. Walking is the most appropriate exercise, and weightlifting should be avoided."
    c. "Your last BMD was normal. Continue to maintain a healthy weight and avoid all alcohol. I'd like to check vitamin D levels to ensure you're getting enough in your diet. Given your age, you should consume at least 1 000 mg of calcium each day."
    d. "Your last BMD was normal. It's important that you continue to eat a healthy diet and maintain a healthy weight. You should exercise at least five times each week and consider a combination of cardiovascular, balance, and strength training."

14. You are assessing a patient for scoliosis. From the list below, which four steps should be followed, and in what order?

Potential Steps
a. Position yourself in front of the patient so their entire torso is visible.
b. Note the level of the shoulders, scapulae, and iliac crests.
c. Position yourself behind the patient so their full spine is visible.
d. Note the level of the shoulders, ribs, and superior iliac spine.
e. Ask the patient to bend at the waist and reach for their toes.
f. Note the level of the superior iliac spine while the patient is bent forward.
g. Note the level of the shoulders, ribs, and iliac crests while the patient is bent forward.

Step 1: _____; step 2: _____; step 3: _____; step 4: _____

15. You are assessing a patient with a suspected rotator cuff tear. What assessment findings do you expect? (Select all that apply.)
    a. upright positioning
    b. hunched position
    c. limited adduction
    d. atrophy of shoulder girdle
    e. fluctuant to palpation
    f. limited abduction
    g. positive arm drop test

Match column A to column B.

Column A—Movement

16. _____ Flexion
17. _____ Extension
18. _____ Abduction
19. _____ Adduction
20. _____ Pronation
21. _____ Supination
22. _____ Circumduction
23. _____ Inversion
24. _____ Eversion
25. _____ Rotation
26. _____ Protraction
27. _____ Retraction
28. _____ Elevation
29. _____ Depression

Column B—Description

a. Turning the forearm so that the palm is up
b. Bending a limb at a joint
c. Lowering a body part
d. Turning the forearm so that the palm is down
e. Straightening a limb at a joint
f. Raising a body part
g. Moving a limb away from the midline of the body
h. Moving a body part backward and parallel to the ground
i. Moving a limb toward the midline of the body
j. Moving the arm in a circle around the shoulder
k. Moving the sole of the foot outward at the ankle
l. Moving a body part forward and parallel to the ground
m. Moving the sole of the foot inward at the ankle
n. Moving the head around a central axis

CRITICAL THINKING EXERCISE

Read the Korownyk et al. article listed at the beginning of this chapter. Next, review the Peer Low Back Pain Calculator at https://pain-calculator.com/calculators/low-back-pain/. Work with a partner practising how you would counsel a patient requesting each of the different treatments listed for low back pain.

SKILLS LABORATORY/CLINICAL SETTING

You are now ready for the clinical component of the musculo-skeletal system. The purpose of the clinical component is to practise the regional examination on a peer in the skills laboratory or a patient in the clinical setting and to achieve the following.

Clinical Objectives

1. Demonstrate knowledge of the symptoms related to the musculo-skeletal system by obtaining a focused health history from a peer or patient.

2. Demonstrate inspection and palpation of the musculo-skeletal system by assessing the muscles, bones, and joints for size, symmetry, swelling, nodules, deformities, atrophy, and active ROM.

3. Assess the person's ability to carry out functional activities of daily living.

4. Record the history and physical examination findings accurately, reach an assessment about the health state, and develop a plan of care.

Instructions

Gather your equipment. Wash your hands. Practise the steps of the examination on a peer or a patient in the clinical setting, giving appropriate instructions as you proceed, and maintaining the safety of the person during movement. Record your findings using the documentation sheet that follows. The first part is intended as a worksheet; the last page is intended for your narrative summary recording using the subjective, objective, assessment, plan (SOAP) format.

Note the student competency checklist that follows the documentation sheet. It lists the essential behaviours you should display as an examiner, and it may be used by your clinical instructor to evaluate your clinical musculo-skeletal examination.

DOCUMENTATION—MUSCULO-SKELETAL SYSTEM

Date _____

Examiner _____

Patient _____ Age _____ **Gender** _____

Occupation _____

I. Health History

	No	Yes, explain
1. Any **pain** in the joints?		
2. Any **stiffness** in the joints?		
3. Any **swelling, heat, redness** in the joints?		
4. Any **limitation of movement**?		
5. Any **muscle pain** or cramping?		
6. Any **deformity** of bone or joint?		
7. Any **accidents or trauma** to bones?		
8. Ever had **back pain**?		
9. Any problems with the activities of daily living: bathing, toileting, dressing, grooming, eating, mobility, communicating?		

II. Physical Examination

A. Temporomandibular joint

1. Inspect size, contour _____ Mass or deformity _____

2. Palpate for temperature _____ Pain _____

   Swelling or mass _____

3. Active ROM

   Flexion _____ Extension _____

B. Cervical spine

1. Inspect size, contour _____ Mass or deformity _____

2. Palpate for temperature _____ Pain _____

   Swelling or mass _____

3. Active ROM

   Flexion _____ Extension _____

   Lateral bending right _____ Left _____

   Right rotation _____ Left _____

C. Shoulders

1. Inspect size, contour _____ Colour, swelling _____

   Mass or deformity _____

2. Palpate for temperature _____ Pain _____

   Swelling or mass _____

3. Active ROM

   Flexion _____ Extension _____

   Abduction _____ Adduction _____

   Internal rotation _____ External rotation _____

D. Elbows

1. Inspect for size, contour _____ Colour, swelling _____

   Mass or deformity _____

2. Palpate for temperature _____ Pain _____

   Swelling or mass _____

3. Active ROM

   Flexion _____ Extension _____

   Pronation _____ Supination _____

E. Wrists and hands

1. Inspect for size, contour _____ Colour, swelling _____

   Mass or deformity _____

2. Palpate for temperature _____ Pain _____

   Swelling or mass _____

3. Active ROM

   Wrist extension _____ Flexion _____

   Finger extension _____ Flexion _____

   Ulnar deviation _____ Radial deviation _____

   Fingers spread _____ Make fist _____

   Touch thumb to each finger _____

F. Hips

1. Inspect size, contour _____ Colour, swelling _____

   Mass or deformity _____

2. Palpate for temperature _____ Pain _____

   Swelling or mass _____

3. Active ROM

   Extension _____ Flexion _____

   External rotation _____ Internal rotation _____

   Abduction _____ Adduction _____

G. Knees

1. Inspect size, contour _____ Colour, swelling _____

   Mass or deformity _____

2. Palpate for temperature _____ Pain _____

   Swelling or mass _____

3. Active ROM

   Flexion _____ Extension _____

   Walk _____ Shallow knee bend _____

H. Ankles and feet

1. Inspect for size, contour _____ Colour, swelling _____

   Mass or deformity _____

2. Palpate for temperature _____ Pain _____

   Swelling or mass _____

3. Active ROM

   Dorsiflexion _____ Plantar flexion _____

   Inversion _____ Eversion _____

I. Spine

1. Inspect for straight spinous processes _____

   Equal horizontal positions for shoulders, scapulae, iliac crests, gluteal folds _____

   Equal spaces between arms and lateral thorax _____

   Knees and feet align with trunk, point forward _____

   From side note curvature: cervical, thoracic, lumbar _____

2. Palpate spinous processes

3. Active ROM

   Flexion _____ Extension _____

   Lateral bending right _____ Left _____

   Rotation right _____ Left _____

J. Functional assessment (if indicated)

   Walk (with shoes on).

   Climb up stairs.

   Walk down stairs.

   Pick up object from floor.

   Rise up from sitting in chair.

   Rise up from lying in bed.

DOCUMENTATION—MUSCULO-SKELETAL SYSTEM

Summarize your findings using the SOAP format.

Subjective (Reason for seeking care, health history)

Objective (Physical examination findings)

Assessment (Assessment of health state or problem, diagnosis)

Plan (Diagnostic evaluation, follow-up care, patient teaching)

STUDENT COMPETENCY CHECKLIST

Musculo-Skeletal System—Essential Behaviours

	Yes	No	Comments
Obtain relevant history, functional and self-care assessments.			
Gather equipment.			
Tape measure			
Goniometer			
Skin marking pen			
Light, if needed			
Provide privacy.			
Wash hands.			
Observe for symmetry.			
Inspect each joint for:			
Size			
Contour			
Range of motion (ROM)/limitation			
Inspect skin and tissue joints for:			
Colour			
Swelling			
Masses			
Deformity			
Palpate each joint for:			
Heat			
Tenderness			
Swelling			
Masses			
Test ROM.			
Grade muscle strength.			
Record findings including notations regarding specific joints.			
Temporomandibular			
Cervical spine			
Shoulders			
Elbow			

	Yes	No	Comments
Wrist			
Phalen test			
Tinel's sign			
Hand			
Hip			
Knee			
Ballottement test			
McMurray test			
Ankle			
Foot			
Document findings.			

NOTES

25 Neurological System

PURPOSE

This chapter reviews the structure and function of the components of the neurological system, including the cranial nerves, cerebellar system, motor system, sensory system, and reflexes; the rationale for and methods of examination of the neurological system; and the accurate recording of the assessment. You will be able to perform a complete assessment of the neurological system at the end of this chapter. It can be combined with the mental status examination presented in Chapter 6.

READING ASSIGNMENT

Jarvis: *Physical Examination and Health Assessment*, 4th Canadian ed., Chapter 25.

Suggested Reading

Washington, H. H., Glaser, K. R., & Ifejika, N. L. (2021). CE: Acute ischemic stroke. *The American Journal of Nursing, 121*(9), 26–33. https://doi:10.1097/01.NAJ.0000790184.66496.1d

GLOSSARY

Study the following terms after reading the corresponding chapter in the text.

Analgesia: loss of pain sensation
Aphasia: loss of power of expression by speech, writing, or signs, or of comprehension of spoken or written language
Ataxia: the inability to perform coordinated movements
Athetosis: a bizarre, slow, twisting, writhing movement, resembling a snake or worm
Chorea: a sudden, rapid, jerky, purposeless movement involving limbs, trunk, or face
Clonus: the rapidly alternating involuntary contraction and relaxation of a muscle in response to sudden stretch
Coma: a state of profound unconsciousness from which a person cannot be aroused
Decerebrate rigidity: arms stiffly extended, adducted, internally rotated; legs stiffly extended, plantar flexed
Decorticate rigidity: arms adducted and flexed, wrists and fingers flexed; legs extended, internally rotated, plantar flexed
Deep tendon reflexes: one of the four types of reflexes
Dysarthria: the imperfect articulation of speech due to problems of muscular control resulting from central or peripheral nervous system damage
Extinction: the disappearance of conditioned response
Fasciculation: a rapid, continuous twitching of a resting muscle without movement of limb
Flaccidity: loss of muscle tone, limpness
Graphaesthesia: the ability to "read" a number by having it traced on the skin
Hemiplegia: loss of motor power (paralysis) on one side of the body, usually caused by a cerebrovascular accident; paralysis occurs on the side opposite the lesion
Lower motor neuron: a motor neuron in the peripheral nervous system with its nerve fibre extending out to the muscle and only its cell body in the central nervous system
Myoclonus: the rapid sudden jerk of a muscle
Nystagmus: back-and-forth oscillation of the eyes
Opisthotonos: prolonged arching of the back, with head and heels bent backward; it indicates meningeal irritation
Paraesthesia: an abnormal sensation; that is, burning, numbness, tingling, prickling, or a crawling skin sensation
Paralysis: a decrease or loss of motor function due to problem with motor nerve or muscle fibres
Paraplegia: impairment or loss of motor or sensory function, or both, in the lower half of the body
Point location: ability of the person to discriminate exactly where on the body the skin has been touched
Proprioception: sensory information concerning body movements and position of the body in space

Spasticity: continuous resistance to stretching by a muscle due to abnormally increased tension, with increased deep tendon reflexes
Stereognosis: the ability to recognize objects by feeling their forms, sizes, and weights while the eyes are closed
Tic: the repetitive twitching of a muscle group at inappropriate times; for example, wink, grimace
Tremor: the involuntary contraction of opposing muscle groups resulting in rhythmic movement of one or more joints
Two-point discrimination: the ability to distinguish the separation of two simultaneous pinpricks on the skin
Upper motor neuron: a nerve located entirely within the central nervous system
Vibration: a sensation conducted by the posterior (dorsal) columns; the ability to feel vibrating objects

STUDY GUIDE

After completing the reading assignment, you should be able to answer the following questions in the spaces provided.

1. List the major function(s) of the following components of the central nervous system (CNS):

   Cerebral cortex—frontal lobe _____

   Cerebral cortex—parietal lobe _____

   Cerebral cortex—temporal lobe _____

   Cerebral cortex—Wernicke's area _____

   Cerebral cortex—Broca's area _____

   Basal ganglia _____

   Thalamus _____

   Hypothalamus _____

   Cerebellum _____

   Midbrain _____

   Pons _____

   Medulla _____

   Spinal cord _____

2. List the primary sensations mediated by the two major sensory pathways of the CNS.

3. Describe three major motor pathways in the CNS, including the type of movements mediated by each.

4. Differentiate an upper motor neuron from a lower motor neuron.

5. List the five components of a deep tendon reflex arc.

6. List the major symptom areas to assess when collecting a health history for the neurological system.

7. List the method of testing for each of the 12 cranial nerves.

8. List and describe three tests of cerebellar function.

9. Describe the method of testing the sensory system for pain, temperature, touch, vibration, and position.

10. Define the five-point grading scale for deep tendon reflexes.

11. State the vertebral level whose intactness is assessed when eliciting each of these reflexes:

    Biceps reflex _____

    Triceps reflex _____

    Brachioradialis reflex _____

    Quadriceps reflex _____

    Achilles reflex _____

12. List the components of the neurological reassessment examination that are performed routinely on hospitalized people being monitored for neurological deficit.

13. List the three areas of assessment on the Glasgow Coma Scale.

14. Describe the gait patterns of the following abnormal gaits:

    Spastic hemiparesis _____
    _____

    Cerebellar ataxia _____
    _____

    Parkinsonian _____
    _____

    Scissors _____
    _____

    Steppage _____
    _____

    Waddling _____
    _____

    Short leg _____
    _____

15. State the type of reflex response you would expect to see with an upper motor neuron lesion versus a lower motor neuron lesion.

16. Describe the method of testing the type of reflexes that are also termed *frontal release signs*.

17. Distinguish *dysphonia* from *dysarthria*.

18. Fill in the labels indicated on the following illustrations.

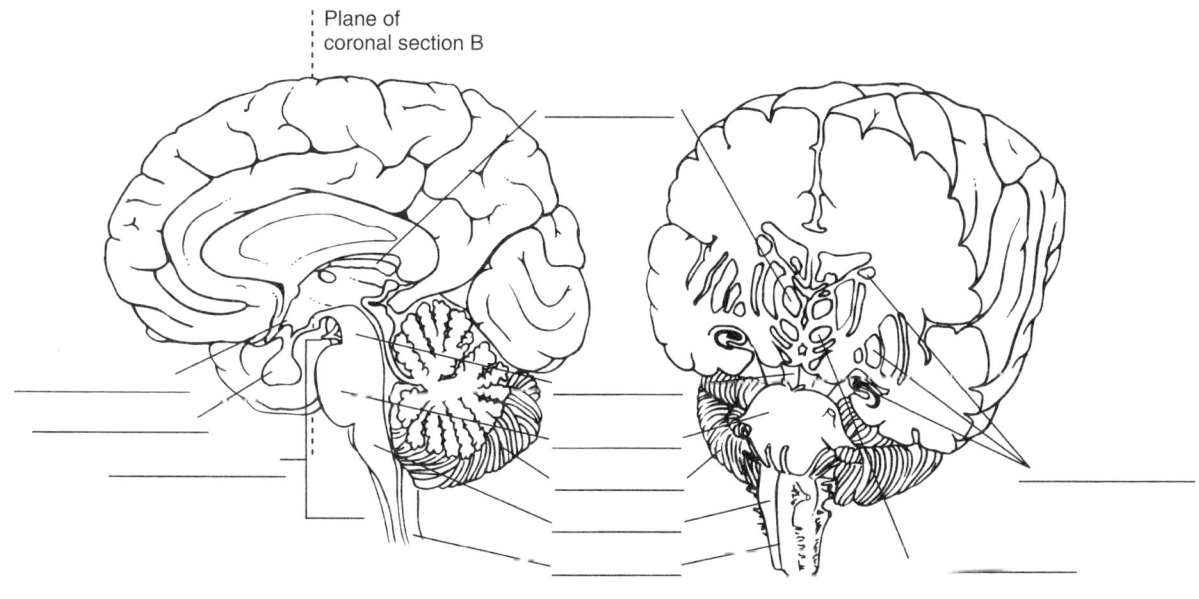

Plane of coronal section B

A. Medial view of right hemisphere

B. Coronal section

CONTENTS OF THE CENTRAL NERVOUS SYSTEM

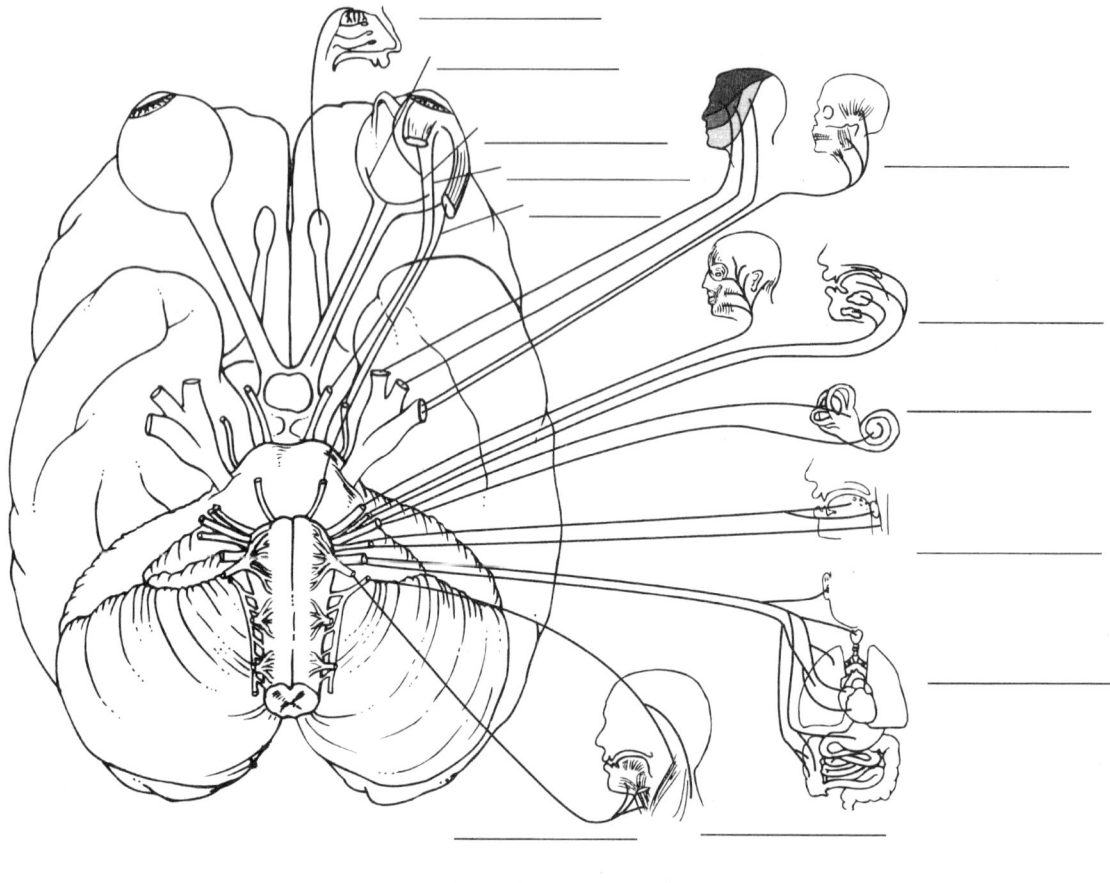

(© Pat Thomas, 2006.)

Fill in the name of each cranial nerve, then write S (sensory), M (motor), or MX (mixed).

REVIEW AND CLINICAL JUDGEMENT QUESTIONS

This test is for you to check your own mastery of the content. Answers are provided on the text's Evolve site.

1. The medical record indicates that a person has an injury to Broca's area. When meeting this person you expect
   a. difficulty speaking.
   b. receptive aphasia.
   c. visual disturbances.
   d. emotional lability.

2. The control of body temperature is located in
   a. Wernicke's area.
   b. the thalamus.
   c. the cerebellum.
   d. the hypothalamus.

3. To test for stereognosis, you would
   a. have the person close his or her eyes, then raise the person's arm and ask the person to describe its location.
   b. touch the person with a tuning fork.
   c. place a coin in the person's hand, and ask him or her to identify it.
   d. touch the person with a cold object.

4. During the examination of an infant, use a cotton-tipped applicator to stimulate the anal sphincter. The absence of a response suggests a lesion of
   a. L2.
   b. T12.
   c. S2.
   d. C5.

5. During a neurological examination, the tendon reflex fails to appear. Before striking the tendon again, the examiner might use the technique of
   a. two-point discrimination.
   b. reinforcement.
   c. vibration.
   d. graphaesthesia.

6. Cerebellar function is assessed by which of the following tests?
   a. muscle size and strength
   b. cranial nerve examination
   c. coordination—hopping on one foot
   d. spinothalamic test

7. To elicit a Babinski reflex, the examiner should
   a. gently tap the Achilles tendon.
   b. stroke the lateral aspect of the sole of the foot from heel to the ball.
   c. present a noxious odour to a person.
   d. observe the person walking heel to toe.

8. A positive Babinski sign is
   a. dorsiflexion of the big toe and fanning of all toes.
   b. plantar flexion of the big toe with a fanning of all toes.
   c. the expected response in healthy adults.
   d. withdrawal of the stimulated extremity from the stimulus.

9. The cremasteric response is
   a. positive when disease of the pyramidal tract is present.
   b. positive when the ipsilateral testicle elevates upon stroking of the inner aspect of the thigh.
   c. a reflex of the receptors in the muscles of the abdomen.
   d. not a valid neurological examination.

10. To examine for the function of the trigeminal nerve in an infant, you would
    a. startle the baby.
    b. hold an object within the child's line of vision.
    c. pinch the nose of the child.
    d. offer the baby a bottle.

11. Senile tremors may resemble parkinsonism, except that senile tremors do not include
    a. nodding the head as if responding "yes" or "no."
    b. rigidity and weakness of voluntary movement.
    c. tremor of the hands.
    d. tongue protrusion.

12. People who have Parkinson's disease usually have which of the following characteristic styles of speech?
    a. a garbled manner
    b. loud, urgent
    c. slow, monotonous
    d. word confusion

Match column A to column B.

Column A—Cranial Nerve

13. _____ Olfactory (I)
14. _____ Optic (II)
15. _____ Oculomotor (III)
16. _____ Trochlear (IV)
17. _____ Trigeminal (V)
18. _____ Abducens (VI)
19. _____ Facial (VII)
20. _____ Acoustic (VIII)
21. _____ Glossopharyngeal (IX)
22. _____ Vagus (X)
23. _____ Spinal (XI)
24. _____ Hypoglossal (XII)

Column B—Function

a. Movement of the tongue
b. Vision
c. Lateral movement of the eyes
d. Hearing and equilibrium
e. Talking, swallowing, carotid sinus, and carotid reflex
f. Smell
g. Extraocular movement, pupil constriction, down and inward movement of the eye
h. Mastication and sensation of face, scalp, cornea
i. Phonation, swallowing, taste in the posterior third of tongue
j. Movement of trapezius and sternomastoid muscles
k. Down and inward movement of the eye
l. Taste in the anterior two thirds of tongue, closing of the eyes

CRITICAL THINKING EXERCISE

Read the Washington et al. article on acute ischemic stroke listed at the beginning of this chapter. Because strokes are so common in North America, and because strokes are potentially so devastating, the improvement of risk factors for stroke is crucial.

1. To understand the impact of risk factors, review the risk and prevention page on the heart and stroke foundation web site at s://www.heartandstroke.ca/stroke/risk-and-prevention. Discuss ways in which you can alter your lifestyle to decrease the risk factors for a stroke when you are older.
2. Apply the assessment tool again, but base the assessment on an older adult in your family or among your acquaintances. How does your personal score compare with that of this older adult?
3. Finally, take on the role of the health care provider and formulate a patient teaching plan that addresses how the older adult can reduce their risk for stroke.

SKILLS LABORATORY/CLINICAL SETTING

You are now ready for the clinical component of the neurological system. The purpose of the clinical component is to practise the regional examination on a peer in the skills laboratory or a patient in the clinical setting and to achieve the following.

Clinical Objectives

1. Demonstrate knowledge of the symptoms related to the neurological system by obtaining a focused health history from a peer or patient.
2. Demonstrate examination of the neurological system by assessing the cranial nerves, motor system, sensory system, deep tendon reflexes, and cerebellar function.
3. Record the history and physical examination findings accurately, reach an assessment of the health state, and develop a plan of care.

Instructions

Gather all equipment for a complete neurological examination. Wash your hands. Practise the steps of the examination on a peer or a patient in the clinical setting, giving appropriate instructions as you proceed. Record your findings using the documentation sheet that follows. The first part is intended as a worksheet; the last page is intended for your narrative summary recording using the subjective, objective, assessment, plan (SOAP) format.

DOCUMENTATION—NEUROLOGICAL SYSTEM

Date _____

Examiner _____

Patient _____ Age _____ Gender _____

Occupation _____

I. Health History

	No	Yes, explain
1. Any unusual frequent or unusually severe **headaches**?		
2. Ever had any **head injury**?		
3. Ever feel **dizziness**?		
4. Ever had any **convulsions**?		
5. Any **tremors** in hands or face?		
6. Any **weakness** in any body part?		
7. Any problem with **coordination**?		
8. Any **numbness or tingling**?		
9. Any problem **swallowing**?		
10. Any problem **speaking**?		
11. Past history of stroke, spinal cord injury, meningitis, congenital defect, alcoholism?		
12. Any environmental or occupational hazards (e.g., insecticide exposure)?		

II. Physical Examination

A. Cranial nerves

I _____

II _____

III, IV, VI _____

V _____

VII _____

VIII _____

IX, X _____

XI _____

XII _____

B. Motor system

1. Muscles:

   Size, strength, tone _____

   Involuntary movements _____

2. Cerebellar function:

   Gait _____

   Romberg test _____

Rapid alternative movements _____

Finger-to-finger test _____

Finger-to-nose test _____

Heel-to-shin test _____

C. Sensory system

1. Spinothalamic tract:

    Pain _____

    Temperature _____

    Light touch _____

2. Posterior column tract:

    Vibration _____

    Position (kinaesthesia) _____

    Tactile discrimination _____

    Stereognosis _____

    Graphaesthesia _____

    Two-point discrimination _____

D. Reflexes

	Bi	Tri	BR	P	A	PL (↑/↓)	Abd	Cre	Bab
R									
L									

Abd = abducens; A = Achilles; Bab = Babinski; Bi = biceps; BR = brachioradialis; Cre = cremasteric; P = patellar; PL = plantar; Tri = triceps.
0 = absent, 1+ = hypoactive, 2+ = normal, 3+ = hyperactive, 4+ = hyperactive with clonus, ↑ = dorsiflexion, ↓ = plantar flexion.

DOCUMENTATION—NEUROLOGICAL SYSTEM

Summarize your findings using the SOAP format.

Subjective (Reason for seeking care, health history)

Objective (Physical examination findings)   Record reflexes on the diagram.

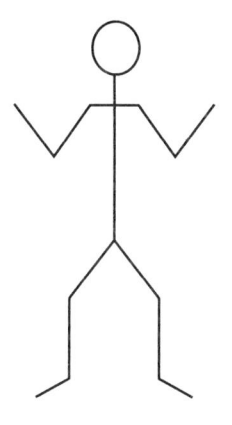

Assessment (Assessment of health state or problem, diagnosis)

Plan (Diagnostic evaluation, follow-up care, patient teaching)

NOTES

26 Male Genitourinary System

PURPOSE

This chapter reviews the structure and function of the male genitalia; the methods of inspection and palpation of these structures; and the accurate recording of the assessment.

READING ASSIGNMENT

Jarvis: *Physical Examination and Health Assessment*, 4th Canadian ed., Chapter 26.

Suggested Reading

Aho, J., Lybeck, C., Tetteh, A., et al. (2022). Rising syphilis rates in Canada, 2011–2020. *Canadian Communicable Disease Report, 48*(23), 52–60. https://doi.org/10.14745/ccdr.v48i23a01

GLOSSARY

Study the following terms after reading the corresponding chapter in the text.

Chancre: a red, round, superficial ulcer with a yellowish serous discharge that is a sign of syphilis
Circumcision: an elective surgical procedure to remove all or part of the foreskin (prepuce) from the penis, usually performed on newborn males
Condylomata acuminate: soft, pointed, fleshy papules that occur on the genitalia and are caused by the human papillomavirus (HPV)
Cryptorchidism: undescended testes
Cystitis: inflammation of the urinary bladder
Epididymis: a structure composed of coiled ducts located over the superior and posterior surface of the testes; it stores sperm
Epispadias: a congenital defect in which the urethra opens on the dorsal (upper) side of the penis instead of at the tip
Genital herpes: a sexually transmitted infection characterized by clusters of small, painful vesicles; caused by a virus
Hernia: a weak spot in abdominal muscle wall (usually in area of inguinal canal or femoral canal) through which a loop of bowel may protrude
Hydrocele: cystic fluid in the tunica vaginalis surrounding the testis
Hypospadias: a congenital defect in which the urethra opens on the ventral (under) side of the penis rather than at the tip
Orchitis: acute inflammation of the testis, usually associated with mumps
Paraphimosis: when the foreskin is retracted and fixed behind the glans penis
Peyronie's disease: nontender, hard plaques on the surface of penis, associated with painful bending of the penis during erection
Phimosis: when the foreskin is advanced and tightly fixed over the glans penis
Prepuce: foreskin; the hood or flap of skin over the glans penis that often is surgically removed after birth by circumcision
Priapism: prolonged, painful erection of the penis without sexual stimulation
Spermatic cord: collection of vas deferens, blood vessels, lymphatics, and nerves that ascends along the testis and through the inguinal canal into the abdomen
Spermatocele: a retention cyst in epididymis filled with milky fluid that contains sperm
Torsion: a sudden twisting of spermatic cord; a surgical emergency
Varicocele: a dilated tortuous varicose veins in the spermatic cord
Vas deferens: a duct carrying sperm from the epididymis through the abdomen and then into the urethra

STUDY GUIDE

After completing the reading assignment, you should be able to answer the following questions in the spaces provided.

1. Describe the function of the cremaster muscle.

2. Identify the structures that provide transport of sperm.

3. Describe the significance of the inguinal canal and the femoral canal.

4. List the pros and cons of circumcision of the male newborn.

5. Discuss ways of creating an environment that will provide psychological comfort for the man and the examiner during examination of male genitalia.

6. List teaching points to include with the teaching of testicular self-examination.

7. Discuss the rationale for making certain that testes have descended in the male infant.

8. Contrast the physical appearance and clinical significance of these scrotal lumps:

   Epididymitis _____

   _____

   Varicocele _____

   _____

   Spermatocele _____

   _____

   Testicular tumour _____

   _____

   Hydrocele _____

   _____

9. Contrast the anatomical course and the clinical significance of these hernias:

   Indirect inguinal _____

   _____

   Direct inguinal _____

   _____

   Femoral _____

   _____

10. Identify the normal bladder capacity, daily total volume of urine output, and the average bladder volume that typically initiates the urge to void.

11. Fill in the labels indicated on the following illustrations.

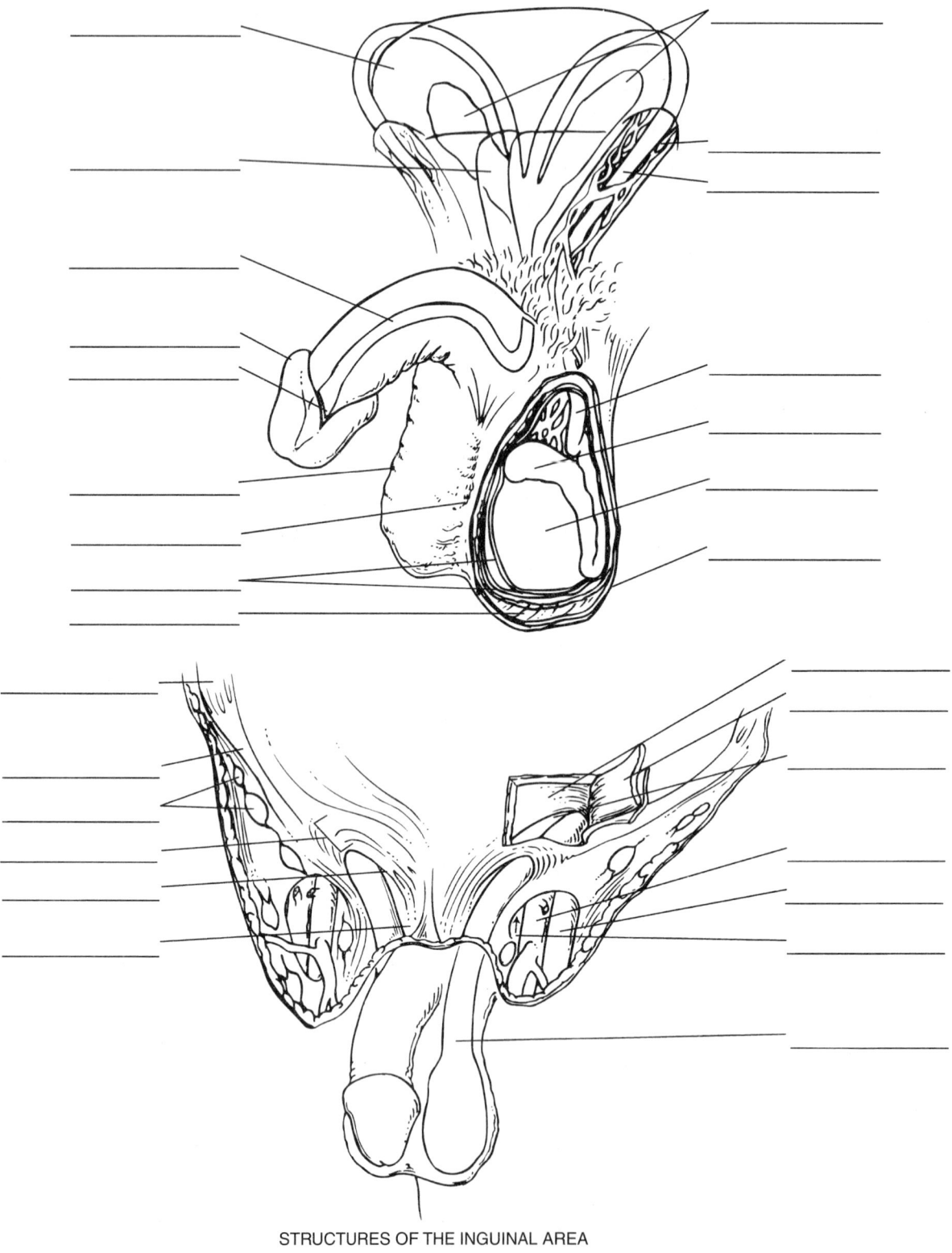

STRUCTURES OF THE INGUINAL AREA
(© Pat Thomas, 2010.)

228
Chapter 26 Male Genitourinary System

REVIEW AND CLINICAL JUDGEMENT QUESTIONS

This test is for you to check your own mastery of the content. Answers are provided on the text's Evolve site.

1. The examiner is going to inspect and palpate for a hernia. During this examination, the man is instructed to
   a. hold his breath during palpation.
   b. cough after the examiner has gently inserted the examination finger into the rectum.
   c. bear down when the examiner's finger is at the inguinal canal.
   d. relax in a supine position while the examiner's finger is inserted into the canal.

2. During examination of the scrotum, a normal finding would be that
   a. the left testicle is firmer to palpation than the right.
   b. the left testicle is larger than the right.
   c. the left testicle hangs lower than the right.
   d. the left testicle is more tender to palpation than the right.

3. H.T. has come to the clinic for a follow-up visit. Six months ago, he was started on a new medication. The class of medication is most likely to cause impotence as a side effect; therefore, medication classes explored by the nurse are
   a. antipyretics.
   b. bronchodilators.
   c. corticosteroids.
   d. antihypertensives.

4. Prostatic hypertrophy occurs frequently in older men. The symptoms that may indicate this problem are
   a. polyuria and urgency.
   b. dysuria and oliguria.
   c. straining, loss of force, and sense of residual urine.
   d. foul-smelling urine and dysuria.

5. A 64-year-old man has come for a health examination. A normal, age-related change in the scrotum would be
   a. testicular atrophy.
   b. testicular hypertrophy.
   c. pendulous scrotum.
   d. increase in scrotal rugae.

6. During palpation of the testes, the normal finding would be
   a. firm to hard, and rough.
   b. nodular.
   c. 2 to 3 cm long by 2 cm wide and firm.
   d. firm, rubbery, and smooth.

7. A 20-year-old man has indicated that he does not perform testicular self-examination. One of the facts that should be shared with him is that testicular cancer, though rare, does occur most commonly in men aged
   a. under 15.
   b. 15 to 49.
   c. 50 to 65.
   d. 65 and older.

8. During the examination of a full-term newborn male, a finding requiring investigation would be
   a. absent testes.
   b. meatus centred at the tip of the penis.
   c. wrinkled scrotum.
   d. penis 2 to 3 cm in length.

9. During transillumination of a scrotum, you note a nontender mass that transilluminates with a red glow. This finding is suggestive of
   a. scrotal hernia.
   b. scrotal edema.
   c. orchitis.
   d. hydrocele.

10. How sensitive to pressure are normal testes?
    a. somewhat
    b. not at all
    c. left more sensitive than right
    d. only when inflammation is present

11. The congenital displacement of the urethral meatus to the inferior surface of the penis is
    a. hypospadias.
    b. epispadias.
    c. hypoaesthesia.
    d. hypophysis.

12. You are about to examine the genitalia of a 93-year-old man who has an adhesion of the prepuce of the head of the penis, making the foreskin impossible to retract. You recognize this as
    a. paraphimosis.
    b. phimosis.
    c. smegma.
    d. dyschezia.

13. The first physical sign associated with puberty in boys is
    a. height spurt.
    b. penis lengthening.
    c. sperm production.
    d. pubic hair development.
    e. testes enlargement.

14. Write a narrative account of an assessment of male genitalia with healthy findings.

CRITICAL THINKING EXERCISE

It may surprise you to learn that there is an alarming and continued increase in the incidence of syphilis in the United States and Canada. Read the Aho et al. article listed at the beginning of this chapter. Consider the risk factors presented in the article concerning groups at higher risk of acquiring syphilis, as well as the assessment factors. Place yourself in the health care provider role of assessing and teaching a person with syphilis. Prepare a script for this teaching. Use the content in this article. Make your script nonjudgmental and free of medical jargon. Practise your delivery on a peer in your lab setting. The role of "patient" should be (1) a young sexually active woman having oral or vaginal sex; (2) a man having oral, anal, or insertive sex; (3) a person using substances, particularly methamphetamine; (4) a pregnant person.

SKILLS LABORATORY/CLINICAL SETTING

You are now ready for the clinical component of the male genitalia examination. Because of the need to maintain personal privacy, you will not practise this examination on a classmate. You will probably practise with a teaching mannequin in the skills laboratory or with a male in the clinical setting under the guidance of a preceptor. Before you proceed, discuss the feelings that may be experienced by the man and the examiner, and methods to increase the comfort of both. Make sure you have discussed the steps of the examination with your instructor before examining a patient.

Clinical Objectives

1. Demonstrate knowledge of the signs and symptoms related to the male genitalia by obtaining a pertinent health history.
2. Inspect and palpate the penis and scrotum.
3. Palpate the inguinal region for hernia.
4. Teach testicular self-examination.
5. Record the history and physical examination findings accurately, reach an assessment of the health state, and develop a plan of care.

Instructions

Prepare the examination setting, and gather your equipment. Wash your hands; wear gloves during the examination. Practise the steps of the examination on a male in the clinical setting, giving appropriate instructions as you proceed. Record your findings using the documentation sheet that follows. The front of the page is intended as a worksheet; the back of the page is intended for your narrative summary recording using the subjective, objective, assessment, plan (SOAP) format.

Note the student competency checklist that follows the documentation sheet. It lists the essential behaviours you should display as an examiner, and it may be used by your clinical instructor to evaluate your clinical teaching of testicular self-examination.

NOTES

NOTES

DOCUMENTATION—MALE GENITOURINARY SYSTEM

Date _____

Examiner _____

Patient _____ Age _____ Gender _____

Occupation _____

I. Health History

	No	Yes, explain
1. Any urinary **frequency, urgency**, or waking during the night to urinate?		
2. Any **pain** or **burning** with urinating?		
3. Any **trouble** starting **urine** stream?		
4. Urine **colour cloudy** or **foul-smelling**? **Red-tinged** or **bloody**?		
5. Any **problem controlling your urine**?		
6. Any **pain** or **sores** on penis?		
7. Any **lump** in testicles or scrotum? Do you perform testicular self-examination?		
8. In a relationship now involving intercourse? Use a contraceptive? Which one?		
9. Any contact with a partner who has a sexually transmitted infection?		

II. Physical Examination

A. Inspect and palpate the penis.

Skin condition _____

Glans _____

Urethral meatus _____

Shaft _____

B. Inspect and palpate the scrotum.

Skin condition _____

Testes _____

Spermatic cord _____

Transillumination (if indicated) _____

C. Inspect and palpate for hernia.

Inguinal canal _____

Femoral area _____

D. Palpate the inguinal lymph nodes.

E. Teach testicular self-examination.

DOCUMENTATION—MALE GENITOURINARY SYSTEM

Summarize your findings using the SOAP format.

Subjective (Reason for seeking care, health history)

Objective (Physical examination findings)

Assessment (Assessment of health state or problem, diagnosis)

Plan (Diagnostic evaluation, follow-up care, patient teaching)

STUDENT COMPETENCY CHECKLIST

Teaching Testicular Self-Examination (TSE)

	S	U	Comments
I. Cognitive			
1. Explain:			
a) Why testicles are examined			
b) Who should perform TSE			
c) Frequency of testicular examination			
2. Describe the technique.			
II. Performance			
1. Explain to males the need for TSE.			
2. Instruct males on technique of TSE by:			
a) Describing method of palpating testicles			
b) Describing normal findings			
c) Describing abnormal findings to look for			
3. Instruct males to report unusual findings promptly.			

NOTES

27 Female Genitourinary System

PURPOSE

This chapter reviews the structure and function of the female genitalia; the methods of inspection and palpation of the internal and external structures; the procedures for collection of cytological specimens; and the accurate recording of the assessment.

READING ASSIGNMENT

Jarvis: *Physical Examination and Health Assessment*, 4th Canadian ed., Chapter 27.

Suggested Readings

Davis, N. J., Wyman, J. F., Gubitosa, S., et al. (2020). Urinary incontinence in older adults. *The American Journal of Nursing, 120*(1), 57–62. https://doi.org/10.1097/01.naj.0000652124.58511.24

Gogineni, V., Waselewski, M. E., Jamison, C. D., et al. (2021). The future of STI screening and treatment for youth. *BMC Public Health*, 21, 1–9. https://doi.org/10.1186/s12889-021-12091-y

GLOSSARY

Study the following terms after reading the corresponding chapter in the text.

Adnexa: accessory organs of the uterus; that is, ovaries and fallopian tubes

Amenorrhea: the absence of menstruation; it is termed *secondary amenorrhea* when menstruation has begun and then ceases; most common cause is pregnancy

Bartholin's glands: vestibular glands located on either side of the vaginal orifice; they secrete a clear lubricating mucus during intercourse

Bloody show: dislodging of the thick cervical mucus plug at the end of pregnancy; it is a sign of beginning of labour

Caruncle: a small, deep-red mass protruding from the urethral meatus, usually due to urethritis

Chadwick's sign: bluish discoloration of the cervix that occurs normally in pregnancy at 6 to 8 weeks' gestation

Chancre: a red, round, superficial ulcer with a yellowish serous discharge that is a sign of syphilis

Clitoris: a small, elongated, erectile tissue in the female, located at the anterior juncture of labia minora

Cystocele: prolapse of urinary bladder and its vaginal mucosa into the vagina

Dysmenorrhea: abdominal cramping and pain associated with menstruation

Dyspareunia: painful intercourse

Dysuria: painful urination

Endometriosis: aberrant growths of endometrial tissue scattered throughout the pelvis

Fibroid: myoma; hard, painless nodules in uterine wall that cause uterine enlargement

Gonorrhea: a sexually transmitted infection (STI) characterized by purulent vaginal discharge, or it may have no symptoms

Hegar's sign: softening of the cervix that is a sign of pregnancy, occurring at 10 to 12 weeks' gestation

Hematuria: bloody urine

Hymen: a membranous fold of tissue partly closing the vaginal orifice

Leukorrhea: whitish or yellowish discharge from vaginal orifice

Menarche: onset of first menstruation, usually between 11 and 13 years of age

Menopause: cessation of the menses, usually occurring around 48 to 51 years of age

Menorrhagia: excessively heavy menstrual flow

Multiparous: condition of having two or more pregnancies

Nulliparous: condition of first pregnancy

Papanicolaou (Pap) test: a test used to detect cervical cancer

Polyp: cervical polyp is a bright-red, soft, pedunculated growth emerging from os

Rectocele: prolapse of the rectum and its vaginal mucosa into vagina

Rectouterine pouch: cul-de-sac of Douglas; the deep recess formed by the peritoneum between the rectum and cervix
Salpingitis: inflammation of the fallopian tubes
Skene's glands: paraurethral glands
Vaginitis: inflammation of the vagina
Vulva: external genitalia of female

STUDY GUIDE

After completing the reading assignment, you should be able to answer the following questions in the spaces provided.

1. List the external structures of the female genitalia.

2. Describe the size, shape, and location of the internal structures of the female genitalia.

3. Outline the changes observed during the perimenopausal period.

4. Discuss ways of creating an environment that will provide psychological comfort for both the person receiving care and practitioner during the female genitalia examination.

5. Discuss selection, preparation, and insertion of the vaginal speculum.

6. Describe the appearance or sketch these normal variations of the cervix and os:

    Nulliparous

    Parous

    Stellate lacerations

    Cervical eversion

    Nabothian cysts

7. List the steps in obtaining the following specimens:

   Cervical scrape using spatula

   Endocervical specimen using cytobrush

8. Discuss the procedure and rationale for bimanual examination, and list normal findings for the cervix, uterus, and adnexa.

9. Discuss infection control precautions taken during examination of female genitalia and procuring of specimens.

10. Describe or sketch the appearance of the following abnormalities of the cervix:

    Chadwick's sign

    Erosion

    Polyp

    Carcinoma

11. List the characteristics of vaginal discharge associated with the following conditions of vaginitis:

    Atrophic vaginitis _____

    Candidiasis _____

    Trichomoniasis _____

    Bacterial vaginosis _____

    Chlamydia _____

    Gonorrhea _____

12. Differentiate the signs and symptoms of these conditions of adnexal enlargement:

    Ectopic pregnancy _____

    Ovarian cyst _____

13. Fill in the labels indicated on the following illustrations.

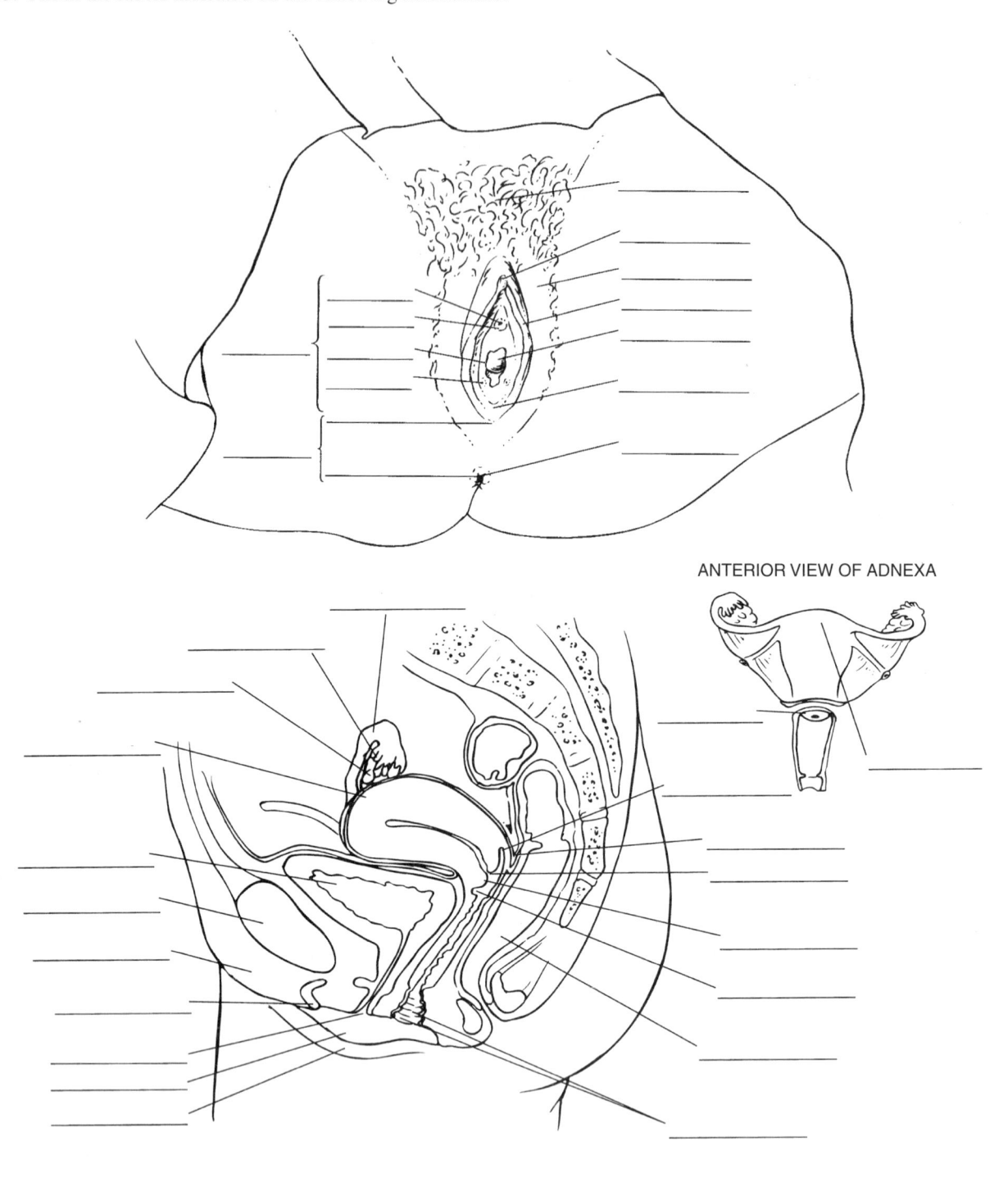

ANTERIOR VIEW OF ADNEXA

REVIEW AND CLINICAL JUDGEMENT QUESTIONS

This test is for you to check your own mastery of the content. Answers are provided on the text's Evolve site.

1. Vaginal lubrication is provided during intercourse by
   a. the labia minora.
   b. sebaceous follicles.
   c. Skene's glands.
   d. Bartholin's glands.

2. A 25 year old female has come for her first gynecological examination. Because the patient has not had any children, the examiner would expect the cervical os to appear
   a. smooth and circular.
   b. irregular and slit like.
   c. irregular and circular.
   d. smooth and enlarged.

3. A 28 year old female has come for an examination because of a missed menstrual period and a positive home pregnancy test. Examination reveals a cervix that appears cyanotic. This is referred to as
   a. Goodell's sign.
   b. Hegar's sign.
   c. Tanner's sign.
   d. Chadwick's sign.

4. During the examination of the genitalia of a 70-year-old female, a normal finding would be
   a. hypertrophy of the mons pubis.
   b. increase in vaginal secretions.
   c. thin and sparse pubic hair.
   d. bladder prolapse.

5. A woman has come for health care complaining of a thick, white vaginal discharge with intense itching. These symptoms are suggestive of
   a. atrophic vaginitis.
   b. trichomoniasis.
   c. chlamydia.
   d. candidiasis.

6. To prepare the vaginal speculum for insertion, the examiner
   a. lubricates it with warm water or a water-soluble lubricant.
   b. lubricates it with petrolatum.
   c. warms it under the light, then inserts it into the vagina.
   d. lubricates it with hot water.

7. To insert the speculum as comfortably as possible, the examiner
   a. opens the speculum slightly and inserts in an upward direction.
   b. presses the introitus down with one hand and inserts the blades obliquely with the other.
   c. spreads the labia with one hand, inserts the closed speculum horizontally with the other.
   d. pushes down on the introitus and inserts the speculum in an upward direction.

8. Select the best description of the uterus.
   a. anteverted, round asymmetrical organ
   b. pear-shaped, thick-walled organ flattened anteroposteriorly
   c. retroverted, almond-shaped asymmetrical organ
   d. midposition, thick-walled oval organ

9. In placing a finger on either side of the cervix and moving it side to side, you are assessing
   a. the diameter of the fallopian tube.
   b. cervical motion tenderness.
   c. the ovaries.
   d. the uterus.

10. Which of the following is (are) normal, common finding(s) on inspection and palpation of the vulva and perineum?
    a. labia majora that are wide apart
    b. palpable Bartholin's glands
    c. clear, thin discharge from paraurethral glands
    d. bulging at introitus during Valsalva's manoeuvre

11. Which of the following is the most common bacterial sexually transmitted infection in Canada?
    a. human papillomavirus
    b. gonorrhea
    c. trichomoniasis
    d. syphilis
    e. bacterial vaginosis

12. Write a narrative account of an assessment of female genitalia with normal findings.

13. When discussing sexuality or sexual feelings with teenagers, a permission statement helps to communicate that it is normal and healthy to think or to feel a certain way. Which of the following would you consider to be a permission statement?
    a. "It's okay for teens your age to have sex."
    b. "Often youth have questions about sex and sexual activity. What questions do you have?"
    c. "Now I want to ask you some questions about sexual activity. I ask all girls these questions."
    d. "Do you use condoms every time you have sex?"

14. You are preparing a female patient for a pelvic examination in the lithotomy position. What measures can you employ to ease her comfort? (Select all that apply.)
    a. Elevate her head and shoulders to keep eye contact during the examination.
    b. Ask her to place her arms up and behind her head.
    c. Position a chaperone standing by the woman's head.
    d. Make sure she has emptied her bladder before the examination.
    e. Position her buttocks 15 cm up from the edge of the table so that she will not feel she will fall off.
    f. State, "now I'm going to . . ." before each step in the examination.
    g. Touch the inner thigh before you directly touch the vulva.

15. You are caring for a 32-year-old female who presents to the clinic with vaginal discharge. She has not had vaginal intercourse for 5 years before arrival. She reports (A) _____. Your physical examination reveals (B) _____. You suspect she has (C) _____.

(A) Subjective Findings	(B) Objective Findings	(C) Condition
1 —No further significant symptoms	1 —Red and swollen vulva and vagina. Thick, white, curdy, nonsmelling discharge	1 —Trichomoniasis
2 —Urinary frequency and painful urination	2 —Reddened vaginal walls with tiny red spots	2 —Chlamydia
3 —Urinary frequency and intense itching	3 —Tenderness on moving cervix	3 —Candidiasis (Moniliasis) Gonorrhea
4 —Intense itching, recent treatment for bronchitis	4 —Purulent vaginal discharge, no further abnormal examination findings	

CRITICAL THINKING EXERCISES

1. Read the Davis et al. article, listed at the beginning of the chapter, on the common condition of urinary incontinence occurring in older adults. One type, stress incontinence, occurs in women of all ages, especially athletes!
   a. Differentiate between urge incontinence and stress incontinence.
   b. How would you frame an assessment by health history for an older adult with incontinence?
   c. Discuss the ways incontinence can lead to social isolation, strain on caregivers, falls, pressure injuries, and depression.

2. Read the Gogineni et al. article, listed at the beginning of this chapter, on screening youth for common STIs (chlamydia and gonorrhea). Study the representative respondent quotes listed in Table 2 of the article.
   a. Answer the research questions yourself:
      - "Would it be hard for you to get TESTED for chlamydia or gonorrhea if you wanted?"
      - "If you tested positive, would it be hard for you to get TREATED for chlamydia or gonorrhea?"
      - "If you thought you had chlamydia or gonorrhea, where would you go to get treatment?"
      - "If you got chlamydia or gonorrhea, would you tell your sexual partner(s)? Why or why not?"
   b. Now discuss these questions as if you were an under-resourced person. What are the barriers to care?
   c. What is the incidence of these common STIs in youth aged 15 to 24 years? What are the risks of untreated infections?
   d. At many sites, a woman can collect her own vaginal swab specimen and bring it in for testing for STIs. What advantages do you see with this technique?

SKILLS LABORATORY/CLINICAL SETTING

You are now ready for the clinical component of the female genitalia examination. Because of the need to maintain personal privacy, you will not practise this examination on a peer. You will probably practise with a teaching mannequin in the skills laboratory or with a woman in the clinical setting under the guidance of a preceptor. Before you proceed, discuss the feelings that may be experienced by the woman and examiner, and methods to increase the comfort of both. With your instructor, discuss methods of positioning the woman, steps in using the vaginal speculum, steps in procuring specimens, and methods of infection control precautions.

Clinical Objectives

1. Demonstrate knowledge of the signs and symptoms related to the female genitourinary system by obtaining a pertinent health history.
2. Demonstrate measures to increase comfort before and during the female genitourinary examination.
3. Demonstrate knowledge of infection control precautions before, during, and after the examination.
4. Inspect and palpate the external genitalia.
5. Using the vaginal speculum, gather materials for cytological study.
6. Inspect and palpate the internal genitalia.
7. Record the history and physical examination findings accurately, reach an assessment of the health state, and develop a plan of care.

Instructions

Prepare the examination setting, and gather your equipment. Collect the health history prior to the patient disrobing for the examination. Wash your hands; wear gloves during the examination; wash hands again after removing gloves. Practise the steps of the examination on a woman in the clinical setting, giving appropriate instructions as you proceed. Record your findings using the documentation sheet that follows. The first part is intended as a worksheet; the last page is intended for your narrative summary recording using the subjective, objective, assessment, plan (SOAP) format. Collection of data for the rectal examination is usually combined with the examination of female genitalia; see Chapter 23 of this study guide for the documentation sheet for the rectal examination.

NOTES

DOCUMENTATION—FEMALE GENITOURINARY SYSTEM

Date _____

Examiner _____

Patient _____ Age _____ Gender _____

Occupation _____

I. Focused Health History

	No	Yes, explain
1. Date of **last menstrual period**? Do you have a period? Age at first period? Usual cycle? Duration? Usual amount of flow? Any pain or cramps with period?		
2. Ever been **pregnant**? How many times? Describe pregnancy(ies) Any complications?		
3. Periods slowed down or **stopped**?		
4. How often do you have a **gynecological checkup**? Date of last Pap test? Results?		
5. Any problem with **urinating**?		
6. Any unusual **vaginal discharge**?		
7. **Sores or lesions** in genitals?		
8. In a relationship now involving intercourse?		
9. Use a contraceptive? Which one?		
10. Any contact with a partner who has a sexually transmitted infection (STI)?		
11. Any precautions to reduce risk for STIs?		
12. Taking any medications? Any hormone therapy?		

II. Physical Examination

A. Inspect the external genitalia.

Skin colour and characteristics _____

Hair distribution _____

Infestations _____

Symmetry _____

Clitoris _____

Labia _____

Urethral opening _____

Vaginal opening _____

Perineum _____

B. Palpate the external genitalia.

Skene's glands _____

Bartholin's glands _____

Perineum _____

Assessment of perineal muscle strength _____

Assess for vaginal wall bulging or urinary incontinence _____

Discharge and characteristics _____

C. Examine with the speculum.

Inspect vaginal vault, cervix, and os.

Colour _____

Moisture _____

Rugae _____

Position _____

Size _____

Surface _____

Discharge and characteristics/odours _____

Obtain cervical smears and cultures.

Vaginal pool _____

Cervical/endocervical specimen _____

Other (if indicated) _____

Acetic acid wash (if indicated/desired) _____

Inspect vaginal wall as speculum is removed _____

D. Perform the bimanual examination.

Cervix:

Consistency _____

Mobility _____

Tenderness with motion _____

Uterus:

Size and shape _____

Consistency _____

Position _____

Mobility _____

Tenderness _____

Adnexa: _____

Able to palpate? (Be honest.) _____

Size and shape of ovaries _____

Tenderness _____

Masses _____

Rectovaginal examination: _____

DOCUMENTATION—FEMALE GENITOURINARY SYSTEM

Summarize your findings using the SOAP format.

Subjective (Reason for seeking care, health history)

Objective (Physical examination findings)

Record your findings on the diagram.

Assessment (Assessment of health state or problem, diagnosis)

Plan (Diagnostic evaluation, follow-up care, patient teaching)

NOTES

UNIT 4 INTEGRATION OF THE HEALTH ASSESSMENT

28 The Complete Health Assessment: Putting It All Together

PURPOSE

This chapter reviews how to integrate focused examinations so that you will be able to conduct a complete, head-to-toe physical examination on an adult patient.

READING ASSIGNMENT

Jarvis: *Physical Examination and Health Assessment*, 4th Canadian ed., Chapter 28.

CLINICAL OBJECTIVES

1. Demonstrate skills of inspection, percussion, palpation, and auscultation during the physical examination.
2. Demonstrate the correct use of instruments, including assembly, manipulation of component parts, and positioning with patient.
3. Use appropriate terminology, and correctly pronounce medical terminology with the clinical instructor and the patient.
4. Complete the head-to-toe examination in a systematic manner, including integration of the assessments for each system throughout the examination (e.g., skin, musculo-skeletal).
5. Coordinate procedures to limit position changes for the examiner and patient.
6. Accurately describe the findings of the examination, including normal and abnormal findings.
7. Demonstrate appropriate infection control measures.
8. Recognize and maintain the privacy and dignity of the patient.
   a. Adequately explain what is being done while limiting small talk.
   b. Consider the patient's anxiety and fears.
   c. Consider your own facial expression; professional, sensitive language use; and comments.
   d. Demonstrate confidence, empathy, and a gentle manner.
   e. Acknowledge and apologize for any discomfort caused.
   f. Provide for privacy.
   g. Determine the patient's comfort level, pausing if the patient becomes tired.
   h. Wash hands, and use gloves appropriately.
   i. Allow adequate time for each step.
   j. Briefly summarize findings to the patient, and thank the patient for their time.

Instructions

The key to developing high-quality health assessment and physical examination skills is practice. You should conduct at least five complete physical examinations in preparation for this final examination. You may be responsible for obtaining a peer or volunteer "patient" for the examination, or you may be assigned a peer or volunteer "patient." You should prepare your own health assessment–physical examination template for the examination and for later use in your clinical experiences. You may refer to these templates minimally during the examination, but overdependence on your notes will decrease your efficiency and constitute failure. You will have 45 minutes in which to conduct the examination (not including setup).

Genitalia, breast, and fundoscopic examinations are not completed on the volunteer patient but are verbalized only.

If you prepare and practise adequately, you should have no difficulty completing the examination in the allotted time.

Prepare the examination setting: Arrange for proper lighting. Arrange adequate patient gown, blankets, and drapes as appropriate.

Gather equipment: The items in the equipment list that follows are needed for a complete physical examination (including the examination of female genitalia). Check with your instructor for any items that you may omit for your own examination proficiency.

Equipment List:

Platform scale with height attachment
Sphygmomanometer with appropriate-size cuff
Stethoscope with bell and diaphragm endpieces or function
Antimicrobial wipes for cleaning equipment
Thermometer
Flashlight or penlight
Otoscope/ophthalmoscope
Tuning fork
Nasal speculum (if a short, broad speculum is not included with the otoscope)
Tongue depressor
Snellen eye chart pocket vision screener
Skin-marking pen
Flexible measuring tape and ruler marked in centimetres
Reflex hammer
Sharp object (split tongue blade or long cotton-tip swab)
Cotton balls or cotton-tip swab
Bivalve vaginal speculum
Disposable gloves
Materials for cytological study and vaginal swabs
Water-soluble lubricant
Fecal occult blood test (FOBT or iFOBT) materials

Record your findings using the documentation sheets that follow. After you have completed the examination and documentation, return your completed documentation to your instructor.

Good luck!

NOTES

COMPLETE PHYSICAL EXAMINATION

Date _____

Examiner _____

Patient _____ Age _____ **Gender** _____

Preferred Pronouns _____ **Occupation** _____

General Survey of Patient
Inspect:

1. Appears stated age _____
2. Level of consciousness _____
3. Apparent nutritional status _____
4. Posture and position _____
5. Obvious physical deformities _____
6. Mobility: gait, use of assistive devices, no involuntary movement _____
   _____
7. Facial expression _____
8. Mood and affect _____
9. Speech: articulation, pattern, content appropriate, first language _____
10. Hearing _____
11. Personal hygiene _____
12. Signs of distress or discomfort _____

Measurement and Vital Signs

1. Weight _____
2. Height _____
3. Body mass index _____
4. Vision using Snellen eye chart _____
   Right eye _____ Left eye _____ Correction? _____
5. Radial pulse, rate, and rhythm _____
6. Respirations, rate, depth _____
7. Blood pressure
   Right arm _____ (sitting or lying down?)
   Left arm _____ (sitting or lying down?)
8. Temperature (if indicated) _____
9. Pain assessment _____

Stand in Front of Patient, Patient Is Sitting

Skin
Inspect and palpate:

1. Hands and nails _____

2. For the rest of the examination, examine the skin of the corresponding region for the following:

   Colour and pigmentation _____

   Temperature _____

   Moisture _____

   Texture _____

   Turgor _____

   Any lesions _____

Head and Face
Inspect and palpate:

1. Scalp, hair, cranium _____

2. Face (cranial nerve VII) _____

3. Temporal artery, temporomandibular joint _____

4. Maxillary sinuses, frontal sinuses _____

Eyes
Inspect and palpate:

1. Visual fields (cranial nerve II) _____

2. Extraocular muscles, corneal light reflex _____

   Cardinal positions of gaze (cranial nerves III, IV, VI) _____

3. External eye structures _____

4. Conjunctivae _____

5. Sclerae _____

6. Corneas _____

7. Irides _____

8. Pupils _____

9. Ophthalmoscopic examination _____

10. Red reflex _____

11. Disc* _____

12. Vessels* _____

13. Retinal background* _____

---

*Fundoscopic examination components are verbalized only. Most programs do not require students to conduct actual ophthalmoscopic examinations using light ophthalmoscopes during their physical examination, for the comfort of volunteer patients who may be volunteering for more than one student in a day. Students are asked to verbalize the fundoscopic examination and demonstrate the skill without use of the light.

Ears
Inspect and palpate:

1. External ear _____
2. Ear canal, with an otoscope _____
3. Tympanic membrane _____
4. Hearing test (cranial nerve VIII, voice test) _____
5. Weber test _____
6. Rinne test _____

Nose
Inspect and palpate:

1. External nose _____
2. Patency of nostrils _____
3. Nasal mucosa, with a speculum _____
4. Septum _____
5. Turbinates _____

Mouth and Throat
Inspect and palpate:

1. Lips and buccal mucosa _____
2. Teeth and gums _____
3. Tongue _____
4. Hard/soft palate _____
5. Tonsils _____
6. Uvula (cranial nerves IX, X) _____
7. Tongue (cranial nerve XII) _____

Neck
Inspect and palpate:

1. Symmetry, lumps, pulsations _____
2. Cervical lymph nodes _____
3. Carotid pulse (bruits if indicated) _____
4. Trachea _____
5. Thyroid _____
6. ROM and muscle strength (cranial nerve XI) _____

Upper Extremities
Inspect and palpate:

1. Symmetry, bulk, and tone _____
2. Skin characteristics, hair distribution _____
3. Temperature, edema, masses _____
4. Pulse–radial _____
5. Epitrochlear lymph nodes _____
6. ROM _____
7. Muscle strength _____

Patient Is Sitting
Palpate

Chest and Lungs, Posterior, Anterior, and Lateral
Inspect:

1. AP diameter _____
2. Skin characteristics _____
3. Symmetrical expansion _____

Palpate:

4. Tactile fremitus _____
5. Lumps or tenderness _____
6. Spinous processes _____

Percuss:

7. Lung fields _____
8. Diaphragmatic excursion _____
9. Costovertebral angle tenderness _____

Auscultate:

10. Breath sounds _____
11. Egophony, bronchophony, or whispered pectoriloquy (student to demonstrate one) _____

Heart—Sitting
Inspect and palpate:

1. Precordium: pulsations, heaves, thrills _____
2. Apical impulse _____

Auscultate:

3. Apical rate and rhythm _____

Patient Is Supine, Stand at Patient's Right
Breasts and Axillae
Palpate:

1. Symmetry, mobility, dimpling, skin changes _____

2. Supraclavicular and infraclavicular areas _____

3. Breast palpation using vertical strip pattern _____

4. Nipple _____

5. Axillae and regional nodes _____

Neck Vessels
Inspect:

1. Jugular venous pulse _____

2. Jugular venous pressure (if indicated) _____

Heart—Supine
Inspect and palpate:

1. Precordium: pulsations, heaves, thrills _____

2. Apical impulse _____

Auscultate:

3. Apical rate and rhythm _____

4. Heart sounds in all listening areas with bell and diaphragm: _____

Abdomen
Inspect:

1. Contour, symmetry _____

    Skin characteristics _____

    Umbilicus and pulsations _____

Auscultate:

2. Bowel sounds _____

3. Aortic, renal, iliac, femoral arteries for bruits (students are not expected to demonstrate femoral bruits and instead can describe their landmarking for this) _____

Percuss:

4. Percussion _____

5. Liver span in right midclavicular line _____

6. Spleen _____

Palpate:

    7. Light and deep palpation _____

    8. Palpation of liver, spleen, kidneys, aorta _____

    9. Abdominal reflexes (if indicated) _____

Inguinal Area
Inspect and palpate (verbalize only):

    1. Femoral pulse _____

    2. Inguinal nodes _____

Lower Extremities
Inspect and palpate:

    1. Symmetry, bulk, and tone _____

    2. Skin characteristics, hair distribution _____

    3. Joint swelling, deformity _____

    4. Temperature _____

    5. Pulses _____

        Popliteal _____

        Posterior tibial _____

        Dorsalis pedis _____

Patient Sits Upright

    6. ROM and muscle strength _____

        Hips _____

        Knees _____

        Ankles and feet _____

Neurological System
Inspect and palpate:

    1. Sensation _____

        Face _____

        Arms and hands _____

        Legs and feet _____

Test:

    2. Position sense _____

    3. Stereognosis _____

    4. Cerebellar function, rapid alternating movements (RAM) test _____

    5. Cerebellar function, finger to nose _____

6. Cerebellar function, heel to shin _____

7. Deep tendon reflexes _____

   Brachioradialis _____

   Biceps _____

   Triceps _____

   Patellar _____

   Achilles _____

8. Babinksi/Plantar reflex _____

Patient Stands Upright
Musculo-Skeletal System
Inspect:

1. Walk across room _____

   Walk, heel to toe (tandem gait) _____

2. Walk on tiptoes, then walk on heels _____

3. Shallow knee bend _____

4. ROM of spine _____

Test:

5. Romberg's sign _____

Male Genitalia (Verbalize Only)
Drape and position patient comfortably, explain procedures, use language sensitively.

Inspect:

1. Penis and scrotum _____

2. Testes and spermatic cord _____

3. Inguinal hernia (if indicated) _____

Educate:

4. Teach testicular self-examination (if indicated) _____

Male Rectum (Verbalize Only)
Drape and position patient comfortably, explain procedures, use language sensitively.

Inspect:

1. Perianal area _____

2. Rectal walls and prostate gland _____

3. Stool for FOBT (if indicated) _____

Female Patient in Lithotomy Position
Female Genitalia and Rectum (Verbalize Only)
Drape and position patient comfortably, explain procedures, use language sensitively.

Inspect:
1. External genitalia and perianal area _____
2. Vaginal speculum: cervix and vaginal walls _____
3. Procure specimens (if indicated) _____
4. Bimanual: cervix, uterus, and adnexa (if indicated) _____
5. Rectovaginal examination (if indicated) _____
6. Stool for FOBT (if indicated) _____

Closure
1. Help patient sit up _____
2. Ensure patient's needs are met and that patient is comfortable _____
3. Thank patient for time, and depart from patient _____

NOTES

29 Bedside Assessment and Reporting

PURPOSE

This chapter helps you learn the methods of integrating focused examinations in a manner that suits the inpatient setting. The selection and sequencing of the techniques included here are intended to provide an assessment that is efficient, thorough, and consistent with the assessments performed by other nurses in the course of 24-hour care.

READING ASSIGNMENT

Jarvis: *Physical Examination and Health Assessment*, 4th Canadian ed., Chapter 29.

Suggested Reading
Oren, G. T., Lazzara, E. H., Keebler, J. R., et al. (2021). Dissecting communication barriers in healthcare: A path to enhancing communication resiliency, reliability, and patient safety. *Journal of Patient Safety, 17*(8), e1465–e1471.

CLINICAL OBJECTIVES

1. Demonstrate the skills of inspection, percussion, palpation, and auscultation.
2. Demonstrate the correct use of instruments (including assembly), manipulation of component parts, and positioning of the patient.
3. Use appropriate terminology, and correctly pronounce medical terminology with the clinical instructor and the patient.
4. Complete the bedside examination in a systematic manner, including integration of certain focused assessments throughout the examination (e.g., skin, musculo-skeletal).
5. Coordinate procedures to limit position changes for the examiner and patient.
6. Accurately describe the findings of the examination, including normal and abnormal findings.
7. Demonstrate appropriate infection control measures.
8. Recognize and maintain the privacy and dignity of the patient.
    a. Adequately explain what is being done while limiting small talk.
    b. Consider the patient's anxiety and fears.
    c. Consider your own facial expression; professional, sensitive language use, and comments.
    d. Demonstrate confidence, empathy, and a gentle manner.
    e. Acknowledge and apologize for any discomfort caused.
    f. Provide for privacy.
    g. Determine the patient's comfort level, pausing if the patient becomes tired.
    h. Wash hands, and use gloves appropriately.
    i. Allow adequate time for each step.
    j. Briefly summarize findings to the patient, and thank the patient for their time.
9. Complete all procedures with attention to specifics of technique, which allows clear and consistent replication of the procedures by other nurses assessing the same patient.
10. Document the assessment and findings in a systematic, efficient, and accurate manner. This includes attending to documentation in paper or electronic health record (EHR) format (or a combination of both).

INSTRUCTIONS

As with other assessments, this particular version of the head-to-toe examination requires a great deal of practice before you feel truly confident. The assessment outlined in this section is directly applicable to any inpatient clinical site in which you provide care. If you have already begun your clinical experiences, you are advised to use this assessment to assess your assigned patients.

You may be responsible for recruiting a peer or volunteer patient for this examination, or you may have a peer or volunteer patient assigned. Create and use a template to complete the assessment. You should not use your template as step-by-step instructions, but rather as a double-check to ensure nothing has been omitted. Once this examination is over, you can use these templates during your clinical learning experiences.

You will have 20 minutes for this examination, not including setup. If you have practised the individual regional and head-to-toe assessments thoroughly and have practised this particular sequence at least five times, you should be able to complete it satisfactorily within the time allotted.

Prepare the examination setting: Arrange the lighting, furniture, and bed to allow for the most efficient and comfortable activity for yourself and your patient. Think carefully about the functions of the patient's hospital bed. It can be useful to raise the bed closer to your eyes and stethoscope, but you cannot expect the patient to get out of bed safely from that height. Position sheets, drapes, and bath blankets strategically to achieve the proper balance of modesty, efficiency, and comfort.

Gather and arrange your equipment before you begin: The following items are needed for this sequence, but your instructor may modify the equipment list slightly for your individual class or exercise.

Equipment List:

Water (in a cup)
Watch with a second hand
Stethoscope
Blood pressure cuff
Pulse oximeter
Penlight
Ruler in millimetres

Oxygen equipment (as indicated by your instructor)
Doppler (as indicated by your instructor)
Bladder scanner (as indicated by your instructor)
Standardized scales to calculate the patient's fall risk and risk for skin breakdown
Documentation forms (as included here, or provided by your instructor)

After you have completed your assessment, document the assessment and submit it to your instructor.
  Good luck!

NOTES

COMPLETE INPATIENT REASSESSMENT

Date _____

Examiner _____

Patient _____ **Age** _____ **Gender** _____

Preferred Pronouns _____ **Occupation** _____

Introduction
1. Check for flags or markers at doorway.
2. Introduce yourself.
3. Perform hand hygiene.
4. Make eye contact.
5. Offer water.
6. Check name band.
7. Ask appropriate interview questions.
8. Elevate the bed to appropriate height.

General Appearance
1. Facial expression _____
2. Body position _____
3. Level of consciousness _____
4. Skin colour _____
5. Nutritional status _____
6. Speech: articulation, pattern, content appropriate _____
7. Hearing _____
8. Personal hygiene _____

Measurement and Vital Signs
1. Measure temperature _____
2. Measure pulse _____
3. Measure respiration _____
4. Measure blood pressure _____
5. Measure pulse oximetry (oxygen saturation) _____
6. Assess weight on admission or if daily weight is indicated _____
7. Rate pain level on 0 to 10 scale; note ability to tolerate pain _____
8. Reassess pain, if appropriate to scenario _____

Skin
1. Inspect hands and nails _____
2. For the rest of the examination, examine the skin of the corresponding region for the following:

   Colour and pigmentation _____

261

Temperature _____

Moisture _____

Texture _____

Turgor _____

Any lesions _____

Neurological System

1. Note whether eyes open

    a. Spontaneously _____

    b. To name _____

2. Note motor response _____

3. Note verbal response _____

4. Measure pupil size in millimetres and inspect reaction

    a. R _____ b. L _____

5. Assess muscle strength, upper

    a. R _____ b. L _____

6. Assess muscle strength, lower

    a. R _____ b. L _____

7. Note any ptosis, facial droop _____

8. Evaluate sensation _____

9. Note communication _____

10. Assess ability to swallow _____

Respiratory System

1. If patient receives oxygen by mask or nasal prongs, check fitting _____

2. Note fraction of inspired oxygen (FiO2) _____

3. Assess respiratory effort _____

4. Auscultate breath sounds

Anterior lobes:

   Right upper _____

   Left upper _____

   Right middle _____

   Right lower _____

   Left lower _____

Posterior lobes:

    Left upper _____

    Right upper _____

    Left lower _____

    Right lower _____

    Instruct patient to cough and breathe deeply; any mucus? Check colour and amount _____

Cardiovascular System

1. Auscultate rhythm at apex: regular, irregular? _____

2. Check apical versus radial pulse _____

3. Assess heart sounds in all auscultatory areas: first with diaphragm, repeat with bell

4. Check capillary refill _____

5. Check pretibial edema

    a. R _____   b. L _____

6. Palpate posterior tibial pulse

    a. R _____   b. L _____

7. Palpate dorsalis pedis pulse

    a. R _____   b. L _____

8. Assess pulses by Doppler, if assigned _____

9. Verify intravenous fluid and rate, if present _____

Skin (May Be Integrated with Rest of Assessment)

1. Note colour _____

2. Palpate skin temperature _____

3. Pinch up a fold of skin under the clavicle or on the forearm _____

4. Complete standardized scale regarding skin breakdown _____

5. Verify the settings and application of air loss or alternating pressure mattresses, if present, _____

Abdomen

1. Assess contour of abdomen: flat, rounded, protuberant _____

2. Listen to bowel sounds in all four quadrants _____

3. Check any tube drainage and site, noting amount and colour _____

4. Inquire if passing flatus or stool _____

Genitourinary

1. Inquire if voiding regularly _____
2. Examine urine for colour, clarity _____
3. Perform bladder scan, if indicated _____

Activity

1. Transfer patient to chair, as appropriate per activity orders _____
2. Note any assistance needed, how movement is tolerated, distance walked to chair, ability to turn _____
_____
3. Note any need for ambulatory aid or equipment _____
4. Complete standardized scale regarding falling _____

Closure

1. Return bed to lowest height.
2. Verify that brakes are locked.
3. Make sure appropriate rails are up.
4. Ensure call bell is available.
5. Verify bed alarm, if indicated.
6. Thank the patient for their time and share plan for the day.
7. Communicate plan for the day and when you plan to return.

NOTES

30 Pregnancy

PURPOSE

This chapter reviews the changes and function of the female reproductive system during pregnancy; the methods of inspection and palpation of the internal and external structures and the pregnant abdomen; and the accurate recording of the assessment.

READING ASSIGNMENT

Jarvis: *Physical Examination and Health Assessment*, 4th Canadian ed., Chapter 30.

Suggested Reading:

MacLean, L. R.-D. (2021). Preconception, pregnancy, birthing, and lactation needs of transgender men. *Nursing for Women's Health, 25*(2), 129–138.

GLOSSARY

Study the following terms after reading the corresponding chapter in the text.

Amniocentesis: the transabdominal perforation of the amniotic sac for the purpose of obtaining a sample of amniotic fluid

Antepartum: the period occurring before childbirth

Attitude: the position of fetal parts in relation to each other; may be flexed, military (straight), or extended

Bi-ischial diameter: the measurement across the perineum between the ischial tuberosities

Blastocyst: the fertilized ovum; a specialized layer of cells around the blastocyst that becomes the placenta

Chadwick's sign: bluish-purple discoloration of the cervix during pregnancy due to venous congestion

Chloasma: the "mask of pregnancy"; a butterfly-shaped pigmentation of the face

Chorionic villi sampling: transabdominal or transvaginal sampling of trophoblastic tissue surrounding the gestational sac

Colostrum: the precursor to milk that contains minerals, proteins, and antibodies

Corpus luteum: "yellow body"; a structure on the surface of the ovary that is formed by the remaining cells in the follicle; it acts as a short-lived endocrine organ that produces progesterone to help maintain the pregnancy in its early stages

Dextrorotation: possible rotation of the pregnant uterus toward the right side as it rises out of the pelvis due to the presence of the descending colon on the left

Diagonal conjugate: it indicates the anteroposterior diameter of the pelvic inlet, measured from the inferior border of the symphysis pubis to the sacral promontory

Diastasis recti: a separation of the abdominal muscles during pregnancy, returning to normal after pregnancy

Effacement: thinning of the cervix in preparation for dilation and labour

Engagement: when the widest diameter of the presenting part (most often the fetal head) has descended into the pelvic inlet

Fetal lie: orientation of the fetal spine to the maternal spine

Goodell's sign: the softening of the cervix due to increased vascularity, congestion, and edema

Hegar's sign: when the uterus becomes globular in shape, softens, and flexes easily over the cervix

Hyperemesis gravidarum: severe and debilitating nausea and vomiting that may persist beyond the fourteenth week of pregnancy and cause dehydration, weight loss, and electrolyte imbalance

Intrapartum: occurring during labour and delivery

Leopold's manoeuvres: external palpation of the maternal abdomen to determine fetal lie, presentation, attitude, position, variety, and engagement

Linea nigra: a median line of the abdomen that becomes pigmented (darkens) during pregnancy

Maternal death: any death that occurs during pregnancy or within 42 days after termination of any pregnancy; it must be a direct or indirect result of the pregnancy or any condition aggravated by the pregnancy

Maternal mortality rate (MMR): the number of maternal deaths per 100 000 live births

"Morning sickness": nausea and vomiting of pregnancy that usually begin between weeks 4 and 5, peak between weeks 8 and 12, and resolve between weeks 14 and 16
Mucous plug: mucus that forms a thick barrier in the cervix that is expelled at various times before or during labour
Multigravida: a pregnant person who has previously carried a fetus to the point of viability (i.e., 20 weeks' gestation or more)
Multipara: a person who has had two or more viable (i.e., 20 weeks' gestation or more) pregnancies and deliveries
Nägele's rule: a rule for calculating the estimated date of delivery; add seven days to the first day of the last menstrual period (LMP), subtract three months, and then add 1 year
Oligohydramnios: a reduced level of amniotic fluid in the amniotic sac
Pelvimetry: assessment of the maternal pelvis bones for shape and size
Pica: a craving for unnatural articles of food, such as cornstarch and ice chips
Piskacek's sign: irregular enlargement of the uterus that may be noted at 8 to 10 weeks' gestation; it occurs when implantation occurs close to a corneal area of the uterus
Placenta: the specialized layer of cells around the blastocyst becomes the placenta; it starts to produce progesterone to support the pregnancy at 7 weeks and takes over this function completely from the corpus luteum at about 10 weeks
Polyhydramnios: an excessive volume of amniotic fluid in the amniotic sac
Position: the location of a fetal part to the right or left of the maternal pelvis
Postpartum: the period occurring after delivery
Presentation: the part of the fetus that is entering the pelvis first
Presumptive signs (of pregnancy): signs and symptoms that the woman experiences, such as amenorrhea, breast tenderness, nausea, fatigue, and increased urinary frequency
Primigravida: a woman (or trans or intersex person) pregnant for the first time
Primipara: a person who has had one pregnancy and given birth at 20 weeks' gestation or more
Probable signs (of pregnancy): signs detected with examination, such as uterine enlargement
Striae gravidarum: "stretch marks" that may be seen on the abdomen and breasts (in areas of weight gain) during pregnancy
Variety: the location of the fetal back to the anterior, lateral, or posterior part of the maternal pelvis
VBAC: vaginal birth after Caesarean

STUDY GUIDE

After completing the reading assignment, you should be able to answer the following questions in the spaces provided.

1. Describe the function of the placenta.

2. Using Nägele's rule, calculate the estimated date of delivery if the last menstrual period (LMP) is August 22.

3. Give examples of the following signs of pregnancy:

    Presumptive _____

    Probable _____

    Positive _____

4. When can serum human chorionic gonadotropin (hCG) be detected in blood? In urine?

5. Describe three physical and physiological changes that are seen in the following:

   First trimester

   Second trimester

   Third trimester

6. Describe the "expected" weight gain during pregnancy.

7. List the major obstetrical risks and psychosocial stressors for pregnant adolescents.

8. List at least three risk factors concerning pregnant people of advanced maternal age.

9. Discuss the importance of the social determinants of health in a person's pregnancy.

10. Discuss how using a relational approach to nursing allows you to provide culturally safe care to a person during pregnancy.

11. True or false: Circle the best answer.

    a. True False The maternal mortality rate represents the risk of dying that a pregnant person faces with each pregnancy.

    b. True False In early fetal development, the corpus luteum plays no significant role.

    c. True False A person who is pregnant for the first time is called a primipara.

    d. True False The fetal period begins after the ninth gestational week.

    e. True False Pre-eclampsia is seen only in the third trimester of pregnancy.

    f. True False Vaginal bleeding in pregnancy always indicates a miscarriage.

    g. True False Cervical incompetence is always accompanied by painful contractions.

12. Describe why it is important to ask a pregnant person if they feel safe in their relationships and environment.

13. Draw on this diagram where the fundal height should be at the twentieth week of gestation.

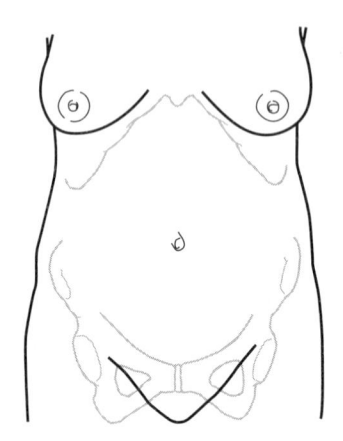

14. Label the following types of pelvis. (Fill in each blank.)

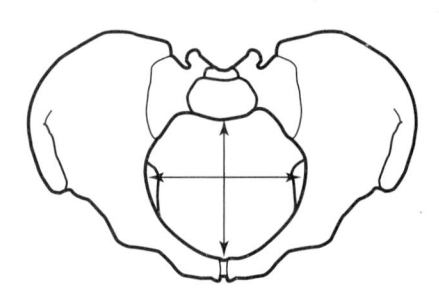

1 _____

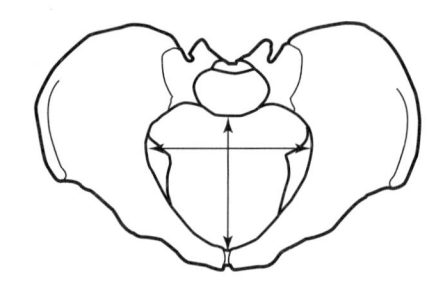

2 _____

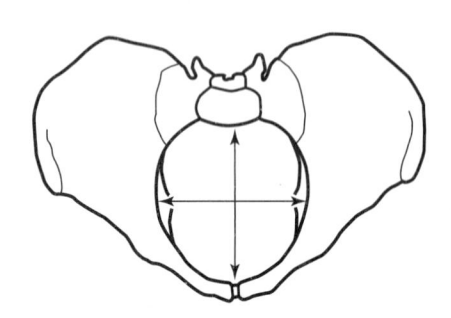

3 _____

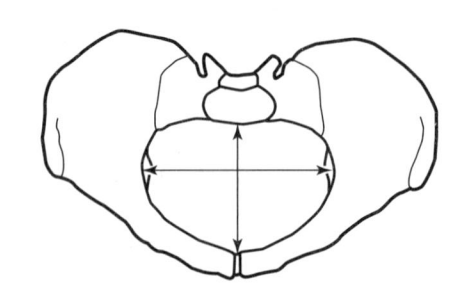

4 _____

15. Label, list the order of, and describe the purpose of the following manoeuvres. (Fill in each blank.)

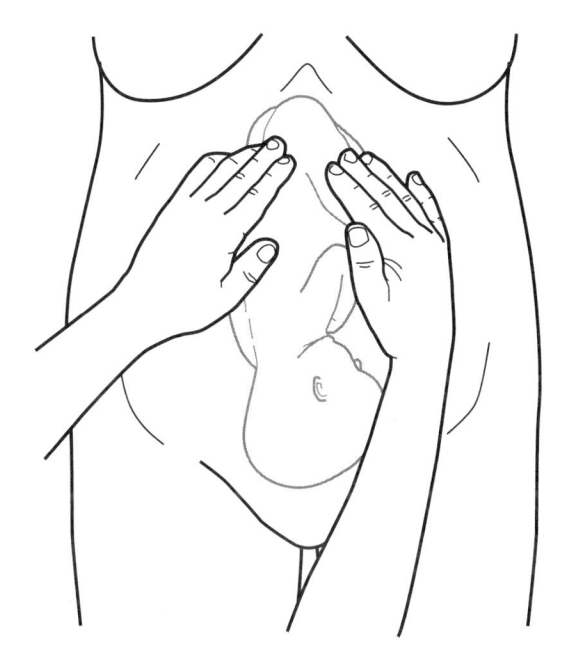

1 _____

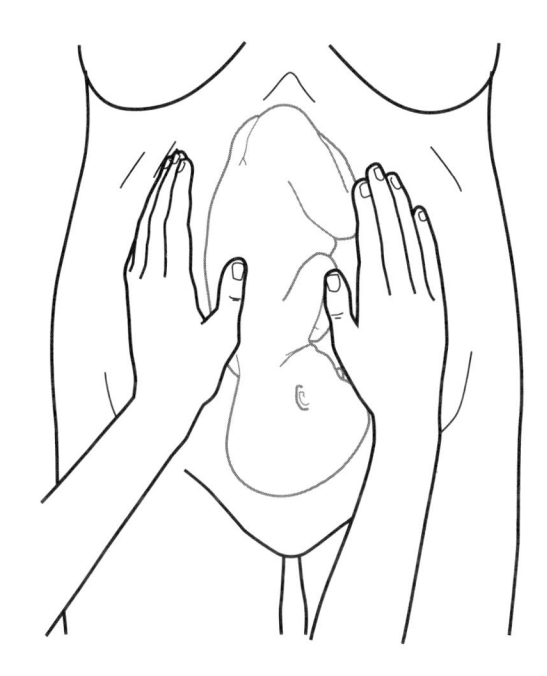

2 _____

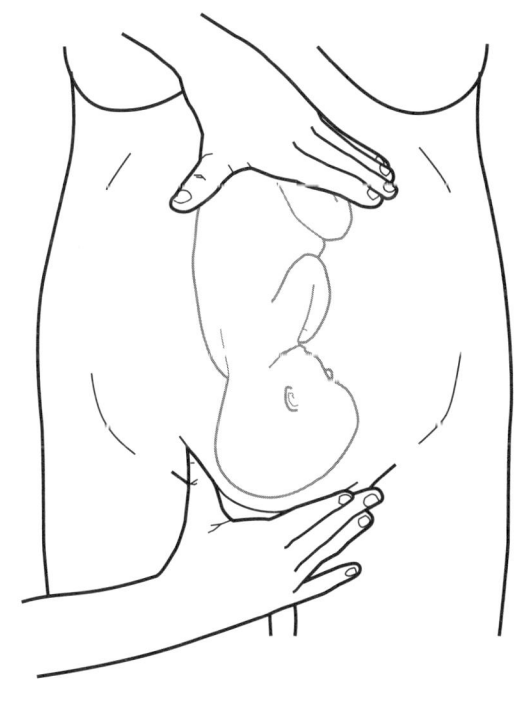

3 _____

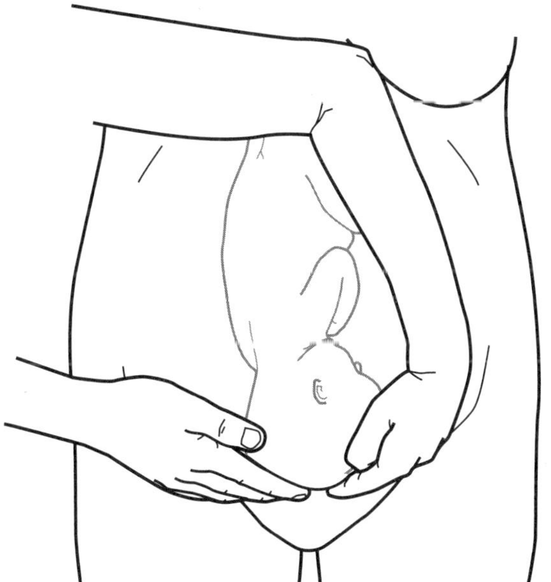

4 _____

16. Describe the following for this figure:

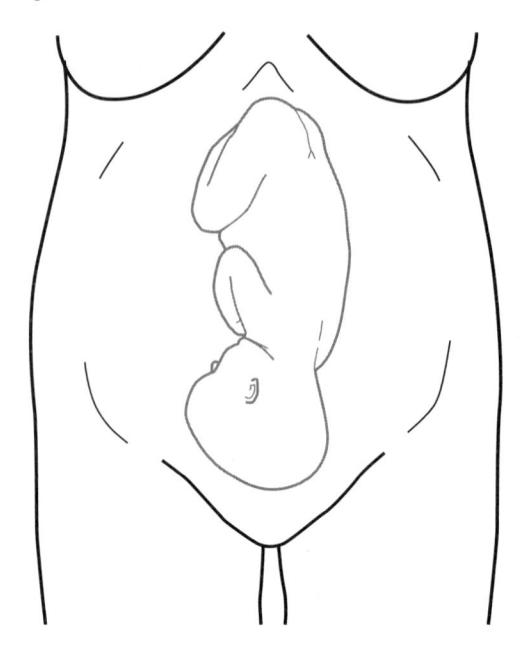

Fetal lie

Fetal presentation

Fetal position

17. List the signs and symptoms of pre-eclampsia.

18. List at least two reasons why fundal height may be small for gestational age.

19. List at least two reasons why fundal height may be large for gestational age.

20. List three risk factors for developing iron deficiency anemia in pregnancy and three risk factors associated with anemia during pregnancy.

21. Describe considerations and additional history questions for transgender men who are pregnant or who wish to become pregnant.

REVIEW AND CLINICAL JUDGEMENT QUESTIONS

This test is for you to check your own mastery of the content. Answers are provided on the text's Evolve site.

1. In the following scenario, underline information that requires follow-up, may indicate potential risk for complications, or is abnormal.

   A nurse is caring for a 38-year-old female who is Grav 8/Para 8. All spontaneous vaginal deliveries were after 38 weeks' gestation. She reports a history of pre-eclampsia with her last two pregnancies, with no long-term sequelae. She states that the pre-eclampsia occurred "right at the end" of each pregnancy, though she does not remember specific information. She is 162 cm and weighs 102 kg. Her pre-pregnancy weight was 81.6 kg. She is 36 weeks' gestation and is in active labour. Her due date was confirmed by ultrasonography (US) at 21 weeks' gestation. Fetal heart tones are 155 bpm with normal accelerations. Vital signs: HR 110 bpm; RR 20/min, unlaboured; BP 146/98 mm Hg; T 36.5°C (97.7°F). Currently she rates pain at 2/10 at rest and 10/10 during contractions. Medical history of postpartum hemorrhage (PPH) with last pregnancy requiring blood transfusion. Routine medications include a prenatal vitamin.

2. Advanced maternal age is increasingly common in Canada. What obstetrical risks are more likely to occur with advanced maternal age? (Select all that apply.)
   a. intrauterine growth restriction (IUGR)
   b. preterm birth
   c. spontaneous vaginal delivery (SVD)
   d. multigravidity
   e. postpartum hemorrhage (PPH)
   f. pre-eclampsia
   g. pain

3. The nurse should recognize that _____ and _____ are classic symptoms of pre-eclampsia, but _____ is not required for diagnosis. Onset and worsening of symptoms may be sudden, and rapid intervention is necessary. A serious variant of pre-eclampsia is HELLP.

   Choose from the words below. Words may be used more than once or not at all.

   | hypertension | elevated liver enzymes | sudden | eclampsia |
   | hypotension | proteinuria | insipidus | HELLP |

4. During pregnancy, the body undergoes a number of normal physiological changes to support the growing fetus. What normal skin changes may occur during pregnancy? (Select all that apply.)
   a. vascular spiders
   b. scars along easily accessed veins
   c. facial edema
   d. butterfly-shaped pigmentation of the face
   e. hyperpigmented line down the abdomen
   f. nevi that darken during pregnancy

5. Identify whether each of the following pregnancy related changes are physiological or pathological.

	Physiological	Pathological
Mammary souffle		
Purulent nipple discharge		
Diastolic murmur 2/6		
Breast enlargement		
Decreased cardiac output		
Blood volume increase by 45%		
Slight hemodilution		
Increased pulse		

6. Select all of the statements that apply to transgender men:
   a. They should be counselled against becoming pregnant due to the increased risks associated with pregnancy after gender-affirming therapy is initiated.
   b. They should receive counselling on the outcomes of gender-affirming hormone therapy and surgery on future fertility.
   c. They should receive high-quality peripartum care that affirms their gender and supports their emotional, physical, and psychological health.
   d. They should be referred to a clinic where resources addressing their specific needs for pregnancy care, birthing, and nursing or feeding their babies are available.

7. A 32-year-old female is in your clinic for their first prenatal appointment. She believes that she is currently 25 weeks' gestation but is uncertain. She has just moved to your city from Calgary. You have received all of her prenatal records. The most reliable method of dating a pregnancy in the absence of an excellent history is
   a. first-trimester ultrasound.
   b. Nägele's rule.
   c. auscultation of fetal heart tones.
   d. "quickening."

8. A 27-year-old female patient comes to your clinic reporting nausea, fatigue, breast tenderness, urinary frequency, and amenorrhea. These are
   a. probable signs of pregnancy.
   b. positive signs of pregnancy.
   c. presumptive signs of pregnancy.
   d. signs of stress.

9. After implantation, what structure makes progesterone to support the pregnancy up until about week 10?
   a. corpus luteum.
   b. blastocyst.
   c. placenta.
   d. ovary.

10. Cardiac output in a pregnant person
    a. drops dramatically.
    b. remains the same.
    c. increases along with stroke volume.
    d. decreases along with stroke volume.

11. Sexually transmitted infections (STIs) place the pregnant person at risk for
    a. infertility.
    b. premature rupture of membranes.
    c. preterm labour.
    d. preterm birth.
    e. all of the above.
    f. b, c, and d only.

12. During a routine prenatal assessment, a patient at approximately 20 weeks' gestation presents with abdominal pain. They deny a fever, chills, urinary frequency, urgency, hematuria, or dysuria. This patient is most likely experiencing
    a. appendicitis.
    b. constipation.
    c. urinary tract infection.
    d. stretching of the round ligament.
    e. none of the above.

13. Fetal heart tones are best auscultated over the fetal
    a. back.
    b. abdomen.
    c. shoulder.
    d. buttocks.

14. You are conducting a pelvic examination on a pregnant person during early pregnancy and note a bluish colour of the cervix and vaginal walls. The term for this finding is
    a. Goodell's sign.
    b. linea nigra.
    c. Hegar's sign.
    d. Chadwick's sign.

15. An obstetrical ultrasound is done to determine
    a. thickness of the uterine wall.
    b. fetal position.
    c. placental location.
    d. amniotic fluid volume.
    e. none of the above.
    f. b, c, and d.

16. Identify the following as presumptive, probable, or positive signs of pregnancy.

	Presumptive	**Probable**	**Positive**
Amenorrhea			
Enlarged uterus			
Fatigue			
Fetal heart tones			
Nausea			
Breast tenderness			
Cardiac activity on ultrasonography			

SKILLS LABORATORY/CLINICAL SETTING

You are now ready for the clinical component of the pregnancy examination. Because of the need to maintain personal privacy, it is unlikely that you will practise this examination on a peer. Some clinical settings may arrange for a pregnant person to participate, or your practice setting may have available a pregnancy simulator that you may use to practise your skills. If you have a pregnant person available, discuss with them, in the presence of your instructor, the methods of examination that will be used. Maintain their comfort and adequate positioning to prevent maternal dizziness, nausea, and hypotension, and to maintain adequate uterine blood flow. If you are unable to work with a pregnant patient, practice the history component of the exam with a peer. Together, discuss what the physical examination entails.

Clinical Objectives
1. Demonstrate knowledge of the physical changes related to pregnancy in the first, second, and third trimesters.
2. Demonstrate knowledge and importance of obtaining a pertinent health history during the first prenatal visit.
3. Demonstrate cultural sensitivity during the examination.
4. Inspect and palpate the pregnant abdomen for uterine size and fetal position.
5. Demonstrate obtaining fetal heart tones.
6. Record the history and physical examination findings accurately; reach an assessment of the health state, estimated gestational age, and fetal position (when appropriate); and develop a plan of care.

Instructions
Prepare the setting and gather any necessary equipment. Working through the Ontario Perinatal Record, take an appropriate history and conduct a focused, relevant perinatal exam.

NOTES

DOCUMENTATION—PREGNANCY

Ontario Ministry of Health and Long-Term Care
Ontario Perinatal Record 1

Last Name	First Name

Address - street number, street name	Apt/Suite/Unit	Buzzer No

City/Town	Province	Postal Code	Partner's First Name	Partner's Last Name

Contact - Preferred	Leave Message ☐Y ☐N	Contact - Alternate/E-mail	Partner's Occupation	Partner's Education Level	Age

Date of Birth YYYY/MM/DD	Age at EDB	Language	Interpreter Required ☐Y ☐N	Occupation	Education Level	Relationship Status	Sexual Orientation

OHIP Number	Patient File Number	Disability Requiring Accommodation ☐Y ☐N	Planned Place of Birth	Planned Birth Attendant

Newborn Care Provider	Family Physician/Primary Care Provider
In Hospital In Community	

Allergies or Sensitivities (include reaction)	Medications (include Rx/OTC, complementary/alternative/vitamins and dosage)

Pregnancy Summary

LMP YYYY/MM/DD	Cycle q ___	Certain ☐Y ☐N	Regular ☐Y ☐N	EDB By LMP YYYY/MM/DD	Dating Method ☐T₁US ☐T₂US ☐LMP
Planned Preg ☐Y ☐N	Contraceptive Type		Last Used YYYY/MM	Final EDB YYYY/MM/DD	☐IUI YYYY/MM/DD ☐Embryo Transfer YYYY/MM/DD
Conception: Assisted ☐Y ☐N	Details				☐Other

Gravida	Term	Preterm	Abortus	Living Children	Stillbirth(s)	Neonatal / Child Death

Obstetrical History

Year/Month	Place of Birth	Gest. (wks)	Labour Length	Type of Birth	Comments regarding abortus, pregnancy, birth, and newborn (e.g. GDM, HTN, IUGR, shoulder dystocia, PPH, OASIS, neonatal jaundice)	Sex M/F	Birth Weight	Breastfed / Duration	Child's Current Health

Medical History (provide details in comments)

Current Pregnancy
1. Bleeding ☐Y ☐N
2. Nausea/vomiting ☐Y ☐N
3. Rash/fever/illness ☐Y ☐N

Nutrition
4. Calcium adequate ☐Y ☐N
5. Vitamin D adequate ☐Y ☐N
6. Folic acid preconception ☐Y ☐N
7. Prenatal vitamin ☐Y ☐N
8. Food access/quality adequate ☐Y ☐N
9. Dietary restrictions ☐Y ☐N

Surgical History
10. Surgery ☐Y ☐N
11. Anaesthetic complications ☐Y ☐N

Medical History
12. Hypertension ☐Y ☐N
13. Cardiac / Pulmonary ☐Y ☐N
14. Endocrine ☐Y ☐N
15. GI / Liver ☐Y ☐N
16. Breast (incl. surgery) ☐Y ☐N
17. Gynecological (incl. surgery) ☐Y ☐N
18. Urinary tract ☐Y ☐N
19. MSK/Rheumatology ☐Y ☐N
20. Hematological ☐Y ☐N
21. Thromboembolic/coag ☐Y ☐N
22. Blood transfusion ☐Y ☐N
23. Neurological ☐Y ☐N
24. Other ☐Y ☐N

Family History
25. Medical Conditions ☐Y ☐N
(e.g. diabetes, thyroid, hypertension, thromboembolic, anaesthetic, mental health).

Genetic History of Gametes
26. Ethnic/racial background:
Egg _____ Age ____ Yrs
Sperm _____
27. Carrier screening: at risk? ☐Y ☐N
- Hemoglobinopathy screening (Asian, African, Middle Eastern, Mediterranean, Hispanic, Caribbean) ☐Y ☐N
- Tay-Sachs disease screening (Ashkenazi Jewish, French Canadian, Acadian, Cajun) ☐Y ☐N
- Ashkenazi Jewish screening panel ☐Y ☐N
28. Genetic Family History
- Genetic conditions (e.g. CF, muscular dystrophy, chromosomal disorder) ☐Y ☐N
- Other (e.g. intellectual, birth defect, congenital heart, developmental delay, recurrent pregnancy loss, stillbirth) ☐Y ☐N
- Consanguinity ☐Y ☐N

Infectious Disease
29. Varicella disease ☐Y ☐N
30. Varicella vaccine ☐Y ☐N
31. HIV ☐Y ☐N
32. HSV Self ☐Y ☐N Partner ☐Y ☐N
33. STIs ☐Y ☐N
34. At risk population (Hep C, TB, Parvo, Toxo) ☐Y ☐N
35. Other ☐Y ☐N

Mental Health / Substance Use
36. Anxiety Past ☐Y ☐N Present ☐Y ☐N
GAD-2 Score ____
37. Depression Past ☐Y ☐N Present ☐Y ☐N
PHQ-2 Score ____
38. Eating disorder ☐Y ☐N
39. Bipolar ☐Y ☐N
40. Schizophrenia ☐Y ☐N
41. Other ☐Y ☐N
(e.g. PTSD, ADD, personality disorders)
42. Smoked cig within past 6 months ☐Y ☐N
Current smoking ____ cig/day
43. Alcohol: Ever drink alcohol? ☐Y ☐N
If Yes: Last drink: (when) ____
Current drinking ____ drinks/wk
T-ACE Score ____
44. Marijuana ☐Y ☐N
45. Non-prescribed substances/drugs ☐Y ☐N

Lifestyle/Social
46. Occupational risks ☐Y ☐N
47. Financial/housing issues ☐Y ☐N
48. Poor social support ☐Y ☐N
49. Beliefs/practices affecting care ☐Y ☐N
50. Relationship problems ☐Y ☐N
51. Intimate partner/family violence ☐Y ☐N
52. Parenting concerns ☐Y ☐N
(e.g. developmental disability, family trauma)
53. Other ☐Y ☐N

Comments

Completed By	Reviewed By
Signature Date	MRP Signature Date

5046-64 (2017/03)   © Queen's Printer for Ontario, 2017   User Guide available at www.pcmch.on.ca

Ontario Perinatal Record 2

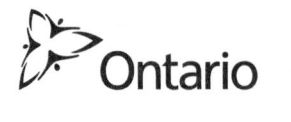

Ministry of Health and Long-Term Care

Last Name	First Name	
Planned Birth Attendant		

Newborn Care Provider
In Hospital   In Community

G	T	P	A	L	S	Final EDB YYYY/MM/DD	Family Physician/Primary Care Provider

Physical Exam

Ht _____ cm   Pre-pregnancy Wt _____ kg
BP _____   Pre-pregnancy BMI _____

Exam As Indicated

Head and neck	N/Abn	MSK	N/Abn
Breast/nipples	N/Abn	Pelvic	N/Abn
Heart/lungs	N/Abn	Other	N/Abn
Abdomen	N/Abn		

Exam Comments

Last Pap YYYY/MM/DD   Result

Initial Laboratory Investigations

Test	Result
Hb	
ABO/Rh(D)	
MCV	
Antibody screen	
Platelets	
Rubella immune	
HBsAg	
Syphilis	
HIV	
GC	
Chlamydia	
Urine C&S	

Second and Third Trimester Lab Investigations

Test	Result
Hb	
Platelets	
ABO/Rh(D)	
Repeat Antibodies	
1hr GCT	
2 hr GTT	

Additional investigations as indicated

TSH, Diabetes screen, Hb Electrophoresis/ HPLC, Ferritin, B12, Infectious diseases (e.g. Hep C, Parvo B19, Varicella, Toxo, CMV), Drug screen, repeat STI screen.

Test	Result	Test	Result

Prenatal Genetic Investigations

Screening Offered ☐ Yes ☐ No   Result

☐ FTS (between 11-13+6wks)
☐ IPS Part 1(between 11-13+6wks) ☐ Part 2(between 15-20+6wks)
☐ MSS (between 15-20+6wks) ☐ AFP (between 15-20+6wks)
Cell-free fetal DNA (NIPT) Offered ☐ Y ☐ N

	Result
CVS/Amnio Offered ☐ Y ☐ N	
Other genetic testing Offered ☐ Y ☐ N	
NT Risk Assessment 11-13+6wk (multiples)	
Abnormal Placental Biomarkers	

No Screening Tests

☐ Counseled and declined   Date YYYY/MM/DD   ☐ Presentation > 20+6wk NIPT offered ☐ Y ☐ N   Date YYYY/MM/DD

Ultrasound

Date	GA	Result
YYYY/MM/DD		
YYYY/MM/DD		NT Ultrasound (between 11-13+6 weeks)
YYYY/MM/DD		Anatomy scan (between 18-22wks) Placental Location Soft Markers
YYYY/MM/DD		
YYYY/MM/DD		
YYYY/MM/DD		
YYYY/MM/DD		
YYYY/MM/DD		
YYYY/MM/DD		
YYYY/MM/DD		
YYYY/MM/DD		Genetic screening result reviewed with pt/client ☐
YYYY/MM/DD		Approx 22 wks: Copy of OPR 1 & 2 to hospital ☐ and/or to pt/client ☐

5046-64 (2017/03) © Queen's Printer for Ontario, 2017   User Guide available at www.pcmch.on.ca

Ontario Perinatal Record 3

Ministry of Health and Long-Term Care

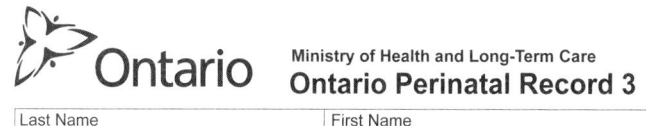

Last Name	First Name

Planned Birth Attendant

Newborn Care Provider		Allergies or Sensitivities (include reaction)
In Hospital	In Community	
Family Physician/Primary Care Provider		Medications (include Rx/OTC, complementary/alternative/vitamins, include dosage)

G	T	P	A	L	S	Final EDB
						YYYY/MM/DD

Issues (abnormal results, medical/social problems)	Plan of Management / Medication Change / Consultations

Special Circumstances

Low dose ASA indicated ☐ Progesterone indicated (PTB Prevention) ☐ HSV supression indicated ☐

Social (e.g. child protection, adoption, surrogacy)

GBS
Rectovaginal swab ☐ pos ☐ neg

Other indications for prophylaxis ☐ Y ☐ N

Recommended Immunoprophylaxis

Rh(D) neg ☐ Rh(D) IG given YYYY/MM/DD Additional dose given YYYY/MM/DD	Influenza Discussed ☐ ☐ Received ☐ Declined	Pertussis Discussed ☐ Up-to-date ☐ Y ☐ N Year _____ Received ☐ Declined ☐	Post-partum vaccines discussed ☐ Rubella ☐ Other _____	Newborn needs ☐ Hep B prophylaxis ☐ HIV prophylaxis

Pre-pregnancy Wt _____ kg   BMI _____

Subsequent Visits

Date	GA (wks/days)	Weight (kg)	BP	Urine Prot.	SFH	Pres.	FHR	FM	Comments	Next Visit	Initial(s)
YYYY/MM/DD											
YYYY/MM/DD											
YYYY/MM/DD											
YYYY/MM/DD											
YYYY/MM/DD											
YYYY/MM/DD											
YYYY/MM/DD											
YYYY/MM/DD											
YYYY/MM/DD											
YYYY/MM/DD											
YYYY/MM/DD											
YYYY/MM/DD											
YYYY/MM/DD											
YYYY/MM/DD											

Discussion Topics

1st Trimester
- ☐ Nausea / Vomiting
- ☐ Routine prenatal care /Emergency contact /On call providers
- ☐ Safety: food, medication, environment, infections, pets
- ☐ Healthy weight gain   ☐ Breastfeeding
- ☐ Physical activity   ☐ Travel
- ☐ Seatbelt use   ☐ Quality information sources
- ☐ Sexual activity   ☐ VBAC counseling

2nd Trimester
- ☐ Prenatal classes
- ☐ Preterm labour
- ☐ PROM
- ☐ Bleeding
- ☐ Fetal movement
- ☐ Mental health
- ☐ VBAC consent

3rd Trimester
- ☐ Fetal movement   ☐ Work plan / Maternity leave
- ☐ Birth plan: pain management, labour support
- ☐ Type of birth, potential interventions, VBAC plan
- ☐ Admission timing   ☐ Mental health
- ☐ Breastfeeding and support   ☐ Contraception
- ☐ Newborn care / Screening tests / Circumcision / Follow-up appt.
- ☐ Discharge planning / Car seat safety   ☐ Postpartum care

Comments

Approx 36 wks: Copy of OPR 2 (updated) & OPR 3 to hospital ☐   and/or to pt/client ☐

1. Name / Initials	2. Name / Initials	3. Name / Initials	4. Name / Initials	5. Name / Initials

5046-64 (2017/03)   © Queen's Printer for Ontario, 2017   User Guide available at www.pcmch.on.ca

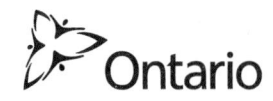

Ontario
Ministry of Health and Long-Term Care
Resources

Last Name	First Name

Anxiety Screening

Generalized Anxiety Disorder scale (GAD-2)   Date YYYY/MM/DD

Over the last 2 weeks, how often have you been bothered by the following problems:	Not at all	Several days	More than half the days	Nearly every day
1. Feeling nervous, anxious or on edge	0	1	2	3
2. Not been able to stop or control worrying	0	1	2	3

A total score of 3 or more warrants consideration of: Using the GAD-7 for further assessment or additional mental health follow-up.

Total Score ____

Depression Screening

The Patient Health Questionnaire-2 (PHQ-2)   Date YYYY/MM/DD

Over the last 2 weeks, how often have you been bothered by the following problems:	Not at all	Several days	More than half the days	Nearly every day
1. Little interest or pleasure in doing things	0	1	2	3
2. Feeling down, depressed or hopeless	0	1	2	3

A total score of 3 or more warrants consideration of: Using the Edinburgh Postnatal Depression Scale (EPDS) or the Patient Health Questionnaire (PHQ) 9 for further assessment or additional mental health follow-up.

Total Score ____

T-ACE Screening Tool (Alcohol)

Response Key
1 Drink is equivalent to:
• 12 oz of beer   • 12 oz of cooler   • 5 oz of wine   • 1.5 oz of hard liquor (mixed drink)

Date YYYY/MM/DD

Question	Response	
1. How many drinks does it take to make you feel high?	≤ 2 drinks = 0	> 2 drinks = 1
2. Have people annoyed you by criticizing your drinking?	No = 0	Yes = 1
3. Have you felt you ought to cut down on your drinking?	No = 0	Yes = 1
4. Have you ever had a drink first thing in the morning to steady your nerves or to get rid of a hangover?	No = 0	Yes = 1

A total score of 2 or greater indicates potential prenatal risk and need for follow-up.

Total Score ____

Edinburgh Perinatal / Postnatal Depression Scale (EPDS) Cox, Holden, Sagovsky, (1987).

In the past 7 days: Date YYYY/MM/DD

Question	Option A	Option B
1. I have been able to laugh and see the funny side of things	☐ As much as I always could = 0 ☐ Not quite so much now = 1	☐ Definitely not so much now = 2 ☐ Not at all = 3
2. I have looked forward with enjoyment to things	☐ As much as I ever did = 0 ☐ Rather less than I used to = 1	☐ Definitely less than I used to = 2 ☐ Hardly at all = 3
3. I have blamed myself unnecessarily when things went wrong	☐ No, never = 0 ☐ No, not very often = 1	☐ Yes, some of the time = 2 ☐ Yes, most of the time = 3
4. I have been anxious or worried for no good reason	☐ No, not at all = 0 ☐ Hardly ever = 1	☐ Yes, sometimes = 2 ☐ Yes, very often = 3
5. I have felt scared or panicky for no very good reason	☐ No, not at all = 0 ☐ No, not much = 1	☐ Yes, sometimes = 2 ☐ Yes, quite a lot = 3
6. Things have been getting on top of me	☐ No, I have been coping as well as ever = 0 ☐ No, most of the time I have coped well = 1	☐ Yes, sometimes I haven't been coping as well as usual = 2 ☐ Yes, most of the time I haven't been able to cope = 3
7. I have been so unhappy that I have had difficulty sleeping	☐ No, not much = 0 ☐ Not very often = 1	☐ Yes, sometimes = 2 ☐ Yes, most of the time = 3
8. I have felt sad or miserable	☐ No, not much = 0 ☐ Not very often = 1	☐ Yes, quite often = 2 ☐ Yes, most of the time = 3
9. I have been so unhappy that I have been crying	☐ No, never = 0 ☐ Only occasionally = 1	☐ Yes, quite often = 2 ☐ Yes, most of the time = 3
10. The thought of harming myself has occurred to me	☐ No, never = 0 ☐ Only occasionally = 1	☐ Yes, quite often = 2 ☐ Yes, most of the time = 3

Total Score ____
- Score of 1-3 on item 10 indicates a risk of self-harm. Patient requires immediate mental health assessment and intervention as appropriate.
- Score > 9 Monitor, support, and offer education
- Score > 12 Follow up with comprehensive bio-psychosocial diagnostic assessment for depression.

Institute of Medicine Weight Gain Recommendations for Pregnancy (2009)

Prepregnancy Weight Category	Body Mass Index	Recommended range of Total Weight in kg (lb)	Rates of Weight Gain in Second and Third Trimesters	
			kg/wk	lb/wk (mean range)
Underweight	Less than 18.5	12.5-18 kg (28-40)	0.5	1 (1-1.3)
Normal Weight	18.5-24.9	11.5-16 kg (25-35)	0.4	1 (0.8-1)
Overweight	25-29.9	7-11.5 kg (15-25)	0.3	0.6 (0.5-0.7)
Obese (includes all classes)	30 and greater	5-9 kg (11-20)	0.2	0.5 (0.4-0.6)

†Calculations assume a 0.5 to 2 kg (1.1-4.4 lb) weight gain in the first trimester.

5046-64 (2017/03)   © Queen's Printer for Ontario, 2017   User Guide available at www.pcmch.on.ca

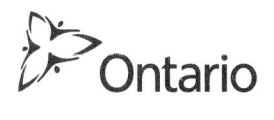

Ontario
Ministry of Health and Long-Term Care

Ontario Perinatal Record
Postnatal Visit

Last Name	First Name				
Date of visit	Date of Delivery	Number of weeks postpartum	GA at Birth	Primary Care Provider	

History

Review of birth	Vaginal:	☐ Spontaneous	☐ Vacuum	☐ Forceps	☐ VBAC	☐ Episiotomy / Lacerations	☐ OASIS
	Caesarean:	☐ Planned	☐ Unplanned				

Details | Birth Attendant

Pregnancy/birth issues requiring follow-up (e.g. diabetes, hypertension, thyroid)

Baby's Name | Baby's Care Provider

Birth Weight (g) | Baby's Health/Concerns

Infant feeding ☐ Breast milk only ☐ Combination of breast milk and breast milk substitute ☐ Breast milk substitute only

Feeding concerns

Current Medications

Bladder function	Emotional wellbeing
Bowel function	Relationship
Sexual function	Postpartum Depression Screen (EPDS or other)
Lochia / Menses	Family Support / Community Resources
Perineum / Incision	

Smoking ☐ No ☐ Yes ____ cig/day | Alcohol ☐ No ☐ Yes If yes: Drinks/wk ____ and If yes: T-ACE score ____

Non-prescribed substances / drugs (e.g. opioids, cocaine, marijuana, party drugs, other) ☐ No ☐ Yes

Rubella Immune ☐ Yes ☐ No ☐ Discussed ☐ Declined ☐ Received | Influenza ☐ Discussed ☐ Declined ☐ Received

Pertussis (TdAP) Up-to-date ☐ Yes ☐ No ☐ Discussed ☐ Declined ☐ Received | Other Immunizations

Last Pap _____ Result

Physical Exam As Indicated

Weight Today	kg	Pre-Delivery Weight	kg	Pre-Pregnancy Weight	kg	BP	mm Hg

Affect	N/Abn	Abdomen	N/Abn	Comments
Thyroid	N/Abn	Perineum	N/Abn	
Breasts	N/Abn	Pelvic	N/Abn	

Discussion Topics | Comments

☐ Transition to parenthood/partner's adjustment
☐ Family violence and safety
☐ Nutrition/physical activity/healthy weight
☐ Plan for management of alcohol / tobacco / substance use
☐ Contraception
☐ Pelvic floor exercises
☐ Community resources (e.g. Healthy Babies Healthy Children)
☐ Advice regarding future pregnancies and risks
☐ Preconception planning (e.g. folic acid, medications)
☐ If CS, future mode of birth and pregnancy spacing
☐ Other comments / concerns

Signature of healthcare provider

5046-64 (2017/03) © Queen's Printer for Ontario, 2017 | User Guide available at www.pcmch.on.ca

NOTES

31 Assessment of the Older Adult

PURPOSE

This chapter describes the functional assessment of the older adult using a systems perspective, including the normal changes of aging and ongoing chronic geriatric syndromes. A number of tools that may be used as part of the functional assessment of the older adult are described.

READING ASSIGNMENT

Jarvis: *Physical Examination and Health Assessment*, 4th Canadian ed., Chapter 31.

Suggested Readings

Gabauer, J. (2020). Mitigating the dangers of polypharmacy in community-dwelling older adults. *American Journal of Nursing, 120*(2), 36–43.

Zonsius, M. C., Cothran, F. A., & Miller, J. M. (2020). Acute care for patients with dementia. *American Journal of Nursing, 120*(4), 34–43.

GLOSSARY

Study the following terms after reading the corresponding chapter in the text.

Activities of daily living (ADLs): tasks that are necessary for self-care, such as eating or feeding, bathing, grooming, toileting, walking, and transferring

Advanced activities of daily living (AADLs): activities that an older adult performs as a family member or as a member of society or community, including occupational and recreational activities

Caregiver assessment: assessment of the health and well-being of an individual's caregiver

Caregiver burden: the perceived strain by the person who cares for a person who is older, chronically ill, or disabled

Delirium: a common, life-threatening disordered mental state characterized by an acute decline in attention and cognition that develops over a short period of time; reversible with appropriate treatment

Dementia: progressive loss of brain function that can occur with several different diseases, such as stroke and brain injury

Depression: persistent feelings of sadness, hopelessness, and/or a loss of interest or pleasure in previously enjoyable activities, cognitive and physical changes (such as trouble with concentration leading to memory problems), disturbed sleep, decreased energy or excessive tiredness, and decreased appetite, present for 2 weeks or longer

Elder abuse: a term used to describe one or more of the following situations: physical abuse, sexual abuse, emotional or psychological abuse, financial or material exploitation, abandonment, neglect, or a combination of these

Environmental assessment: assessment of an individual's home environment and community system, including hazards in the home

Functional ability: the ability of a person to perform activities necessary to live in modern society; may include driving, using the telephone, or performing personal tasks such as bathing and toileting

Functional assessment: a systematic assessment that includes assessment of an individual's ADLs, instrumental activities of daily living, and mobility

Functional status: a person's actual performance of activities and tasks associated with current life roles

Instrumental activities of daily living (IADLs): functional abilities necessary for independent community living, such as shopping, meal preparation, housekeeping, laundry, managing finances, taking medications, and using transportation

Katz Index of Activities of Daily Living: an instrument that is used to measure physical function in older adults and the chronically ill

Lawton Instrumental Activities of Daily Living: an instrument that is used to measure an individual's ability to perform IADLs; it may assist in assessing one's ability to live independently

MAiD: medical assistance in dying; legislation (Bill C-14) that provides an exemption in the Criminal Code to allow physicians and nurse practitioners to provide medical assistance in dying services. Bill C-14 also allows nurses, along with family members (or other people who are asked by the individual) and other health care providers to participate in the MAiD process.

Physical performance measures: tests that measure balance, gait, motor coordination, and endurance

Polypharmacy: the prescription and use of multiple medications (usually five or more) to deal with concomitant multiple diseases

Social domain: the domain that focuses on an individual's relationships within family, social groups, and the community

Social networks: informal supports that are accessed by older adults, such as family members and close friends, neighbours, church societies, neighbourhood groups, and older adult centres

Spiritual assessment: assessment of an individual's spirituality underlying the meaning and purpose of one's own life; highly individual.

Timed Up and Go Test: a screening test to identify the probability of falls in older adults

STUDY GUIDE

After completing the reading assignment, you should be able to answer the following questions in the spaces provided.

1. Explain the differences between functional ability and functional status.

2. Differentiate the following and provide at least three examples of each:

    a. ADLs

    b. IADLs

    c. AADLs

3. Describe at least two instruments that may be used to assess the following:

    a. ADLs

    b. IADLs

    c. Physical performance

4. What are the disadvantages of self-answered ADL and IADL instruments?

5. What are the advantages and disadvantages of instruments that measure physical performance?

6. Discuss at least two disorders that may alter an older adult's cognition.

7. Differentiate between formal and informal social supports and give three examples of each.

8. List at least three clues that elder abuse is occurring.

9. List at least five risk factors for elder abuse.

10. Explain the best way to document findings in cases of suspected elder abuse.

11. Define *polypharmacy*, and list at least four risks associated with polypharmacy.

12. Define an environmental assessment, and list at least four common environmental hazards that may be found in an individual's home.

13. Discuss the best approach when performing a spiritual assessment.

14. Describe special considerations that may affect the assessment of an older adult's functional status.

15. State the priority when assessing an older adult who is in pain.

ADDITIONAL LEARNING ACTIVITIES

1. Accompany an advanced-practice nurse or nurse practitioner who specializes in the care of older adults as she or he makes rounds in the hospital setting or a long-term care facility.
2. In a clinical setting that focuses on older adults, such as a geriatric or psychiatric unit, a daytime geriatric psychiatric program, or an older adult centre, observe a nurse, occupational therapist, or social worker perform various assessments of older adults.

REVIEW AND CLINICAL JUDGEMENT QUESTIONS

This test is for you to check your own mastery of the content. Answers are provided on the text's Evolve site.

1. An appropriate tool to assess an individual's IADLs would be a tool by
   a. Katz.
   b. Lawton.
   c. Tinetti.
   d. Norbeck.

2. Which of the following statements is true regarding an individual's functional status?
   a. Functional status refers to one's ability to care for another person.
   b. An older adult's functional status is usually static over time.
   c. An older adult's functional status may vary from independence to disability.
   d. Dementia is an example of functional status.

3. An older adult is experiencing an acute change in cognition. The nurse recognizes that this disorder is
   a. Alzheimer's dementia.
   b. attention deficit disorder.
   c. depression.
   d. delirium.

4. Assessment of the social domain includes
   a. family relationships.
   b. the ability to cook meals.
   c. the ability to balance the cheque book and pay bills.
   d. hazards found in the home.

5. An older adult has extensive bruising on her back and arms. Her caregiver, who is her son, explains that she fell in the stairs. When performing an assessment, the nurse's best action would be to
   a. ask the patient what happened in the presence of her son.
   b. arrange time to interview the patient and the son separately.
   c. notify authorities of elder abuse.
   d. document the assessment on the admission history form.

6. The nurse will use which technique when assessing an older adult who has cognitive impairment?
   a. asking open-ended questions
   b. completing the entire assessment in one session
   c. asking the family members for information instead of the older adult
   d. asking simple questions that have "yes" or "no" answers

7. Which of the following is an example of an informal social network for the aging adult?
   a. a close friend and neighbour who drops by with newspapers and magazines on a regular basis
   b. the area church that offers a weekly activity and luncheon for older adults in the neighbourhood
   c. the home health care agency that provides weekly blood pressure screenings at the church luncheon
   d. the older adult chess club whose members hold classes at a local community centre

8. The nurse is assessing an older adult who has a history of dementia and had surgery for a fractured hip. The nurse should keep in mind that older adults with cognitive impairment
   a. experience less pain.
   b. can provide a self-report of pain.
   c. cannot be relied on to self-report pain.
   d. will not express pain sensations.

9. An appropriate use for the Caregiver Strain Index would be which situation?
   a. a daughter who is taking her older adult father home to live with her
   b. an older patient who lives alone
   c. a wife who has cared for her husband for the past 4 years at home
   d. a son whose parents live in an long-term care facility

Match column A to column B.

Column A—Examples or Indicators

10. _____ Verbal assaults, insults, or threats
11. _____ Failure to provide necessaries of life such as food and water
12. _____ Bruised skin and broken bones
13. _____ An older adult's report of unwanted touching
14. _____ An older adult's report of being left alone for long periods without adequate support
15. _____ Misusing or stealing money or possession

Column B—Type of Elder Abuse

a. Physical abuse
b. Abandonment
c. Financial or material exploitation
d. Neglect
e. Emotional or psychological abuse
f. Sexual abuse

Use the following case study to answer questions 16 to 19.
The nurse is caring for an 86-year-old patient who was hospitalized with a urinary tract infection and acute confusion for 2 days. The patient was admitted for IV antibiotics. The nurse receives the following information during shift report:
   A.K. is an 86-year-old gentleman who lives at home with his wife. His brother died in the 1970s, and his son died in the Gulf War, in 1990. He has a history of arthritis, and he had a myocardial infarction (MI) 15 years ago. He has no history of dementia or cognitive impairment. He is alert and oriented to person and place only, but his cognition is improving. Upon admission, he was only oriented to person. His Timed Up and Go Test was 14 seconds. His wife reports that he has fallen at home twice in the past 2 months. Upon physical examination, vital signs are as follows: HR 101 bpm; RR 26/min, shallow; BP 110/60 mm Hg. Lungs are clear and equal bilaterally; normal S_1S_2 with no extra sounds, no murmur. Deep tendon reflexes (DTRs) 1+ and equal. Difficulty with whispered voice test.

16. Underline the findings of concern.

17. Circle the changes expected with normal aging.

18. Early discharge planning is a crucial part of any hospitalization. Which of the following accurately describes the discharge for A.K.?
    a. A.K. can discharge home with his spouse. Social work should be consulted to ensure they have adequate housing, meals, and social support, but it should not be an issue.
    b. A.K. will need a functional assessment to identify any areas of concern prior to discharge. Including his caregiver will be important to ensure adequate support at home.
    c. A.K. will likely need a long-term care facility upon discharge. He has declined significantly, and his spouse is also an older adult, so she may not be able to care for him.
    d. A.K. should cease driving and consider moving to a long-term care facility where he can have adequate transportation, meals, and social support. Returning home is not a good option.

19. Given the information in the case study, which of the following is true regarding hospital at-home care for A.K.
    a. A.K. would not be a candidate for hospital at-home care. Any person over 85 years old with an older adult spouse is not appropriate given the lack of younger social support and care required during a home stay.
    b. A.K. would not benefit from hospital at-home care. His acute confusion places him at risk to himself and others. A hospital environment with a sitter and restraints will ensure his safety throughout his hospitalization.
    c. A.K. is a candidate for hospital at-home care given his diagnoses and the lack of high-acuity needs, but a full assessment would be required to ensure he meets qualifications and that it is an amenable choice for him and his caregiver.
    d. A.K. is a candidate for hospital at-home care and should not be admitted inpatient. Hospital at-home care can be used to avoid some in-hospital complications, such as health care–associated infection, and should be considered for all older adult patients, regardless of diagnosis.

20. You are caring for an older adult woman with early dementia. Her family is concerned about her driving ability, reporting that she "sometimes gets lost on the way home," drives "really slow," and "can't seem to see very well." Given your knowledge of warning signs for cessation of driving, you recommend:
    a. As long as she can still pass her driving test, she can continue to drive safely. There is no need to take her car away as it will only upset her further.
    b. Driving requires executive function, good sensory perception, and good physical abilities. It is likely time to discuss cessation of driving.
    c. Driving requires good sensory perception. I would recommend having her eyes tested. As long as she gets new glasses, she can keep driving.
    d. Cessation of driving is never easy. I may recommend that she only drive during the day when it is light out so she can see better, and have her drive in familiar areas only.

21. The nurse is caring for a 78-year-old female who reports difficulty sleeping. She says she wakes at least twice to urinate each night. She always goes to bed at a different time but wakes up promptly at 0700 without an alarm. Which of the following are recommended interventions to promote sleep? (Select all that apply.)
    a. Avoid all alcohol.
    b. Limit caffeine to 2 caffeinated drinks per day.
    c. Avoid caffeine after lunch.
    d. Take frequent naps up to 1 hour in length.
    e. Eat a large meal before bed.
    f. Adhere to a schedule.
    g. Open drapes/blinds during the day.
    h. Have a light snack before bed.
    i. Be active during the day.

22. Underline the areas of environmental assessment below that are concerning for your 89-year-old patient who lives alone, has limited mobility, and uses a walker.

    M.K. lives in a single-story home in a safe neighbourhood. Streetlights are present, though functionality was not assessed because it is daytime. The neighbourhood has sidewalks, and the nearest fire station is four blocks away. M.K. no longer drives, and the nearest bus stop is approximately 1 km away. There is a grocery store within 2 km. The house has no steps to enter. There are throw rugs in the entry way, the kitchen, and in each of the two bathrooms. The toilet is lower than standard, and there are no grab bars. Curtains are open, and the home is well-lit. Old magazines and books are neatly stacked all over the floor.

23. Given the concerns identified in question 23, which changes would you recommend to promote safety and independent living?
    a. Remove the throw rugs, since they are a tripping hazard.
    b. Ask M.K. about social support and transportation. Provide referral to resources as appropriate.
    c. Recommend reorganization of magazines to get them off the floor, as they are trip hazards.
    d. Consider a renovation to place a standard height toilet or use a raised toilet seat addition.
    e. Put grab bars in the bathroom.
    f. All of the above.

SKILLS LABORATORY/CLINICAL SETTING

You are now ready for the clinical component of functional assessment of the older adult. The purpose of the clinical component is to practise portions of a functional assessment either in a clinical setting with older adults (such as a geriatric inpatient unit or a long-term care facility) or in the home of an older adult (such as a neighbour or family member). In addition, the following should be achieved.

Clinical Objectives
1. Using the Katz Index of Activities of Daily Living instrument, assess the ADLs of an older adult.
2. Assess the safety of the environment of an older adult by using the Public Health Agency of Canada's "Keeping Your Home Safe" Checklist.

Instructions

Katz Index of ADL

Review the questions on the assessment form. In a clinical setting (such as a geriatric inpatient unit or a long-term care facility), use the Katz Index of ADL form to assess at least three older individuals. Compare the results of the three assessments. Did you identify any areas of dependence? Did you actually observe the areas, or did the older adult self-report?

Activities Points (1 or 0)	Independence (1 point) NO supervision, direction, or personal assistance	Dependence (0 points) WITH supervision, direction, personal assistance, or total care
Bathing Points _____	(1 Point) Bathes self completely or needs help in bathing only a single part of the body such as the back, genital area, or disabled extremity	(0 Points) Needs help with bathing more than one part of the body or getting in or out of the tub or shower. Requires total bathing
Dressing Points _____	(1 Point) Gets clothes from closet and drawers and puts on clothes and outer garments complete with fasteners. May have help tying shoes	(0 Points) Needs help with dressing self or needs to be completely dressed
Toileting Points _____	(1 Point) Gets to toilet, gets on and off, arranges clothes, cleans genital area without help	(0 Points) Needs help transferring to the toilet, cleaning self, or using bedpan or commode
Transferring Points _____	(1 Point) Moves in and out of bed or chair unassisted. Mechanical transferring aids are acceptable	(0 Points) Needs help in moving from bed to chair or requires a complete transfer
Continence Points _____	(1 Point) Exercises complete self-control over urination and defecation	(0 Points) Is partially or totally incontinent of bowel or bladder
Feeding Points _____	(1 Point) Gets food from plate into mouth without help. Preparation of food may be done by another person	(0 Points) Needs partial or total help with feeding or requires parenteral feeding
Total points = _____	6 = High (patient independent)	0 = Low (patient very dependent)

Katz Activities of Daily Living

Modified from Gerontological Society of America. Katz, S., Down, T.D., Cash, H.R., & Grotz, R.C. (1970). Progress in the development of the index of ADL. *The Gerontologist, 10,* 20–30.

Home Safety Checklist

Review the questions on the checklist, then practise the assessment in your own home. Did you identify any areas of concern? After practising at your home, perform this assessment in the home of an older adult, such as a neighbour or a family member. Review the results, and provide suggestions for improving safety as indicated by the assessment.

THE PUBLIC HEALTH AGENCY OF CANADA'S "KEEPING YOUR HOME SAFE" CHECKLIST

Outside
- Do all your entrances have an outdoor light?
- Do your outdoor stairs, pathways, or decks have railings and provide good traction (i.e., textured surfaces)?
- Are the front steps and walkways around your house in good repair and free of clutter, snow, and leaves?
- Do the doorways to your balcony or deck have a low sill or threshold?
- Can you reach your mailbox safely and easily?
- Is the number of your house clearly visible from the street and well lit at night?

Inside
- Are all rooms and hallways in your home well lit?
- Are all throw rugs and scatter mats secured in place to keep them from slipping?
- Have you removed scatter mats from the top of the stairs and high-traffic areas?
- Are your high-traffic areas clear of obstacles?
- Do you always take steps to ensure that your pets are not underfoot?
- If you use floor wax, do you use the nonskid kind?
- Do you have a first aid kit and know where it is?
- Do you have a list of emergency numbers near all phones?

© All rights reserved. The Safe Living Guide: A guide to home safety for seniors. The Public Health Agency of Canada, 2015. Adapted and reproduced with permission from the Minister of Health, 2018.

NOTES

32 Next Generation NCLEX® (NGN) Examination–Style Unfolding Case Studies

Use the following case studies to apply the knowledge and skills learned in Jarvis *Physical Examination and Health Assessment*, 4th Canadian edition. There will be 2 questions per section of the unfolding case study for a total of 6 questions per case study. Please note that questions are formatted in a style to represent those found on the Next Generation NCLEX® (NGN) Examination. Answers are provided in the Answer Key on the text's Evolve site.

UNFOLDING CASE STUDY 1: PEDIATRIC HEALTH ASSESSMENT

Question 1: Highlight/Recognize Cues

Highlight any important cues in the Nurses' Notes and Vital Signs that require **immediate** follow-up by the nurse.

| Health History | Nurses' Notes | Vital Signs | Laboratory Results |

1000: 10-year-old male patient arrives at the emergency department (ED) via private car with his mother, who is his legal guardian. Mother reports patient was riding his bicycle without a helmet when the front tire entered a drain grid. Patient hit handlebars and then flew over top of bicycle to ground. Event was witnessed by mother who denies patient loss of consciousness. Mother brought patient directly from scene to ED. Patient is alert and acting appropriate for age. Patient is crying, holding his stomach. Scrapes noted to bilateral forearms oozing blood, as well as an obvious deformity to his right lower leg. Immunizations up to date per mother. NKDA. Denies significant PMH.

| Health History | Nurses' Notes | Vital Signs | Laboratory Results |

1000: Initial vital signs in triage:

T 36.8°C (98.2°F); HR 140 bpm, regular; RR 22/min, crying; BP 142/72 mm Hg; SpO_2 97% on room air (RA)

Pain: 6/10 on Faces Pain Scale

Weight: 27.2 kg (59.9 lb)

Question 2: Select All That Apply/Analyze Cues

The nurse is concerned about the patient's crying and reported pain level of 6/10. What factors may be the cause of the reported pain? **(Select all that apply.)**

1. Fear of the hospital environment
2. Right lower leg injury
3. Abdominal pain
4. Fracture to arm
5. Pain to face and head

Question 3: Drag and Drop Table/Recognize and Analyze Cues

Drag the cues in the Nurses' Notes and Glasgow Score Options to calculate the Glasgow Coma Scale below.

| Health History | Nurses' Notes | Vital Signs | Laboratory Results |

1015: Patient moved to bay 18, placed on stretcher supine, report given by triage nurse to RN who assumed care of patient. Side rails raised ×2, call bell given. Primary trauma survey as follows:

(A) Airway intact; (B) breathing WNL; (C) capillary refill 2 seconds with pulses +2 bilaterally; (D) disability—alert and age appropriate, patient opens eyes spontaneously, answers most questions appropriately but at times is confused, obeys commands with purposeful movement; (E) environment—clothes are damp from sweat and blood, patient clothing cut off with gown placed and warm blankets applied; (F) family presence—mother is worried and at patient's bedside; (G) give comfort—right lower leg splinted, patient reassured with plan of care updated to both mother and patient. C-spine cleared by ED physician.

Glasgow Score Options: 1, 2, 3, 4, 5, 6, 7, 8

Cues	Associated Score
1.	1.
2.	2.
3.	3.
Glasgow Score Calculation: _____	

Question 4: Multiple Response Select Analyze Cues

The nurse prepares to start the secondary survey of the patient. In addition to a head-to-toe examination, and using findings identified prior, the nurse will plan to perform focused assessments on which **4** of the following?

- ☐ Abdomen
- ☐ Heart
- ☐ Neurological
- ☐ Thorax and lungs
- ☐ Peripheral vascular
- ☐ Musculo-skeletal
- ☐ Skin
- ☐ Neck

Question 5: Highlight in Text/Recognize Cues

The nurse prepares to speak with the provider about the patient's assessment findings. From the 1045 h note, **highlight the 3 symptoms from the Nurses' Notes** and **highlight any abnormal vital signs in the flowsheet** to relay to the provider.

| Health History | Nurses' Notes | Vital Signs | Laboratory Results |

1045: Head-to-toe secondary survey complete. Patient log rolled. Back and spine WNL. IV established. IVF bolus initiated and labs sent. Patient with increased complaints of nausea and dry heaving. Abdominal distension noted, bowel sounds hypoactive with tenderness in right upper quadrant upon palpation. X-ray of right leg at bedside.

| Health History | Nurses' Notes | Vital Signs | Laboratory Results |

1000: T 36.8°C (98.2°F); HR 140 bpm, regular; RR 22/min, crying; BP 142/72 mm Hg; SpO_2 97% on RA

1015: T 36.1°C (97.0°F); HR 122 bpm; RR 20/min; BP 120/78 mm Hg; SpO_2 96% on RA

1030: T 36.6°C (97.8°F); HR 138 bpm; RR 20/min; BP 118/72 mm Hg; SpO_2 96% on RA

1045: T 36.6°C (97.8°F); HR 138 bpm; RR 22/min; BP 99/70 mm Hg; SpO_2 96% on RA

Question 6: Matrix Multiple Response/Analyze Cues/Prioritize Hypotheses

Select the **most likely** involved organ with the assessment finding in the table below. Each column must have at least one selection, and each row may have more than one response option.

Symptoms	Liver	Spleen	Kidney(s)
Abdominal distension			
Nausea, dry heaving			
Tenderness RUQ abdomen with palpation			

Conclusion

Health History	Nurses' Notes	Vital Signs	Laboratory Results

1100: Provider at bedside with FAST (focused assessment with sonography) performed. Findings suspicious of internal bleeding. Patient to radiology for CT of abdomen/pelvis. CT abdomen positive for liver laceration. X-ray of right lower leg showing nondisplaced fibula fracture. IVF bolus finishing. Patient will remain NPO. Surgeon at bedside for consult.

Bonus Questions to Level Up with Critical Thinking

1. What could the vital sign trend be indicative of?

2. What lab values from a CBC, electrolytes, LFTs, Cr GRF, type and cross-match, coagulation profile, and lactate level are important for this patient and why?

UNFOLDING CASE STUDY 2: ADULT HEALTH ASSESSMENT

Question 1: Drag and Drop Cloze/Analyze Cues

Health History	Nurses' Notes	Vital Signs	Laboratory Results

0830, October 10: 41-year-old female arrives at clinic today as a follow-up visit for wound check. Patient reports she was "getting ramen soup out of the microwave when it splashed on her arms." Accident occurred 10 days prior. Patient was seen in the ED with treatment for first- and second-degree splash burns.

Bandages to bilateral arms intact, dry, and clean. Patient has been applying over-the-counter (OTC) antibiotic ointment to the areas and dressing twice per day. Complains of a "throbbing" pain, reports it as 5 out of 10. Describes pain as constant, nonradiating focused to round wound areas on bilat arms, worse over the past 2 days. Patient has not been changing the dressing the past 2 days as it seemed to make the pain worse.

Vital signs: T 37.8°C (100.0°F), HR 86 bpm, RR 18/min, BP 138/78 mm Hg, SpO$_2$ 97% on RA

The nurse wants to ensure they have assessed the patient's pain completely. Drag and drop from the items below to finish what the nurse should document for the PQRST acronym related to pain: **P**_____, **Q**_____, **R**_____, **S**_____, **T**_____.

Answer Options

10 days	Nonradiating	Throbbing
Changing the dressing	Pain: 5/10 on 0–10 numerical scale	Constant
First- and second-degree burns	T 37.8°C (100.0°F)	Bilateral arms

Question 2: Drag and Drop Rationale/Prioritize Hypotheses

Drag 1 potential risk and 1 assessment finding to complete the sentence for this patient.

The nurse knows the patient is at risk for _____ due to _____.

Potential Risk	Assessment Finding
sleep deprivation	wounds
infection	scarring from burn
poor self-image	pain
poor pain control	lack of proper dressing changes

Question 3: Highlight/Recognize Cues

Highlight the cues in the Health History note that put the patient at an increased health risk.

Health History | Nurses' Notes | Vital Signs | Laboratory Results

1300: Immunizations: unknown; allergies: NKDA; height: 167.5 cm (5'6"); weight: 81.65 kg (180 lb)

Surgical hx: tonsils and adenoids, age 4; C-section ages 33 and 35

Health conditions: type 2 diabetes, high cholesterol

Hospitalizations: diabetic ketoacidosis, age 36

Denies alcohol use presently or in past. Denies recreational drugs presently or in the past. Patient currently uses e-cigarettes on and off throughout the day; smoked cigarettes (1 ppd) for 10 years prior.

Current medications: metformin 1000 mg PO BID; lispro insulin SQ before meals, sliding scale; antibiotic ointment to burns OTC BID; atorvastatin 80 mg qhs

Question 4: Select All That Apply/Analyze Cues

Health History | **Nurses' Notes** | Vital Signs | Laboratory Results

0900, October 10: Patient discharged with verbal and written instructions given with verbalized understanding from patient. Wound consult ordered and home visit scheduled with the nurse in 2 days for wound check. Patient advised to continue with antibiotic ointment to wounds and dressing changes twice a day.

The nurse, in preparation for discharge, would add which items for patient education handouts? **(Select all that apply.)**

1. Smoking cessation
2. Medication adherence
3. Nonpharmacological and pharmacological pain options
4. Wound care
5. Daily nutrition charts

Question 5: Drag and Drop Table/Analyze Cues

Subjective and objective data were obtained from the wound nurse's focused assessment.

Health History	Nurses' Notes	Vital Signs	Laboratory Results

1200, October 12:

S (situation): Wound nurse visit to patient's home for a wound follow-up assessment.

B (background): Patient at day 12 from occurrence of accidental burn. Had follow-up visit at day 10 with primary health care clinic. Patient has been treating bilat arm burn with antibiotic ointment and dressings twice per day. Reports taking OTC ibuprofen (Advil) for pain.

A (assessment): Bilateral arms with full range of motion. +2 radial pulses bilaterally, 2 second cap refill bilaterally. Varying degrees of healing to skin on both arms. Some blisters have popped and are oozing yellow drainage. Red streaks from the burns on right arm extending up to right elbow. Right arm is warm to touch.

Vital signs: T 38.6°C (101.5°F), HR 100 bpm, RR 22/min, BP 145/90 mm Hg, SpO$_2$ 97% on RA

Patient reports blood sugars at home running "high," and she is "running out of her insulin and is waiting for the refill to come via mail delivery."

R (recommendation): Patient sent to ED for evaluation of possible infection of wound.

Drag and drop items from the "Subjective and Objective Findings" list below to the corresponding normal or abnormal finding column.

Normal Finding	Abnormal Finding

Subjective and Objective Findings

OTC ibuprofen (Advil) for pain
Varying degrees of healing to skin on both arms
Bilat arms with full range of motion
+ 2 radial pulses
2 second capillary refill
Blisters with yellow drainage
Red streaks from burn on right arm extending to right elbow

Right arm warm to touch
T 38.6°C (101.5°F)
HR 100 bpm
RR 22/min
BP 145/90 mm Hg
SpO$_2$ 97% on RA
Blood sugars running "high"

Question 6: Multiple Response Select Analyze Cues/Recognize Hypotheses

Using the "Subjective and Objective Findings" list from Question 5, select **7** assessments that correspond with the wound nurse's R (recommendation) to send the patient to the ED for evaluation of possible infection of wound.

- ☐ OTC ibuprofen (Advil) for pain
- ☐ Varying degrees of healing to skin on both arms
- ☐ Bilat arms with full range of motion
- ☐ +2 radial pulses
- ☐ 2 second capillary refill
- ☐ Blisters with yellow drainage
- ☐ Red streaks from burn on right arm extending to right elbow
- ☐ Right arm warm to touch
- ☐ T 38.6°C (101.5°F)

☐ HR 100 bpm
☐ RR 22/min
☐ BP 145/90 mm Hg
☐ SpO$_2$ 97% on RA
☐ Blood sugars running "high"

Bonus Questions to Level Up with Critical Thinking

1. Describe why pathophysiologically a patient with diabetes is at an increased risk for poor, delayed wound healing.

2. What labs do you think would be ordered for the patient once they are sent to the ED in relation to the wound nurse's recommendation for evaluation of possible infection?

UNFOLDING CASE STUDY 3: OLDER ADULT HEALTH ASSESSMENT

Question 1: Drop Down Cloze/Recognize Cues/Analyze Cues

Health History	Nurses' Notes	Vital Signs	Laboratory Results

0800: Day 1 of admission to cardiac floor, General Hospital, 83-year-old admitted for shortness of breath, chest pain, and positive for COVID-19.

Per family, patient is alert and oriented to person and place for baseline mental status. Lives with daughter due to advanced dementia. Upon admission, patient is confused, only alert to person at this time. Positive COVID-19 test 6 days prior to admission. Progression of illness and weakness brought patient via ambulance to the hospital for evaluation and care.

Vital signs: T 37.2°C (99.0°F); HR 105 bpm, irregular; RR 20/min; BP 122/68 mm Hg; SpO$_2$ 95% on 2 L nasal cannula

Fill in the blanks by choosing from the list of options.

The nurse wants to assess the patient's pain score to complete the vital signs. Using the information from the Nurses' Notes, the nurse identifies 2 cues (options 1 and 2) that determine the pain assessment tool (option 3) that should be used for this patient: ____1____, ____2____, ____3____.

Options for 1	Options for 2	Options for 3
confused	progression of illness	numeric rating scale
weakness	positive COVID-19 test	Faces Pain Scale
shortness of breath	advanced dementia	Visual Analogue Scale
chest pain	HR 105 bpm, irregular	PAINAD scale

Question 2: Drop Down Cloze/Recognize Cues/Analyze Cues

Complete the following sentences by choosing from the list of options.

When taking vital signs, the nurse noted the ____1____ pulse to be irregular. The nurse knows to follow up by auscultating the ____2____ rate for ____3____ minute(s).

Options for 1	Options for 2	Options for 3
carotid	carotid	one
apical	apical	two
radial	radial	three
pedal	aortic	four

Question 3: Select All That Apply/Analyze Cues

| Health History | Nurses' Notes | Vital Signs | Laboratory Results |

0430: Day 2 of admission to cardiac floor, General Hospital, 83-year-old.

Daughter remains at bedside. Patient A&O x1 with increase work of breathing, clutching her chest. Focused assessment of the thorax, lungs, and heart performed. Patient lifted upright in a high Fowler's position with oxygen increased to 5 L nasal cannula. Symmetrical lung expansion, lungs with bilateral inspiratory crackles auscultated. No crepitus. S_1S_2 normal, not accentuated or diminished, S_3 gallop present. No carotid bruit.

Vital signs: T 38.3°C (101.0°F); HR 122 bpm, irregular; RR 36/min; BP 101/70 mm Hg; SpO_2 90% on 5 L nasal cannula

Provider notified of patient status. New orders received for STAT portable chest X-ray, EKG, troponin, BNP, and arterial blood gas. Call respiratory to place patient on heated high-flow oxygen. Transfer patient to Critical Care Unit.

What **significant changes** in the patient status from day 1 admission notes to day 2 admission notes will the nurse include in their report? **(Select all that apply.)**

1. Clutching her chest
2. Patient A&O x1
3. Increased work of breathing, RR 36/min
4. Oxygen increased to 5 L nasal cannula, SpO_2 90%
5. Bilateral inspiratory crackles auscultated
6. S_3 gallop present
7. T 38.3°C (101.0°F)
8. HR 122 bpm, irregular; BP 101/70 mm Hg
9. Symmetrical lung expansion
10. COVID-19 positive

Question 4: Multiple Response Grouping/Recognize Cues/Analyze Cues

Choose the normal assessment finding(s) and abnormal assessment finding(s) that correspond with each body system.

A. Body System	B. Normal Assessment Findings	C. Abnormal Assessment Finding
Thorax and lungs	• BP 105/70 mm Hg • Confusion • Symmetrical lung expansion • Clutching of chest • No crepitus	• Bilateral inspiratory crackles • SpO_2 90% on 5 L nasal cannula • HR in the 120s, irregular • S_3 gallop • T 38.3°C
Heart	• BP 105/70 mm Hg • Bilateral inspiratory crackles • Symmetrical lung expansion • Clutching chest • No carotid bruit	• Confusion • RR 36/min • HR 122 bpm, irregular • S_3 gallop • BP 105/70 mm Hg

Question 5: Highlight in Text/Recognize Cues

Highlight the cues the nurse should make note to follow up on in the Nurses' Notes.

| Health History | Nurses' Notes | Vital Signs | Laboratory Results |

0930: Day 8 Follow-up visit post discharge from hospital, Primary Care Office.

Patient follow-up visit after a 7-day hospitalization for COVID-19 pneumonia and new onset atrial fibrillation. Daughter is with patient. Daughter reports she has hired someone to help with her mother until the patient regains some of her strength. Using walker with gait belt.

Patient is alert and oriented to person and place, which daughter reports is her baseline. Denies any complaints of pain. Skin tear noted to right lower extremity. Lungs with fine crackles bilaterally. Heart S_1S_2, not accentuated or diminished, regular rhythm, 74 bpm. Grade 2/6 murmur heard at apex. +1 pitting edema to bilateral lower extremities. Appetite slowly improving. Daughter denies recent fever. Denies any falls. Denies any issues with current medications.

Question 6: Drop Down Cloze/Analyze Cues

Complete the following sentence by choosing from the list of options.
The nurse knows a murmur heard at the apex suggests a problem with the _____.

Drop Down Options
mitral valve
aortic valve
tricuspid valve
pulmonary valve

Bonus Questions to Level Up with Critical Thinking

1. Describe what pneumonia versus heart failure would look like in a patient (i.e., pathophysiology of condition, subjective findings, assessment findings).

2. The patient had baseline confusion from dementia history. What else can cause acute confusion or an increase in confusion from baseline?

Appendix

APPENDIX A

Summary of Infant Growth and Development

Age (Months)	Physical Competency	Intellectual Competency	Emotional–Social Competency
1 to 2	Holds head in alignment when prone; Moro reflex to loud sound; follows objects; smiles.	Reflex activity; vowel sounds produced.	Gratification through sucking and basic needs being promptly met; smiles at people.
2 to 4	Turns back to side; raises head and chest 45 to 90 degrees off bed and supports weight on arms; reaches for objects; follows object through midline; drools; begins to localize sounds; prefers configuration of face.	Reproduces behaviour initially achieved by random activity; imitates behaviour previously done. Visually studies objects; locates sounds; makes cooing sounds; does not look for objects removed from presence.	Social responsiveness; awareness of those who are not primary caregiver; smiles in response to familiar face.
4 to 6	Birth weight doubled; teeth eruption may begin; sits with stable head and back control; rolls from abdomen to back; picks up object with palmar grasp.	Some intentional actions; some sense of object permanence, looks on same path for vanished object; recognizes partially hidden objects; more systematic in imitative behaviour; babbles.	Prefers primary caregiver; sucking needs decrease; laughs in pleasure.
6 to 8	Turns back to stomach; sits alone; crawls; transfers objects hand to hand; turns to sound behind.	Continued development as in 4 to 6 months.	Differentiated response to nonprimary caregivers; evidence of "stranger" or "separation" anxiety.
8 to 10	Creeps; pulls to stand; pincer grasp.	Actions more goal-directed; able to solve simple problems by using previously mastered responses; actively searches for an object that disappears.	Attachment process complete.
10 to 12	Birth weight tripled; cruises; stands by self; may use spoon.	Begins to imitate behaviour done before by others but not by self. Understands words being said; may say one to four words; intentionality is present.	Begins to explore and separate briefly from parent.

Continued

Summary of Infant Growth and Development—cont'd

Age (Months)	Nutrition	Play	Safety
1 to 2	Breastfed or fortified formula.	Variety of positions. Caregiver should hold and talk to infant; large, brightly coloured objects.	Car carrier; proper use of infant seat.
2 to 4	As for 1 to 2 months.	Talk to and hold; musical toys; rattle, mobile; variety of objects of different colour, size, and texture; mirror, crib toys, variety of settings.	Do not leave unattended on couch, bed, etc. Remove any small objects that infant could choke on.
4 to 6	Introduction of solids; initial store of iron depletion.	Talk and hold provide open space to move and objects to grasp.	Keep environment free of safety hazards; check toys for sharp edges and small pieces that might break.
6 to 8	As for 4 to 6 months.	Provide place to explore; stack toys, blocks; nursery rhymes.	
8 to 10	As for 4 to 6 months.	Games: hide-and-seek, peek-a-boo, pat-a-cake, looking at pictures in a book.	Check infant's expanding environment for hazards. Keep: electrical outlets plugged, cords out of reach, stairs blocked, coffee and end tables cleared of hazards. Do not leave alone in bathtub. Keep poisons out of reach and locked up. Continue use of safety seat in car.
10 to 12	More solids than liquids; increasing use of cup; begin to wean.	Increase space; read to infant. Name and point to body parts. Water; sand play; ball.	As for 8 to 10 months.

Adapted from Betz, C., Hunsberger, M., & Wright, S. (1994). *Family-centered nursing care of children* (2nd ed., pp. 148–149). Philadelphia: W.B. Saunders.

APPENDIX B

Summary of Toddler Growth, Development, and Health Maintenance

Age	Physical Competency	Intellectual Competency	Emotional–Social Competency
General: 1 to 3 years	Gains 5 kg (11 lb). Grows 20.3 cm (8 in.). Twelve teeth erupt. Nutritional requirements: Energy: 100 kcal/kg/day Fluid: 115 to 125 mL/kg/day Protein: 1.8 g/kg/day Ask care provider about vitamins and minerals.	Learns by exploring and experimenting. Learns by imitating. Progresses from a vocabulary of 3 or 4 words at 12 months to about 900 words at 36 months.	Central crisis: to gain a sense of experimenting autonomy vs. doubt and shame. Demonstrates independent behaviours. Exhibits attachment behaviour strongly and regularly until third birthday. Fears persist of strange people, objects, and places and of aloneness and being abandoned. Egocentric in play (parallel play). Imitates parents in household tasks and activities of daily living.
15 months	Legs appear bowed. Walks alone, climbs, slides downstairs backward; stacks two blocks; scribbles spontaneously; grasps spoon but rotates it, holds cup with both hands. Takes off socks and shoes.	Trial-and-error method of learning; experiments to see what will happen. Says at least three words; uses expressive jargon.	Shows independence by trying to feed self and helps in undressing.
18 months	Runs but still falls. Walks upstairs with help. Slides downstairs backward. Stacks three to four blocks. Clumsily throws a ball. Unzips a large zipper. Takes off simple garments.	Begins to maintain a mental image of an absent object. Concept of object permanence fully develops. Has vocabulary of 10 or more words. Holophrastic speech (one word used to communicate whole ideas).	Fears the water. Temper tantrums may begin. Negativism and dawdling predominate. Bedtime rituals begin. Awareness of gender identity begins. Helps with undressing.
24 months	Runs quickly and with fewer falls. Pulls toys and walks sideways. Walks downstairs hanging on a rail (does not alternate feet). Stacks six blocks. Turns pages of a book. Imitates vertical and circular strokes. Uses spoon with little spilling. Can feed self. Puts on simple garments. Can turn doorknobs.	Enters into preconceptual phase of preoperational period: symbolic thinking and symbolic play. Egocentric thinking, imagination, and pretending are common. Has vocabulary of about 300 words. Uses two-word sentences (telegraphic speech). Engages in monologue.	Fears the dark and animals. Temper tantrums may continue. Negativism and dawdling continue. Bedtime rituals continue. Sleep resisted overtly. Usually shows readiness to begin bowel and bladder control. Explores genitalia. Brushes teeth with help. Helps with dressing and undressing.

Continued

Summary of Toddler Growth, Development, and Health Maintenance—cont'd

Age	Physical Competency	Intellectual Competency	Emotional–Social Competency
36 months	Has set of deciduous teeth at about 30 months. Walks downstairs alternating feet. Rides tricycle. Walks with balance and runs well. Stacks 8 to 10 blocks. Can pour from a pitcher. Feeds self completely. Dresses self almost completely (does not know front from back). Cannot tie shoes.	Preconceptual phase of preoperational period as for 24 months. Uses around 900 words. Constructs complete sentences and uses all parts of speech.	Temper tantrums subside. Negativism and dawdling subside. Bedtime rituals subside. Self-care in feeding, elimination, and dressing enhances self-esteem.

Age	Nutrition	Play	Safety
General: 1 to 3 years	Milk 473–709 mL (16–24 oz.). Appetite decreases. Wants to feed self. Has food jags. Caregiver should never force food but should give nutritious snacks. Iron and vitamin supplementation should be given only if there is poor intake.	Books at all stages are enjoyed. Needs physical and quiet activities; does not need expensive toys.	Never leave alone in tub. Keep poisons, including detergents and cleaning products, out of reach. Use car seat.
15 months	Vulnerable to iron-deficiency anemia. Can have table foods except for tough meat and hard vegetables. Wants to feed self.	Stuffed animals, dolls, music toys; peek-a-boo, hide-and-seek; water and sand play; stacking toys; Roll ball on floor. push toys on floor. Caregiver can read to toddler.	Keep small items off floor (pins, buttons, clips). Child may choke on hard food. Cords and tablecloths are a danger. Keep electrical outlets plugged and poisons locked away. Risk of kitchen accidents with toddler underfoot increases.
18 months	Negativism may interfere with eating. Encourage self-feeding. Child is easily distracted while eating. May play with food. High activity level interferes with eating.	Rocking horse; nesting toys; shape-sorting cube; pencil or crayon; pull toys; four-wheeled toy ride; throw ball; running and chasing games; roughhousing; puzzles; blocks; hammer and peg board.	Falls: from riding toy, in bathtub, from running too fast. Climbs up to get dangerous objects. Keep dangerous things out of wastebasket.
24 months	Requests certain foods; therefore, snacks should be controlled. Imitates eating habits of others. May still play with food and especially with utensils and dish (pouring, stacking).	Clay and Play-Doh; finger paint; brush paint; music player with storybook and songs to sing along; toys to take apart; toy tea sets; puppets; puzzles.	May fall from outdoor large play equipment. Can reach farther than expected (knives, razors, and matches must be kept out of reach).
36 months	Sits in booster seat rather than high chair. Verbal about likes and dislikes.	Likes playing with other children, building toys, drawing and painting, doing puzzles; imitation household objects for doll play; nurse and doctor kits; carpenter kits.	Protect from turning on hot water, falling from tricycle, striking matches.

Adapted from Betz, C., Hunsberger, M., & Wright, S. (1994). *Family-centered nursing care of children* (2nd ed., pp. 190–191). Philadelphia: W.B. Saunders.

APPENDIX C

Growth, Development, and Health Promotion for Preschoolers

Age (Years)	Physical Competency	Intellectual Competency	Emotional–Social Competency
General: 3 to 5	Gains 4.5 kg (10 lb). Grows 15 cm (6 in.). Twenty teeth present Nutritional requirements: Energy: 1250 to 1600 cal/day (or 90 to 100 kcal/kg/day) Fluid: 100 to 125 mL/kg/day Protein: 30 g/day (or 3 g/kg/day) Iron: 10 mg/day	Becomes increasingly aware of self and others. Vocabulary increases from 900 to 2100 words. Piaget's preoperational and intuitive period.	Freud's phallic stage Oedipus complex—boy. Electra complex—girl. Erikson's stage of initiative vs. guilt.
3	Runs, stops suddenly; walks backward; climbs steps; jumps; pedals tricycle; undresses self; unbuttons front buttons; feeds self well.	Knows own sex; sense of humour; desires to please. Language—900 words. Follows simple direction. Uses plurals. Names figure in picture. Uses adjectives and adverbs.	Shifts between reality and imagination. Bedtime rituals. Negativism decreases. Animism and realism: anything that moves is alive.
4	Runs well, skips clumsily; hops on one foot; heel–toe walks. Climbs up and down steps without holding rail. Jumps well. Dresses and undresses. Buttons well, needs help with zippers, bows. Brushes teeth. Bathes self. Draws with some form and meaning.	More aware of others. Uses alibis to excuse behaviour; bossy. Language—1500 words. Talks in sentences. Knows nursery rhymes. Counts to five. Highly imaginative; name calling.	Focuses on present. Egocentrism; unable to see the viewpoint of others, unable to understand another's inability to see own viewpoint. Does not comprehend anticipatory explanation. Sexual curiosity. Oedipus complex. Electra complex.
5	Runs skillfully. Jumps three to four steps. Jumps rope, hops, skips. Begins dance. Roller skates. Dresses without assistance. Ties shoelaces. Hits nail on head with hammer. Draws person—six parts. Prints first name.	Aware of cultural differences. Knows name and address. More independent. More sensible, less imaginative. Copies triangle, draws rectangle. Knows four or more colours. Language—2100 words, meaningful sentences. Understands kinship. Counts to 10.	Continues in egocentrism. Fantasy and daydreams. Resolution of Oedipus/Electra complex, girls identify with mother, boys with father. Body image and body boundary especially important in illness. Shows tension in nail-biting, nose-picking, whining, snuffling.

Continued

Growth, Development, and Health Promotion for Preschoolers—cont'd

Age (Years)	Nutrition	Play	Safety
General: 3 to 5	Carbohydrate intake approximately 40% to 50% of calories. Good food sources of essential vitamins and minerals. Regular tooth brushing. Parents are seen as examples; if parent will not eat it, neither will the child.	Reading books is important at all ages. Balance highly physical activities with quiet times. Quiet rest period takes the place of nap time. Provide sturdy play materials. Limit screen time to less than 1 hour a day (https://caringforkids.cps.ca/handouts/behavior-anddevelopment/screen-time-andyoung-children)	Never leave alone in bath or swimming pool. Keep poisons in locked cupboard; learn what household things are poisonous. Use car seats and seatbelts. Never leave child alone in car. Remove doors from abandoned refrigerators.
3	1250 kcal/day. Due to increased sex identity and imitation, child copies parents at table and will eat what they eat. Different colours and shapes of foods can increase interest.	Participates in simple games. Cooperates, takes turns. Plays with group. Uses scissors, paper. Likes crayons, colouring books. Enjoys being read to and "reading." Plays "dress-up" and "house." Likes fire engines.	Teach safety habits early. Let water out of bathtub; don't allow child to stand in tub. Caution against climbing in unsafe areas, onto or under cars, unsafe buildings, drainage pipes. Insist on seatbelts worn at all times in cars.
4	Good nutrition. 1400 kcal/day. Nutritious between-meal snacks essential. Emphasis on quality not quantity of food eaten. Mealtime should be enjoyable, not for criticism. As dexterity improves, neatness increases.	Longer attention span with group activities. "Dress-up" with more dramatic play. Draws, pounds, paints. Likes making paper chains, sewing cards. Scrapbooks. Likes being read to, listening to music, and rhythmic play. "Helps" adults.	Teach child to stay out of streets, alleys. Continually teach safety; child understands. Teach how to handle scissors. Teach what poisons are and why to avoid. Never allow child to stand in moving car.
5	Good nutrition. 1600 kcal/day. Encourage regular tooth brushing. Encourage quiet time before meals. Can learn to cut own meat. Frequent illnesses from increased exposure, increased nutritional needs.	Plays with trucks, cars, soldiers, dolls. Likes simple games with letters or numbers. Much gross motor activity: water, mud, snow, leaves, rocks. Matching picture games. Limit screen time to less than 1 hour a day (https://caringforkids.cps.ca /handouts/behavior-and-development/screen-time-and-young-children)	Teach child how to cross streets safely. Teach child not to speak to strangers or get into cars of strangers. Insist on seatbelts. Teach child to swim.

Adapted from Betz, C., Hunsberger, M., & Wright, S. (1994). *Family-centered nursing care of children* (2nd ed., pp. 235–236). Philadelphia: W.B. Saunders.

APPENDIX D

Competency Development of the School-Age Child

Age (Years)	Physical Competency	Intellectual Competency	Emotional–Social Competency
General: 6 to 12	Gains an average of 2.5 to 3.2 kg/year (5½ to 7 lb/year). Overall height gains of 5.5 cm (2 in.) per year; growth occurs in spurts and is mainly in trunk and extremities. Loses deciduous teeth; most of permanent teeth erupt. Progressively more coordinated in both gross and fine motor skills. Caloric needs increase with growth spurts.	Masters concrete operations. Moves from egocentrism; learns he or she is not always right. Learns grammar and expression of emotions and thoughts. Vocabulary increases to 3 000 words or more; handles complex sentences.	Central crisis: industry vs. inferiority; wants to do and make things. Progressive sex education needed. Wants to be like friends; competition important. Fears body mutilation, alterations in body image; earlier phobias may recur, nightmares; fears death. Nervous habits common.
6 to 7	Gross motor skill exceeds fine motor coordination. Balance and rhythm are good—runs, skips, jumps, climbs, gallops. Throws and catches ball. Dresses self with little or no help.	Vocabulary of 2500 words. Learning to read and print; beginning concrete concepts of numbers, general classification of items. Knows concepts of right and left; morning, afternoon, and evening; coinage. Intuitive thought process. Verbally aggressive, bossy, opinionated, argumentative. Likes simple games with basic rules.	Boisterous, outgoing, and a know-it-all, whiney; parents should sidestep power struggles, offer choices. Becomes quiet and reflective during seventh year; very sensitive. Can use telephone. Likes to make things: starts many, finishes few. Caregiver should give child some responsibility for household duties.
8 to 10	Myopia may appear. Secondary sex characteristics begin in girls. Hand–eye coordination and fine motor skills well established. Movements are graceful, coordinated. Cares for own physical needs completely. Constantly on move; plays and works hard; caregiver should enforce balance in rest and activity.	Learning correct grammar and to express feelings in words. Likes books he or she can read alone; will read comics, scan newspaper. Enjoys making detailed drawings. Mastering classification, seriation, spatial and temporal, numerical concepts. Uses language as a tool; likes riddles, jokes, chants, word games. Rules are guiding force in life now. Very interested in how things work, what and how weather, seasons, etc., are made.	Strong preference for same-sex peers; antagonizes opposite-sex peers. Self-assured and pragmatic at home; questions parental values and ideas. Has a strong sense of humour. Enjoys clubs, group projects, outings, large groups, camp. Modesty about own body increases over time; sex conscious. Works diligently to perfect skills he or she does best. Happy, cooperative, relaxed, and casual in relationships. Increasingly courteous and well-mannered with adults. Gang stage at a peak; secret codes and rituals prevail. Responds better to suggestion than dictatorial approach.

Continued

Competency Development of the School-Age Child—cont'd

Age (Years)	Physical Competency	Intellectual Competency	Emotional–Social Competency
11 to 12	Vital signs approximate adult norms. Growth spurt for girls now; inequalities between sexes are increasingly noticeable; boys have greater physical strength. Eruption of permanent teeth is complete except for third molars. Secondary sex characteristics begin in boys. Menstruation may begin.	Able to think about social problems and prejudices; sees others' points of view. Enjoys reading mysteries, love stories. Begins playing with abstract ideas. Shows interest in whys of health measures and understands human reproduction. Very moralistic; religious commitment often made during this time.	Intense team loyalty; boys begin teasing girls, and girls flirt with boys for attention; best friend period. Wants unreasonable independence. Rebellious about routine; wide mood swings; needs some time daily for privacy. Very critical of own work. Hero worship prevails. "Facts of life" chats with friends prevail; masturbation increases. Appears under constant tension.

Age (Years)	Nutrition	Play	Safety
General: 6 to 12	Fluctuations in appetite due to uneven growth pattern and tendency to get involved in activities. Tendency to neglect breakfast owing to rush of getting to school. Though school lunch is provided in most schools, child does not always eat it.	Plays in groups, mostly of same sex; "gang" activities predominate. Books for all ages. Bicycles important. Sports equipment. Cards, board and table games. Most of play is active games requiring little or no equipment.	Enforce continued use of safety belts during car travel. Bicycle safety must be taught and enforced. Teach safety related to hobbies, handicrafts, mechanical equipment.
6 to 7	Preschool food dislikes persist. Tendency for deficiencies in iron, vitamin A, and riboflavin. Should drink 100 mL/kg of water per day. Should eat 3 g/kg of protein daily.	Still enjoys dolls, cars, and trucks. Plays well alone but enjoys small groups of both sexes; begins to prefer same-sex peer during seventh year. Ready to learn how to ride a bicycle. Prefers imaginary, dramatic play with real costumes. Begins collecting for quantity, not quality. Enjoys active games such as hide-and-seek, tag, jump-rope, roller skating, kickball. Ready for lessons in dancing, gymnastics, music. Caregiver should restrict Limit screen time to less than 2 hours a day. https://cps.ca/en/documents/position/digital-media.	Teach and reinforce traffic safety to child. Still needs adult supervision of play. Teach child to avoid strangers and never to take anything from strangers. Teach illness prevention and reinforce continued practice of other health habits. Restrict bicycle use to home ground; no traffic areas; teach bicycle safety. Teach the harmful use of drugs, alcohol, smoking. Set a good example.
8 to 10	Needs about 2100 calories/day; give nutritious snacks. Tends to be too busy to bother to eat. Tendency for deficiencies in calcium, iron, and thiamine. Problem of obesity may begin now. Good table manners. Able to help with food preparation.	Likes hiking, sports. Enjoys cooking, woodworking, crafts. Enjoys cards and table games. Likes radio and music. Begins qualitative collecting now. Continue restriction on TV time.	Stress safety with firearms. Keep them out of reach, and allow use only with adult supervision. Know who the child's friends are; parents should still have some control over friend selection. Teach water safety; swimming should be supervised by an adult.

Competency Development of the School-Age Child—cont'd

Age (Years)	Nutrition	Play	Safety
11 to 12	Male needs 2500 calories/day; female needs 2250/day (70 kcal/kg/day). Should drink 75 mL/kg of water per day. Should eat 2 g/kg of protein daily.	Enjoys projects and working with hands. Likes to do errands and jobs to earn money. Very involved in sports, dancing, talking on phone. Enjoys all aspects of acting and drama.	Continue monitoring friends; stress bicycle safety on streets and in traffic.

Adapted from Betz, C., Hunsberger, M., & Wright, S. (1994). *Family-centered nursing care of children* (2nd ed., pp. 281–282). Philadelphia: W.B. Saunders.

APPENDIX E

Characteristics of Adolescents

Early Adolescence (12 to 14 Years)	Middle Adolescence (15 to 16 Years)	Late Adolescence (17 to 21 Years)
Becomes comfortable with own body; egocentric. Difficulty solving problems; thinks in present; cannot use past experience to control behaviour; sense of invulnerability—society's rules do not apply to him or her. Struggle between dependent and independent behaviour; begins forming peer alliance. Parent–child conflict begins; teen argues, but without logic.	"Tries out" adultlike behaviour. Begins to solve problems, analyze, and abstract. Established peer group alliance with associated risk-taking behaviour. Peak turmoil in child–family relations; able to debate issues and use some logic, but not continuously.	Aware of own strengths and limitations; establishes own value system. Able to verbalize conceptually: deals with abstract moral concepts; makes decisions regarding future. Peer group diminishes in importance; may develop first intimate relationship. Turbulence subsides. May move away from home. More adultlike friendship with parents.

From Foster, R., Hunsberger, M., & Anderson, J. J. (1989). *Family-centered nursing care of children* (p. 359). Philadelphia: W.B. Saunders.

APPENDIX F

Functional Health Patterns Guide

The following table is a general guide for programs employing a functional health patterns approach to assessment.

Functional Health Patterns	Potential Correlating Chapters in the Text
Health Perception—Health Management	• Chapter 2, Health Promotion in the Context of Health Assessment • Chapter 4, The Interview • Chapter 5, The Complete Health History • Chapter 31, Assessment of the Older Adult
Nutritional—Metabolic	• Chapter 12, Nutritional Assessment and Nursing Practice • Chapter 10, General Survey, Measurement, and Vital Signs • Chapter 13, Skin, Hair, and Nails • Chapter 17, Nose, Mouth, and Throat • Chapter 22, The Abdomen
Elimination	• Chapter 22, The Abdomen • Chapter 23, Anus, Rectum, and Prostate • Chapter 26, Male Genitourinary System • Chapter 27, Female Genitourinary System
Activity—Exercise	• Chapter 19, Thorax and Lungs • Chapter 20, Heart and Neck Vessels • Chapter 21, Peripheral Vascular System and Lymphatic System • Chapter 24, Musculo-skeletal System
Sleep—Rest	• Chapter 5, The Complete Health History
Cognitive—Perception	• Chapter 6, Mental Health Assessment • Chapter 11, Pain Assessment • Chapter 14, Head, Face, and Neck, Including Regional Lymphatic System • Chapter 15, Eyes • Chapter 16, Ears • Chapter 17, Nose, Mouth, and Throat • Chapter 25, Neurological System • Chapter 31, Assessment of the Older Adult
Self-Perception—Self-Concept	• Chapter 6, Mental Health Assessment • Chapter 31, Assessment of the Older Adult
Role—Relationship	• Chapter 3, A Relational Approach to Cultural and Social Considerations in Health Assessment • Chapter 8, Interpersonal Violence and Health Assessment • Chapter 31, Assessment of the Older Adult
Sexuality—Reproductive	• Chapter 18, Breasts and Regional Lymphatic System • Chapter 26, Male Genitourinary System • Chapter 27, Female Genitourinary System • Chapter 30, Pregnancy
Coping—Stress Tolerance	• Chapter 7, Substance Use and Health Assessment • Chapter 31, Assessment of the Older Adult
Values—Beliefs	• Chapter 3, A Relational Approach to Cultural and Social Considerations in Health Assessment